EVERY LIVING THING

James Herriot grew up in Glasgow and qualified as a veterinary surgeon at Glasgow Veterinary College. Shortly afterwards, he took up a position as an assistant in a North Yorkshire practice where he remained, with the exception of his wartime service in the RAF, until his death in 1995.

Other titles available by the same author

If Only They Could Talk

It Shouldn't Happen to a Vet

Let Sleeping Vets Lie

Vet in Harness

Vets Might Fly

Vet in a Spin

The Lord God Made Them All

JAMES HERRIOT

EVERY LIVING THING

with illustrations by
VICTOR AMBRUS

PAN BOOKS

First published 1992 by Michael Joseph Ltd

First published in paperback 1993 by Pan Books

This edition published 2006 by Pan Books
an imprint of Pan Macmillan Ltd
Pan Macmillan, 20 New Wharf Road, London N1 9RR
Basingstoke and Oxford
Associated companies throughout the world
www.panmacmillan.com

ISBN-13: 978-0-330-44345-6
ISBN-10: 0-330-44345-3

3 5 7 9 8 6 4 2

A CIP catalogue record for this book is available from
the British Library.

Printed and bound in Great Britain by
Mackays of Chatham plc, Chatham, Kent

To my revered and elderly friends,

Polly and Bodie

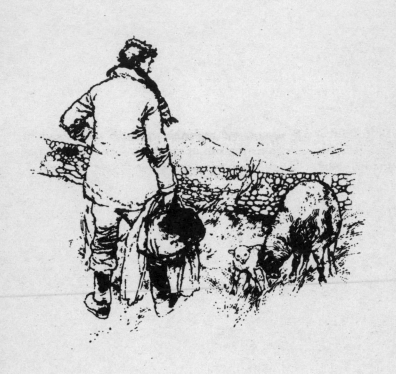

Be fruitful and multiply, and replenish the earth and subdue it: and have dominion over the fish of the sea and over the fowl of the air, and over every living thing that moveth upon the earth.

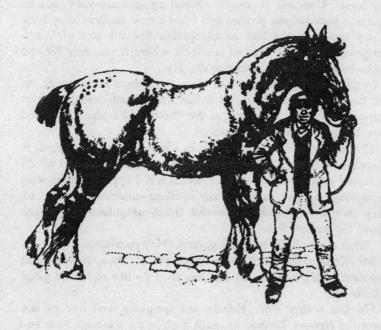

I

I am never at my best in the early morning, especially the cold mornings you get in the Yorkshire spring when a piercing March wind sweeps down from the fells, finding its way inside clothing, nipping at noses and ears. It was a cheerless time, and a particularly bad time to be standing in this cobbled farmyard watching a beautiful horse dying because of my incompetence.

It had started at eight o'clock. Mr Kettlewell telephoned as I was finishing my breakfast.

'I 'ave a fine big cart 'oss here and he's come out in spots.'

'Really? What kind of spots?'

'Well, round and flat, and they're all over 'im.'

'And it started quite suddenly?'

'Aye, he were right as rain last night.'

'All right, I'll have a look at him right away.' I nearly rubbed my hands. Urticaria. It usually cleared up spontaneously, but an injection hastened the process and I had a new antihistamine drug to try out – it was said to be specific for this sort of thing. Anyway, it was the kind of situation where it was easy for the vet to look good. A nice start to the day.

In the fifties, the tractor had taken over most of the work on the farms, but there was still a fair number of draught horses around, and when I arrived at Mr Kettlewell's place I realised that this one was something special.

The farmer was leading him from a loose box into the yard. A magnificent Shire, all of eighteen hands, with a noble head which he tossed proudly as he paced towards me. I appraised him with something like awe, taking in the swelling curve of the neck, the deep-chested body, the powerful limbs abundantly feathered above the massive feet.

'What a wonderful horse!' I gasped. 'He's enormous!'

Mr Kettlewell smiled with quiet pride. 'Aye, he's a right smasher. I only bought 'im last month. I do like to have a good 'oss about.'

He was a tiny man, elderly but sprightly, and one of my favourite farmers. He had to reach high to pat the huge neck and was nuzzled in return. 'He's kind, too. Right quiet.'

'Ah well, it's worth a lot when a horse is good-natured as well as good-looking.' I ran my hand over the typical plaques in the skin. 'Yes, this is urticaria, all right.'

'What's that?'

'Sometimes it's called nettle rash. It's an allergic condition. He may have eaten something unusual, but it's often difficult to pinpoint the cause.'

'Is it serious?'

'Oh no. I have an injection that'll soon put him right. He's well enough in himself, isn't he?'

'Aye, right as a bobbin.'

'Good. Sometimes it upsets an animal, but this fellow's the picture of health.'

As I filled my syringe with the antihistamine I felt that I had never spoken truer words. The big horse radiated health and well-being.

He did not move as I gave the injection, and I was about to put my syringe away when I had another thought. I had always used a proprietary preparation for urticaria and it had invariably worked. Maybe it would be a good idea to supplement the antihistamine, just to make sure. I wanted a good, quick cure for this splendid horse.

I trotted back to my car to fetch the old standby and injected the usual dose. Again the big animal paid no attention and the farmer laughed.

'By gaw, he doesn't mind, does 'e?'

I pocketed the syringe. 'No, I wish all our patients were like him. He's a grand sort.'

This, I thought, was vetting at its best. An easy, trouble-free case, a nice farmer and a docile patient who was a picture of equine beauty, a picture I could have looked at all day. I didn't want to go away although other calls were waiting. I just stood there, half listening to Mr Kettlewell's chatter about the imminent lambing season.

'Ah well,' I said at length, 'I must be on my way.' I was turning to go when I noticed that the farmer had fallen silent.

The silence lasted for a few moments, then, 'He's dotherin' a bit,' he said.

I looked at the horse. There was the faintest tremor in the muscles of the limbs. It was hardly visible, but as I watched, it began to spread upwards, bit by bit, until the skin over the neck, body and rump began to quiver. It was very slight, but there was no doubt it was gradually increasing in intensity.

'What is it?' said Mr Kettlewell.

'Oh, just a little reaction. It'll soon pass off.' I was trying to sound airy, but I wasn't so sure.

With agonising slowness the trembling developed into a gener- alised shaking of the entire frame and this steadily increased in violence as the farmer and I stood there in silence. I seemed to have been there a long time, trying to look calm and unworried, but I couldn't believe what I was seeing. This sudden inexplicable transition – there was no reason for it. My heart began to thump and my mouth turned dry as the shaking was replaced by great shuddering spasms which racked the horse's frame, and his eyes, so serene a short while ago, started from his head in terror, while foam began to drop from his lips. My mind raced. Maybe I shouldn't have mixed those injections, but it couldn't have this fearful effect. It was impossible.

As the seconds passed, I felt I couldn't stand much more of this. The blood hammered in my ears. Surely he would start to recover soon – he couldn't get worse.

I was wrong. Almost imperceptibly the huge animal began to sway. Only a little at first, then more and more until he was tilting from side to side like a mighty oak in a gale. Oh, dear God, he was going to go down and that would be the end. And that end had to come soon. Even the cobbles seemed to shake under my feet as the great horse crashed to the ground. For a few moments he lay there, stretched on his side, his feet pedalling convulsively, then he was still.

Well, that was it. I had killed this magnificent horse. It was impossible, unbelievable that a few minutes ago that animal had been standing there in all his strength and beauty and I had come along with my clever new medicines and now there he was, dead.

What was I going to say? I'm terribly sorry, Mr Kettlewell, I just can't understand how this happened. My mouth opened, but nothing came out, not even a croak. And, as though looking at a picture from the outside I became aware of the square of farm buildings with the dark, snow-streaked fells rising behind under a lowering sky, of the biting wind, the farmer and myself, and the motionless body of the horse.

I felt chilled to the bone and miserable, but I had to say my piece. I took a long, quavering breath and was about to speak when the horse raised his head slightly. I said nothing, nor did Mr Kettlewell, as the big animal eased himself onto his chest, looked around him for a few seconds then got to his feet. He shook his head, then walked across to his master. The recovery was just as quick, just as incredible, as the devastating collapse, and he showed no ill effects from his crashing fall onto the cobbled yard.

The farmer reached up and patted the horse's neck. 'You know, Mr Herriot, them spots have nearly gone!'

I went over and had a look. 'That's right. You can hardly see them now.'

Mr Kettlewell shook his head wonderingly. 'Aye, well, it's a wonderful new treatment. But I'll tell tha summat. I hope you don't mind me sayin' this, but,' he put his hand on my arm and looked up into my face, 'ah think it's just a bit drastic.'

I drove away from the farm and pulled up the car in the lee of a dry-stone wall. A great weariness had descended upon me. This sort of thing wasn't good for me. I was getting on in years now – well into my thirties – and I couldn't stand these shocks like I used to. I tipped the driving mirror down and had a look at myself. I was a bit pale, but not as ghastly white as I felt. Still, the feeling of guilt and bewilderment persisted, and with it the recurring thought that there must be easier ways of earning a living than as a country veterinary surgeon. Twenty-four hours a day, seven days a week, rough, dirty and peppered with traumatic incidents like that near catastrophe back there. I leaned back against the seat and closed my eyes.

When I opened them a few minutes later, the sun had broken through the clouds, bringing the green hillsides and the sparkling ridges of snow to vivid life, painting the rocky outcrops with gold. I wound down the window and breathed in the cold clean air drifting down, fresh and tangy, from the moorland high above. A curlew cried, breaking the enveloping silence, and on the grassy bank by the roadside I saw the first primroses of spring.

Peace began to steal through me. Maybe I hadn't done anything wrong with Mr Kettlewell's horse. Maybe antihistamines did sometimes cause these reactions. Anyway, as I started the engine and drove away, the old feeling began to well up in me and within moments it was running strong: it was good to be able to work with animals in this thrilling countryside; I was lucky to be a vet in the Yorkshire Dales.

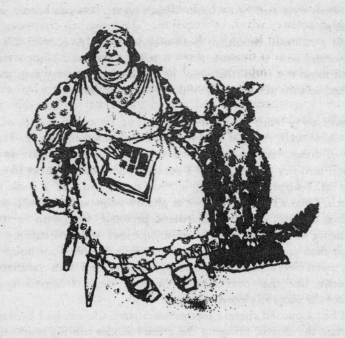

2

There is no doubt that a shock to the system heightens the perception, because as I drove away from Mr Kettlewell's with my heart still fluttering to begin the rest of my morning round, it was as though I were seeing everything for the first time. In my daily work I was always aware of the beauty around me and had never lost the sense of wonder which had filled me when I had had my first sight of Yorkshire, but this morning the magic of the Dales was stronger than ever.

My eyes strayed again and again over the towering flanks of the fells, taking in the pattern of walled green fields won from the yellow moorland grass, and I gazed up at the high tops with the thrill of excitement which always came down to me from that untrodden land.

After visiting the isolated farm, I couldn't resist pulling my car off the unfenced road and climbing with my beagle, Dinah, to the high country which beckoned me. The snow had disappeared almost overnight leaving only runnels of white lying behind the walls and it was as though all the scents of the earth and growing things had been imprisoned and were released now by the spring sunshine in waves of a piercing sweetness. When I reached the summit I was breathless and gulped the crystal air greedily as though I could never get enough of it.

Here there was no evidence of the hand of man and I walked with my dog among miles of heather, peat hags and bog pools with the black waters rippling and the tufts of rushes bending and swaying in the eternal wind.

As the cloud shadows, racing on the wind, flew over me, trailing ribbons of shade and brightness over the endless browns and greens, I felt a rising exhilaration at just being up there on the roof of Yorkshire. It was an empty landscape where no creature stirred and it was silent except for the cry of a distant bird, yet I felt a further surge of excitement in the solitude, a tingling sense of the nearness of all creation.

As always, the siren song of the lonely uplands tempted me to stay, but the morning was wearing on and I had several more farms to visit.

It was with a lingering feeling of fulfilment that I finished my last call and headed for Darrowby, the town where I lived. Its square church tower had been pushing above the tumbled roofs of the little town as I came down the dale and soon I was driving through the cobbled market place with the square of fretted roofs above the shops and pubs which served its three thousand inhabitants.

In the far corner I turned down Trengate, the street where our surgery was, and drew up at the three storeys of mellow brick and climbing ivy of Skeldale House, my work place and happy home where my wife, Helen, and I had brought up our children.

The memories came back of the unforgettable times when my partner, Siegfried Farnon, and his inimitable brother, Tristan, had lived and laughed there with me in our bachelor days, but they were both married and lived with their families in their own homes. Tristan had joined the Ministry of Agriculture, but Siegfried was still my partner and for the thousandth time I thanked heaven that both the brothers were still my close friends.

My son, Jimmy, was ten now and daughter, Rosie, was six, and they were at school, but Siegfried was coming down the steps, stuffing bottles into his pockets.

'Ah, James,' he cried, 'I've just taken a message for you. One of your most esteemed clients – Mrs Bartram. Puppy is in need of your services.' He was grinning as he spoke.

I smiled ruefully in reply. 'Oh, fine. You didn't fancy going there yourself, did you?'

'No, no, my boy. Wouldn't dream of depriving you of the pleasure.' He waved cheerfully and climbed into his car.

I looked at my watch. I still had half an hour before lunch and Puppy was only walking distance away. I got my bag and set off.

The heavenly aroma of fish and chips drifted out on the spring air and I felt a quick stab of hunger as I looked through the shop window at the white-coated figures with their wire scoops, lifting out the crisply battered haddocks and laying them out to drain by the golden mounds of chips.

The lunchtime trade was brisk and the queue moved steadily round the shop, gathering up the newspaper-wrapped parcels, some customers hurrying home with them, others shaking on salt and vinegar before an alfresco meal in the street.

I always had my gastric juices titillated when I visited Mrs Bartram's dog in the flat above the fish and chip shop and I took another rewarding breath as I went down the alley and climbed the stairs.

Mrs Bartram was in her usual chair in the kitchen; fat, massive, deadpan, the invariable cigarette dangling from her lips. She was throwing chips from a bag in her lap to her dog, Puppy, sitting opposite. He caught them expertly one after the other.

Puppy belied his name. He was an enormous, shaggy creature of doubtful ancestry and with a short temper. I always treated him with respect.

'He's still rather fat, Mrs Bartram,' I said. 'Haven't you tried to change his diet as I advised? Remember I said he shouldn't really be fed solely on fish and chips.'

She shrugged and a light shower of ash fell on her blouse. 'Oh aye, ah did for a bit. I cut out the chips and just gave 'im fish every day, but he didn't like it. Loves his chips, 'e does.'

'I see.' I couldn't say too much about the diet because I had the feeling that Mrs Bartram herself ate very little else and it would have been tactless to point out that big chunks of battered fried fish didn't constitute a slimming regime, because her figure, like her dog's, bore witness to the fact.

In fact, as I looked at the two, they had a great similarity sitting there, bolt upright, facing each other. Both huge, immobile, but giving an impression of latent power.

Fat dogs are often lazy and good-natured, but a long succession of postmen, newsboys and door-to-door salesmen had had to take desperate evasive action as Puppy turned suddenly into a monster baying at their heels, and I had one vivid memory of a brush vendor cycling unhurriedly down the alley with his wares dangling from the handle bars, slowing down outside the flat, then, as Puppy catapulted into the street, taking off like the winner of the Tour de France.

'Well, what's the trouble, Mrs Bartram?' I asked, changing the subject.

'It's 'is eye. Keeps runnin'.'

'Ah yes, I see.' The big dog's left eye was almost completely closed, and a trickle of discharge made a dark track down the hair of his face. It made his appearance even more sinister. 'There's some irritation there, probably an infection.'

It would have been nice to find the cause. There could be a foreign body in there or just a spot of conjunctivitis. I reached out my hand to pull the eyelid down but Puppy, without moving, fixed me with his good eye and drew his lips back from a row of formidable teeth.

I withdrew my hand. 'Yes ... yes ... I'll have to give you some antibiotic ointment and you must squeeze a little into his eye three times a day. You'll be able to do that, won't you.'

'Course, I will. He's as gentle as an awd sheep.' Expressionlessly, she lit another cigarette from the old one and drew the smoke down deeply. 'Ah can do anything with 'im.'

'Good, good.' As I rummaged in my bag for the ointment I

had the old feeling of defeat, but there was nothing else for it. It was always long-range treatment with Puppy. I had never tried anything silly like taking his temperature; to be honest, I'd never laid a finger on him in my life.

I heard from Mrs Bartram again two weeks later. Puppy's eye was no better; in fact, it was worse.

I hurried round to the flat, inhaling the delicious vapours from the shop as I went down the alley. Puppy was in the same position as before, upright, facing his mistress and there was no doubt there was an increased discharge from the eye. But this time I fancied I could see something else and I leaned forward, peering closely into the dog's face as a faint but menacing growl warned me not to take any more liberties. And it was there, all right, the cause of the trouble. A tiny papilloma growing from the margin of the eyelid and rubbing on the cornea.

I turned to Mrs Bartram. 'He's got a little growth in there. It's irritating his eye and causing the discharge.'

'Growth?' The lady's face seldom registered any emotion, but one eyebrow twitched upward and the cigarette trembled briefly in her mouth. 'Ah don't like the sound 'o that.'

'Oh, it's quite benign,' I said. 'Nothing to worry about. I'll be able to remove it easily and he'll be perfectly all right afterwards.'

I spoke lightly because indeed these things were quite common and a little injection of local anaesthetic and a quick snip with a pair of curved scissors did the trick effortlessly, but as I looked at the big dog regarding me coldly with his one eye I felt a twinge of anxiety. Things might not be so easy with Puppy.

My misgivings proved to be well founded when Mrs Bartram brought him round to the surgery next morning and left him in the small consulting room. He would obviously have to be sedated before we could do anything and among the rush of new drugs were excellent tranquillisers like acetylpromazine. There was, however, the small matter of one of us grasping that leonine head while the other lifted a fold of skin and inserted the needle. Puppy made it very clear that such things were not on the agenda. Being on strange ground and feeling threatened he came roaring, open-mouthed, at Siegfried and me as soon as we tried to enter the room. We retreated hastily and locked the door.

'Dog catcher?' suggested Siegfried without conviction.

I shook my head. The dog catcher was a snare of soft flex on the end of a long pole and was a handy instrument to slip over a difficult dog's head and steady it while the injection was made, but with Puppy it would be like trying to lasso a grizzly bear. If we ever managed to get the loop over his head it would be the prelude to a fearsome wrestling match.

However, we'd had tough dogs before and we had a little trick in reserve.

'Looks like one for the nembutal,' Siegfried murmured and I nodded agreement. For unapproachable cases we kept a supply of succulent minced beef in the fridge. It was a delicacy which no dog could resist and it was a simple matter to break a few capsules of Nembutal among the meat and wait while the animal drifted into a state of blissful somnolence. It always worked.

However, it was time-consuming. Removing the tiny growth should have been a few minutes' job but we'd have to wait for twenty minutes or so until the stuff took effect. I tried not to think of the urgent cases all over the countryside needing our attention as I prepared the medicated mince.

The consulting room looked onto the garden through a sash window which was open a few inches at the bottom. I threw the meat through this aperture and the two of us went into the office to prepare for our rounds.

When we came back we expected to find Puppy slumbering peacefully, but when we peered in he threw himself at the window, snarling like a starving wolf. On the floor the meat lay untouched.

'Look at that!' I cried. 'I don't believe it. No dog's ever refused that lovely stuff before!'

Siegfried slapped his forehead. 'What a damn nuisance! Do you think he can smell the nembutal? Better try him with a bigger proportion of mince.'

I made up another supply and threw it again through the opening. We retreated to allay the dog's suspicions, but when we crept up ten minutes later the picture hadn't changed. Puppy had not eaten a single mouthful.

'What the hell are we going to do?' Siegfried burst out. 'It's going to be lunch time before we get out!'

It was indeed getting on towards lunch time because a gentle breeze was carrying the first fragrance from the fish and chip shop down the street.

'Just hang on for a minute,' I said. 'I think I know the answer.'

I galloped along Trengate and returned with a bag of chips. It was the work of a moment to insert a capsule in a chip and flick it through the aperture. Puppy was on it like flash and swallowed it without hesitation. Another chip, another capsule, and so on until he had received the requisite dose.

Even as we watched, the big dog's ferocity was gradually replaced by an amiable goofiness and when he took a few uncertain steps then flopped on to his side we knew we had won. When we finally unlocked the door and entered the room, Puppy was in a happy trance and we performed the operation in a couple of minutes.

He was still dopey and unusually peaceful when his mistress called to collect him later that day. When she brought him into the office, his huge head was level with my desk and he almost smiled at me as I sat down.

'We've removed that little thing, Mrs Bartram,' I said. 'His eye will be fine now, but I'm prescribing a course of Lincocin tablets to stop any further infection.'

As I reached for a pen to write the instructions I glanced at some of the other labels I had written. In those days, before injections became the general procedure, many of our medicines were given by mouth. The instructions on the other labels were varied: 'Mixture for bullock. To be given in a pint of treacle water.' 'Drench for calf. To be given in half a pint of flour gruel.'

I poised my pen for a moment, then, for the first time in my life, I wrote, 'Tablets for dog. One to be given three times daily inserted in chips.'

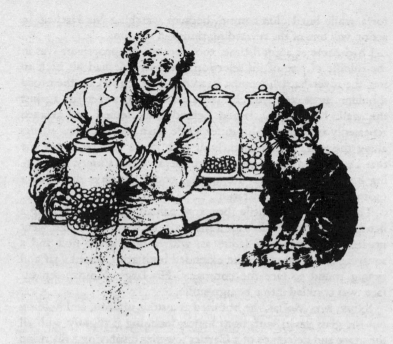

3

My throat was killing me. Three successive nocturnal lambings on the windswept hillsides in my shirt-sleeves had left me with the beginnings of a cold and I felt in urgent need of a packet of Geoff Hatfield's cough drops. An unscientific treatment, perhaps, but I had a childish faith in those powerful little candies which exploded in the mouth, sending a blast of medicated vapour surging through the bronchial tubes.

The shop was down a side alley, almost hidden away, and it was so tiny – not much more than a cubby hole – that there was hardly room for the sign, GEOFFREY HATFIELD, CONFECTIONER above the window. But it was full. It was always full, and, this being market day, it was packed out.

The little bell went 'ching' as I opened the door and squeezed into the crush of local ladies and farmers' wives. I'd have to wait for a while but I didn't mind, because watching Mr Hatfield in action was one of the rewarding things in my life.

I had come at a good time, too, because the proprietor was in the middle of one of his selection struggles. He had his back to me, the silver-haired, leonine head nodding slightly on the broad shoulders as he surveyed the rows of tall glass sweet jars against the wall. His hands, clasped behind him, tensed and relaxed repeatedly as he fought his inner battle, then he took a few strides along the row, gazing intently at each jar in turn. It struck me that Lord Nelson pacing the quarterdeck of the *Victory*, wondering how best to engage the enemy, could not have displayed a more portentous concentration.

The tension in the little shop rose palpably as he reached up a hand, then withdrew it with a shake of the head, but a sigh went up from the assembled ladies as, with a final grave nod and a squaring of the shoulders, he extended both arms, seized a jar and swung round to face the company. His large, Roman senator face, was crinkled into a benign smile.

'Now, Mrs Moffat,' he boomed at a stout matron, and holding out the glass vessel with both hands, inclining it slightly with all the grace and deference of a Cartier jeweller displaying a diamond necklace, 'I wonder if I can interest you in this.'

Mrs Moffat, clutching her shopping basket, peered closely at the paper-wrapped confections in the jar. 'Well, ah don't know . . .'

'If I remember rightly, madam, you indicated that you were seeking something in the nature of a Russian caramel, and I can thoroughly recommend these little sweetmeats. Not quite a Russian, but nevertheless a very nice, smooth-eating toffee.' His expression became serious, expectant.

The fruity tones rolling round his description made me want to grab the sweets and devour them on the spot, and they seemed to have the same effect on the lady. 'Right, Mr Hatfield,' she said eagerly, 'I'll 'ave half a pound.'

The shopkeeper gave a slight bow. 'Thank you so much, madam, I'm sure you will not regret your choice.' His features relaxed into a gracious smile and, as he lovingly trickled the toffees on to his scales before bagging them with a professional twirl, I felt a renewed desire to get at the things.

Mr Hatfield, leaning forward with both hands on the counter, kept his gaze on his customer until he had bowed her out of the shop with a courteous, 'Good day to you, madam', then he turned to face the congregation. 'Ah, Mrs Dawson, how very nice to see you. And what is your pleasure this morning?'

The lady, obviously delighted, beamed at him. 'I'd like some of them fudge chocolates I 'ad last week, Mr Hatfield. They were lovely. Have you still got some?'

'Indeed I have, madam, and I am delighted that you approve of my recommendation. Such a deliciously creamy flavour. Also, it so happens that I have just received a consignment in a special presentation box for Easter. He lifted one from the shelf and balanced it on the palm of his hand. 'Really pretty and attractive, don't you think?'

Mrs Dawson nodded rapidly. 'Oh aye, that's real bonny. I'll take a box and there's summat else I want. A right big bag of nice boiled sweets for the family to suck at. Mixed colours, you know. What 'ave you got?'

Mr Hatfield steepled his fingers, gazed at her fixedly and took a long, contemplative breath. He held this pose for several seconds then he swung round, clasped his hands behind him, and recommenced his inspection of the jars.

That was my favourite bit and, as always, I was enjoying it. It was a familiar scene. The tiny, crowded shop, the proprietor wrestling with his assignment and Alfred sitting at the far end of the counter.

Alfred was Geoff's cat and he was always there, seated upright and majestic on the polished boards near the curtained doorway which led to the Hatfield sitting room. As usual, he seemed to be taking a keen interest in the proceedings, his gaze moving from his master's face to the customer's and though it may have been my imagination I felt that his expression registered a grave involvement in the negotiations and a deep satisfaction at the outcome. He never left his place or encroached on the rest of the counter, but occasionally one or other of the ladies would stroke his cheek and he would respond with a booming purr and a gracious movement of the head towards them.

It was typical that he never yielded to any unseemly display of emotion. That would have been undignified, and dignity was an unchanging part of him. Even as a kitten he had never indulged in immoderate playfulness. I had neutered him three years earlier — for which he appeared to bear me no ill will — and he had grown into a massive, benevolent tabby. I looked at him now, sitting in his place. Vast, imperturbable, at peace with his world. There was no doubt he was a cat of enormous presence.

And it had always struck me forcibly that he was exactly like his master in that respect. They were two of a kind and it was no surprise that they were such devoted friends.

When it came to my turn I was able to reach Alfred and I tickled him under his chin. He liked that and raised his head high while the purring rumbled up from the furry rib cage until it resounded throughout the shop.

Even collecting my cough drops had its touch of ceremony. The big man behind the counter sniffed gravely at the packet then clapped his hand a few times against his chest. 'You can smell the goodness, Mr Herriot, the beneficial vapours. These will have you right in no time.' He bowed and smiled and I could swear that Alfred smiled with him.

I squeezed my way out through the ladies and as I walked down the alley I marvelled for the umpteenth time at the phenomenon of Geoffrey Hatfield. There were several other sweet shops in Darrowby, big double-fronted places with their wares attractively displayed in the windows, but none of them did anything like the trade of the poky establishment I had just left. There was no doubt that it was all due to Geoff's unique selling technique and it was certainly not an act on his part, it was born of a completely sincere devotion to his calling, a delight in what he was doing.

His manner and 'posh' diction gave rise to a certain amount of ribald comment from men who had left the local school with him at the age of fourteen, and in the pubs he was often referred to as 'the bishop', but it was good-natured stuff because he was a well-liked man. And, of course, the ladies adored him and flocked to bask in his attentions.

*

About a month later I was in the shop again to get some of Rosie's favourite liquorice all-sorts and the picture was the same – Geoffrey smiling and booming, Alfred in his place, following every move, the pair of them radiating dignity and well-being. As I collected my sweets, the proprietor whispered in my ear.

'I'll be closing for lunch at twelve noon, Mr Herriot. Would you be so kind as to call in and examine Alfred?'

'Yes, of course.' I looked along the counter at the big cat. 'Is he ill?'

'Oh, no, no . . . but I just feel there's something not right.'

Later I knocked at the closed door and Geoffrey let me into the shop, empty for once, then through the curtained doorway into his sitting room. Mrs Hatfield was at a table, drinking tea. She was a much earthier character than her husband. 'Now then, Mr Herriot, you've come to see t'little cat.'

'He isn't so little,' I said, laughing. And indeed, Alfred looked more massive than ever seated by the fire, looking calmly into the flames. When he saw me he got up, stalked unhurriedly over the carpet and arched his back against my legs. I felt strangely honoured.

'He's really beautiful, isn't he?' I murmured. I hadn't had a close look at him for some time and the friendly face with the dark stripes running down to the intelligent eyes appealed to me as never before. 'Yes,' I said, stroking the fur which shone luxuriantly in the flickering firelight, 'you're a big beautiful fellow.'

I turned to Mr Hatfield. 'He looks fine to me. What is it that's worrying you?'

'Oh, maybe it's nothing at all. His appearance certainly has not altered in the slightest, but for over a week now I've noticed that he is not quite so keen on his food, not quite so lively. He's not really ill . . . he's just different.'

'I see. Well, let's have a look at him.' I went over the cat carefully. Temperature was normal, mucous membranes a healthy pink. I got out my stethoscope and auscultated heart and lungs – nothing abnormal to hear. Palpation of the abdomen produced no clue.

'Well, Mr Hatfield,' I said, 'there doesn't seem to be anything obviously wrong with him. He's maybe a bit run down, but he doesn't look it. Anyway, I'll give him a vitamin injection. That should buck him up. Let me know in a few days if he's no better.'

'Thank you indeed, sir. I am most grateful. You have set my mind at rest.' The big man reached out a hand to his pet. The confident resonance of his voice was belied by the expression of concern on his face. Seeing them together made me sense anew the similarity of man and cat – human and animal, yes, but alike in their impressiveness.

I heard nothing about Alfred for a week and assumed that he had returned to normal, but then his master telephoned. 'He's just the same, Mr Herriot. In fact, if anything, he has deteriorated slightly. I would be obliged if you would look at him again.'

It was just as before. Nothing definite to see even on close examination. I put him on to a course of mixed minerals and vitamin tablets. There was no point in launching into treatment with our new antibiotics – there was no elevation of temperature, no indication of any infectious agent.

I passed the alley every day – it was only about a hundred yards from Skeldale House – and I fell into the habit of stopping and looking in through the little window of the shop. Each day, the familiar scene presented itself; Geoff bowing and smiling to his customers and Alfred sitting in his place at the end of the counter. Everything seemed right, and yet . . . there *was* something different about the cat.

I called in one evening and examined him again. 'He's losing weight,' I said.

Geoffrey nodded. 'Yes, I do think so. He is still eating fairly well, but not as much as before.'

'Give him another few days on the tablets,' I said, 'and if he's no better I'll have to get him round to the surgery and go into this thing a bit more deeply.'

I had a nasty feeling there would be no improvement and there wasn't, so one evening I took a cat cage round to the shop. Alfred was so huge that there was a problem fitting him into the container, but he didn't resist as I bundled him gently inside.

At the surgery I took a blood sample from him and X-rayed

him. The plate was perfectly clear and when the report came back from the laboratory it showed no abnormality.

In a way, it was reassuring, but that did not help because the steady decline continued. The next few weeks were something like a nightmare. My anxious peering through the shop window became a daily ordeal. The big cat was still in his place, but he was getting thinner and thinner until he was almost unrecognisable. I rang the changes with every drug and treatment I could think of, but nothing did any good. I had Siegfried examine him, but he thought as I did. The progressive emaciation was the sort of thing you would expect from an internal tumour, but further X-rays still showed nothing. Alfred must have been thoroughly fed up of all the pushing around, the tests, the kneading of his abdomen, but at no time did he show any annoyance. He accepted the whole thing placidly as was his wont.

There was another factor which made the situation much worse. Geoff himself was wilting under the strain. His comfortable coating of flesh was dropping steadily away from him, the normally florid cheeks were pale and sunken and, worse still, his dramatic selling style appeared to be deserting him. One day I left my viewpoint at the window and pushed my way into the press of ladies in the shop. It was a harrowing scene. Geoff, bowed and shrunken, was taking the orders without even a smile, pouring the sweets listlessly into their bags and mumbling a word or two. Gone was the booming voice and the happy chatter of the customers and a strange silence hung over the company. It was just like any other sweet shop.

Saddest sight of all was Alfred, still sitting bravely upright in his place. He was unbelievably gaunt, his fur had lost its bloom and he stared straight ahead, dead-eyed, as though nothing interested him any more. He was like a feline scarecrow.

I couldn't stand it any longer. That evening I went round to see Geoff Hatfield.

'I saw your cat today,' I said, 'and he's going rapidly downhill. Are there any new symptoms?'

The big man nodded dully. 'Yes, as a matter of fact. I was going to ring you. He's been vomiting a bit.'

I dug my nails into my palms. 'There it is again. Everything points to something abnormal inside him and yet I can't find a thing.' I bent down and stroked Alfred. 'I hate to see him like this. Look at his fur. It used to be so glossy.'

'That's right,' replied Geoff, 'he's neglecting himself. He never washes himself now. It's as though he can't be bothered. And before, he was always at it – lick, lick lick for hours on end.'

I stared at him. His words had sparked something in my mind. 'Lick, lick lick.' I paused in thought. 'Yes . . . when I think about it, no cat I ever knew washed himself as much as Alfred . . .' The spark suddenly became a flame and I jerked upright in my chair.

'Mr Hatfield,' I said, 'I want to do an exploratory laparotomy!'

'What do you mean?'

'I think he's got a hair-ball inside him and I want to operate to see if I'm right.'

'Open him up, you mean?'

'That's right.'

He put a hand over his eyes and his chin sank onto his chest. He stayed like that for a long time, then he looked at me with haunted eyes. 'Oh, I don't know. I've never thought of anything like that.'

'We've got to do something or this cat is going to die.'

He bent and stroked Alfred's head again and again, then without looking up he spoke in a husky voice. 'All right, when?'

'Tomorrow morning.'

Next day, in the operating room, as Siegfried and I bent over the sleeping cat, my mind was racing. We had been doing much more small-animal surgery lately, but I had always known what to expect. This time I felt as though I was venturing into the unknown.

I incised through skin, abdominal muscles and peritoneum and when I reached forward towards the diaphragm I could feel a doughy mass inside the stomach. I cut through the stomach wall and my heart leaped. There it was, a large, matted hair-ball, the cause of all the trouble. Something which wouldn't show up on an X-ray plate.

Siegfried grinned. 'Well, now we know!'

'Yes,' I said as the great waves of relief swept over me. 'Now we know.'

And there was more. After I had evacuated and stitched the stomach, I found other, smaller hair-balls, bulging the intestine along its length. These had all to be removed and the bowel wall stitched in several places. I didn't like this. It meant a bigger trauma and shock to my patient, but finally all was done and only a neat row of skin sutures was visible.

When I returned Alfred to his home, his master could hardly bear to look at him. At length he took a timid glance at the cat, still sleeping under the anaesthetic. 'Will he live?' he whispered.

'He has a good chance,' I replied. 'He has had some major surgery and it might take him some time to get over it, but he's young and strong. He should be all right.'

I could see Geoff wasn't convinced, and that was how it was over the next few days. I kept visiting the little room behind the shop to give the cat penicillin injections and it was obvious that Geoff had made up his mind that Alfred was going to die.

Mrs Hatfield was more optimistic, but she was worried about her husband.

'Eee, he's given up hope,' she said. 'And it's all because Alfred just lies in his bed all day. I've tried to tell 'im that it'll be a bit o' time before the cat starts runnin' around, but he won't listen.'

She looked at me with anxious eyes. 'And, you know, it's gettin' him down, Mr Herriot. He's a different man. Sometimes I wonder if he'll ever be the same again.'

I went over and peeped past the curtain into the shop. Geoff was there, doing his job like an automaton. Haggard, unsmiling, silently handing out the sweets. When he did speak it was in a listless monotone and I realised with a sense of shock that his voice had lost all its old timbre. Mrs Hatfield was right. He was a different man. And, I thought, if he stayed different, what would happen to his clientele? So far they had remained faithful, but I had a feeling they would soon start to drift away.

It was a week before the picture began to change for the better. I entered the sitting room, but Alfred wasn't there.

Mrs Hatfield jumped up from her chair. 'He's a lot better, Mr Herriot,' she said eagerly. 'Eating well and seemed to want to go into t'shop. He's in there with Geoff now.'

Again I took a surreptitious look past the curtain. Alfred was back in his place, skinny but sitting upright. But his master didn't look any better.

I turned back into the room. 'Well, I won't need to come any more, Mrs Hatfield. Your cat is well on the way to recovery. He should soon be as good as new.' I was quite confident about this, but I wasn't so sure about Geoff.

At this point, the rush of spring lambing and post lambing troubles overwhelmed me as it did every year, and I had little time to think about my other cases. It must have been three weeks before I visited the sweet shop to buy some chocolates for Helen. The place was packed and as I pushed my way inside all my fears came rushing back and I looked anxiously at man and cat.

Alfred, massive and dignified again, sat like a king at the far end of the counter. Geoff was leaning on the counter with both hands, gazing closely into a lady's face. 'As I understand you, Mrs Hird, you are looking for something in the nature of a softer sweetmeat.' The rich voice reverberated round the little shop. 'Could you perhaps mean a Turkish Delight?'

'Nay, Mr Hatfield, it wasn't that . . .'

His head fell on his chest and he studied the polished boards of the counter with fierce concentration. Then he looked up and pushed his face nearer to the lady's. 'A pastille, possibly . . ?'

'Nay . . . nay.'

'A truffle? A soft caramel? A peppermint cream?'

'No, nowt like that.'

He straightened up. This was a tough one. He folded his arms across his chest and as he stared into space and took the long inhalation I remembered so well I could see that he was a big man again, his shoulders spreading wide, his face ruddy and well fleshed.

Nothing having evolved from his cogitations, his jaw jutted and he turned his face upwards, seeking further inspiration from the ceiling. Alfred, I noticed, looked upwards, too.

There was a tense silence as Geoff held this pose, then a smile crept slowly over his noble features. He raised a finger. 'Madam,' he said, 'I do fancy I have it. Whitish, you said . . . sometimes pink . . . rather squashy. May I suggest to you . . . marshmallow?'

Mrs Hird thumped the counter. 'Aye, that's it, Mr Hatfield. I just couldn't think of t'name.'

'Ha-ha, I thought so,' boomed the proprietor, his organ tones rolling to the roof. He laughed, the ladies laughed, and I was positive that Alfred laughed, too.

All was well again. Everybody in the shop was happy – Geoff, Alfred, the ladies and, not least, James Herriot.

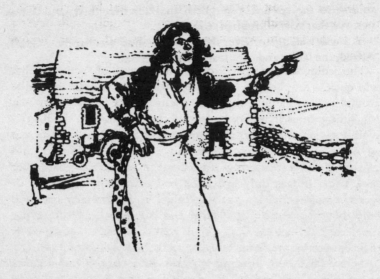

4

'You call yourself a vet, but you're nowt but a robber!'

Mrs Sidlow, her fierce little dark eyes crackling with fury, spat out the words and as I looked at her, taking in the lank, black hair framing the haggard face with its pointed chin, I thought, not for the first time, how very much she resembled a witch. It was easy to imagine her throwing a leg over a broomstick and zooming off for a quick flip across the moon.

'All t'country's talkin' about you and your big bills,' she continued. 'I don't know how you get away with it, it's daylight robbery – robbin' the poor farmers and then you come out here bold as brass in your flash car.'

That was what had started it. Since my old vehicle was dropping to bits I had lashed out on a second-hand Austin 10. It had done twenty thousand miles but had been well maintained and looked like new with its black bodywork shining in the sun and the very sight of it had sparked off Mrs Sidlow.

The purchase of a new car was invariably greeted with a bit of leg pulling by most of the farmers. 'Job must be payin' well,' they would say with a grin. But it was all friendly, with never a hint of the venom which seemed to be part of the Sidlow ménage.

The Sidlows hated vets. Not just me, but all of them and that was quite a few because they had tried every practice for miles around and had found them all wanting. The trouble was that Mr Sidlow himself was quite simply the only man in the district who knew anything about doctoring sick animals – his wife and all his grown-up family knew this as an article of faith and whenever illness struck any of his cattle, it was natural that father took over. It was only when he had exhausted his supply of secret remedies that the vet was called in. I personally had seen only dying animals on that farm and had been unable to bring them back to life, so the Sidlows were invariably confirmed in their opinion of me along with the rest of my profession.

Today I had been viewing with the old feeling of hopelessness an emaciated little beast huddled in a dark corner of the fold yard taking its last few breaths after a week of pneumonia while the family stood around breathing hostility, shooting the usual side glances at me from their glowering faces. I had been trailing wearily back to my car on the way out when Mrs Sidlow had spotted me from the kitchen window and catapulted into the yard.

'Aye, it's awright for you,' she went on. 'We 'ave to work hard to make a livin' on this spot and then such as you come and take our money away from us without doin' anythin' for it. Ah know what it is, your idea is to get rich quick!'

Only my long training that the customer is always right stopped me from barking back. Instead I forced a smile.

'Mrs Sidlow,' I said, 'I assure you that I'm anything but rich. In fact, if you could see my bank balance, you would see what I mean.'

'You're tellin' me you haven't much money?'

'That's right.'

She waved towards the Austin and gave me another searing glare. 'So this fancy car's just a lot o' show on nowt!'

I had no answer. She had me both ways – either I was a fat cat or a stuck-up poseur.

As I drove away up the rising road I looked back at the farm with its substantial house and wide sprawl of buildings. There were five hundred lush acres down there, lying in the low country at the foot of the dale. The Sidlows were big, prosperous farmers with none of the worries of the hill men who struggled to exist on the bleak smallholdings higher up, and it was difficult to understand why my imagined affluence should be such an affront to them.

It occurred to me, too, that this latest attack had come at a time when my finances were at their lowest ebb. As I changed gear I caught a glimpse of pink flesh through the knee of my old corduroys. Oh hell, these trousers had just about had it as indeed had a lot of my clothes, but the needs of two growing children came a long way before my own. Not that there was any point in going round my work looking like a male fashion plate – I had one of the roughest, dirtiest jobs in the world and could only aim at reasonable respectability – and I always had the comforting knowledge that I did have one 'good suit' which had lasted for many years simply because it was hardly ever worn.

But it was indeed strange that I should be perpetually hard up. Siegfried and I had built up a good, successful practice. I worked nearly all the time, seven days a week, in the evenings and often during the night and it was hard work, too – rolling about on cobbled floors fighting with tough calvings to the point of exhaustion, getting kicked, crushed, trodden on and sprayed with muck. Often, I spent days with every muscle in my body aching. But I still had only a niggling and immovable overdraft of £1,000 to show for it all.

Of course, much of my time was spent driving a car. You didn't get paid for that, and maybe it was the reason for my situation. Yet the driving, the work and the whole rich life was spent out in this glorious countryside. I really loved all of it and it was only when I was accused of being a kind of agricultural con man that the contradiction came home to me.

As the road climbed higher I began to see the church tower and roofs of Darrowby and, at last, on the edge of the town, the gates of Mrs Pumphrey's beautiful home lay beckoning. I looked at my watch – twelve noon. Long practice had enabled me to time my visits here just before lunch when I could escape the rigours of country practice and wallow for a little while in the hospitality of the elderly widow who had brightened my life for so long.

As my tyres crunched on the gravel of the drive I smiled as Tricki Woo appeared at the window to greet me. He was old now, but he could still get up there to his vantage point and his Pekingese face was split as always by a panting grin of welcome.

Mounting the steps between the twin pillars of the doorway, I could see that he had left the window and I heard his joyous barking in the hall. Ruth, the long-serving maid, answered my ring, beaming with pleasure as Tricki flung himself at my knees.

'Eee, he's glad to see you Mr 'erriot,' she said and, laying a hand on my arm, 'we all are!'

She ushered me into the gracious drawing room where Mrs Pumphrey was sitting in an armchair by the fire. She raised her white head from her book and cried out in delight. 'Ah, Mr Herriot, how very very nice! Tricki, isn't it wonderful to have Uncle Herriot visiting again!'

She waved me to the armchair opposite. 'I have been expecting you for Tricki's check-up, but before you examine him you must sit down and warm yourself. It is so terribly cold. Ruth, my dear, will you bring Mr Herriot a glass of sherry. You will say yes, won't you, Mr Herriot.'

I murmured my thanks. I always said yes to the very special sherry which came in enormous glasses and was deeply heartening at all times but on cold days in particular. I sank into the cushions and stretched my legs towards the flames which leaped in the fireplace, and as I took my first sip and Ruth deposited a plate of tiny biscuits by my side while the little dog climbed on to my knee, the last of the hostile Sidlow vibes slipped gently away from me.

'Tricki has been awfully well since your last visit, Mr Herriot,' Mrs Pumphrey said. 'I know he is always going to be a little stiff with his arthritis but he does get around so well, and his little heart cough is no worse. And, best of all,' she clasped her hands together and her eyes widened, 'he hasn't gone flop-bott at all. Not once! So perhaps you won't have to squeeze the poor darling.'

'Oh no, I won't. Certainly not. I only do that if he really needs it.' I had been squeezing Tricki Woo's bottom for many years because of his anal gland trouble so graphically named by his mistress and the little animal had never resented it. I stroked his head as Mrs Pumphrey went on.

'There is something very interesting I must tell you. As you know, Tricki has always been deeply knowledgeable about horse racing, a wonderful judge of form, and wins nearly all his bets. Well now,' she raised a finger and spoke in a confidential murmur, 'just recently he has become very interested in greyhound racing!'

'Is that so?'

'Yes, indeed, he has begun to cover the meetings at the Middlesbrough greyhound track and has instructed me to place bets for him and, you know, he has won quite a lot of money already!'

'Gosh!'

'Yes, only this morning Crowther, my chauffeur, collected twelve pounds from the bookmaker after last evening's races.'

'Well, well, how wonderful.' My heart bled for Honest Joe Prendergast, the local turf accountant who must be suffering after losing money on horse-racing to a dog for years and then having to pay out on the greyhounds, too. 'Quite remarkable.'

'Isn't it, isn't it!' Mrs Pumphrey gave me a radiant smile, then she became serious. 'But I do wonder, Mr Herriot, just what is responsible for this new interest. What is your opinion?'

I shook my head gravely. 'Difficult to say. Very difficult.'

'However, I have a theory,' she said. 'Do you think perhaps that as he grows older he is more drawn to animals of his own species and prefers to bet on doggy runners like greyhounds?'

'Could be . . . could be . . .'

'And, after all, you would think with this affinity it would give him more insight and a better chance of winning.'

'Well, yes, that's possible. That's another point.'

Tricki, well aware that we were talking about him, waved his fine tail and looked up at me with his wide grin and lolling tongue.

I settled deeper in the cushions as the sherry began to send warm tendrils through my system. This was a happily familiar situation, listening to Mrs Pumphrey's recitals of Tricki Woo's activities. She was a kind, highly intelligent and cultivated lady, admired by all and a benefactress to innumerable charities. She sat on committees and her opinion was sought on many important matters, but where her dog was concerned her conversation never touched on weighty topics, but was filled with strange and wondrous things.

She leaned forward in her chair. 'There is something else I would like to talk to you about, Mr Herriot. You know that a Chinese restaurant has set up in Darrowby?'

'Yes, very nice, too.'

She laughed. 'But who would have thought it? A Chinese restaurant in a little place like Darrowby – it's amazing!'

'Very unexpected, I agree. But this last year or two they have been popping up all over Britain.'

'Yes, but what I want to discuss with you is that this has affected Tricki.'

'What!'

'Yes, he has been most upset over the whole business.'

'How on earth . . . ?'

'Well, Mr Herriot,' she frowned and gazed at me, solemn faced, 'I told you many years ago and you have always known that Tricki is descended from a long line of Chinese Emperors.'

'Yes, yes, of course.'

'Well, I think I can explain the whole problem if I start at the beginning.'

I took a long swallow at my sherry with the pleasant sensation that I was floating away in a dream world. 'Please do.'

'When the restaurant first opened,' she went on, 'there was a surprising amount of resentment among some of the local people. They criticized the food and the very nice little Chinese man and his wife, and put it about that there was no place for such a restaurant in Darrowby and that it should not be patronised. Now it so happened that when Tricki and I were out on our little walks, he overheard these remarks in the street, and he was furious.'

'Really?'

'Yes, quite affronted. I can tell when he feels like this. He stalks about with an insulted expression and it is so difficult to placate him.'

'Dear me, I'm sorry.'

'And after all, one can fully understand how he felt when he heard his own people being denigrated.'

'Quite, quite, absolutely – only natural.'

'However . . . however, Mr Herriot,' she raised a finger again and gave me a knowing smile, 'the clever darling suggested the cure himself.'

'He did?'

'Yes, he told me that we ourselves should start to frequent the restaurant and sample their food.'

'Ah.'

'And that is what we did. I had Crowther drive us there for lunch and we did enjoy it so much. Also, we found we could take the food home all nice and hot in little boxes – what fun! Now that we have started, Crowther often pops out in the evening and brings us our supper and, you know, the restaurant seems quite busy now. I feel we have really helped.'

'I'm sure you have,' I said, and I meant it. The Lotus Garden, tucked in a corner of the market place, wasn't much more than a shop front with four small tables inside and the sight of the gleaming black length of the limousine and liveried chauffeur parked frequently at its door must have given it a tremendous lift. I was struggling unsuccessfully to picture the locals peering through the window at Mrs Pumphrey and Tricki eating at one of those tiny tables when she went on.

'I'm so glad you think so. And we have enjoyed it so much. Tricki adores the char sui and my favourite is the chow mein. The little Chinese man is teaching us how to use the chop sticks, too.'

I put down my empty glass and dusted the tasty biscuit crumbs from my jacket. I hated to interrupt these sessions and return to reality, but I looked at my watch. 'I'm so glad things turned out so nicely, Mrs Pumphrey, but I think I'd better give the little chap his check-up.'

I lifted Tricki on to a settee and palpated his abdomen thoroughly. Nothing wrong there. Then I fished out my stethoscope and listened to his heart and lungs. There was the heart murmur I knew about and some faint bronchitic sounds which I expected. In fact I was totally familiar with all my old friend's internal workings after treating him over the years. Teeth now – maybe could do with another scale next time. Eyes with the beginnings of the lens opacity of the old dog, but not too bad at all.

I turned to Mrs Pumphrey. Tricki was on prednoleucotropin for his arthritis and oxytet for the bronchitis but I never elaborated on his ailments to her – too many medical terms upset her. 'He's really wonderful for his age, Mrs Pumphrey. You have his tablets to use when necessary and you know where I am if ever you need me. Just one thing. You have been very good with his diet lately so don't give him too many titbits – not even extra char sui!'

She giggled and gave me a roguish look. 'Oh, please don't scold me, Mr Herriot. I promise I'll be good.' She paused for a moment. 'I must mention one more thing with regard to Tricki's arthritis. You know that Hodgkin has been throwing rings for him for years?'

'Yes, I do.' Her words raised an image of the dour old gardener under duress casting the rubber rings on the lawn while the little dog, barking in delight, brought them back to him again. Hodgkin, who clearly didn't like dogs, invariably looked utterly fed up and his lips always seemed to be moving as he muttered either to himself or Tricki.

'Well, I thought in view of Tricki's condition that Hodgkin was throwing the rings too far and I told him to throw them for just a few feet. The little darling would have just as much fun with much less exertion.'

'I see.'

'Unfortunately,' here her expression became disapproving, 'Hodgkin has been rather mean about it.'

'In what way?'

'I wouldn't have known anything about it,' she said, lowering her voice, 'but Tricki confided in me.'

'Did he really?'

'Yes, he told me that Hodgkin had complained bitterly that it meant he had to bend down a lot more often to pick up the rings and that he had arthritis too. I wouldn't have minded,' her voice sank to a whisper, 'but Tricki was deeply shocked; he said Hodgkin used the word "bloody" several times.'

'Oh dear, dear, yes, I see the difficulty.'

'It has made the whole thing so embarrassing for Tricki. What do you think I should do?'

I nodded sagely and after some cogitation gave my opinion. 'I do think, Mrs Pumphrey, that it would be a good idea to have the throwing sessions less often and for a shorter time. After all, both Tricki and Hodgkin are no longer young.'

She gazed at me for a few moments, then smiled fondly. 'Oh, thank you, Mr Herriot, I'm sure you are right, as always. I shall follow your advice.'

I was about to make my farewells when Mrs Pumphrey put a hand on my arm. 'Before you go, Mr Herriot, I would like you to see something.'

She led the way to a room off the hall and opened the doors of a massive wardrobe. I looked at a long row of opulent suits – I had never seen so many outside a shop.

'These,' she said, running her hand slowly along jackets of all kinds, dark and dressy, light and tweed, 'belonged to my late husband.' For a few moments she was silent as she fingered one sleeve after another, then she became suddenly brisk and turned to me with a bright smile. 'He did love good clothes and went to London for all his suits. Now this one,' she reached up and lifted down a jacket and trousers of Lovat tweed, 'this one was made by one of the best tailors in Savile Row. Ooh, it's so heavy, will you hold it, please?' She gasped as she laid it on my outstretched arm and I, too, was amazed at its weight.

'Yes,' she went on, 'it is the most beautiful country suit and, do you know, he never wore it.' She shook her head and her eyes softened as she stroked the lapels. 'No, he never did. He died a few days after it was made and he was so looking forward to it. He was such an outdoor man, but he did like to be smartly dressed.' Then she said somewhat abruptly, looking up at me with a resolute expression, 'Now, Mr Herriot, would you like to have this suit?'

'Eh?'

'I wish you would have it. I'm sure it would be of great use to you and it is being wasted just hanging here in this wardrobe.'

I didn't know what to say, but my mind went back to various pauses in our conversation by the fire when I had noticed her eyes lingering briefly on the fringe of material on my frayed cuff as I raised my glass, and at my threadbare knees.

As I stood silent she looked suddenly worried. 'Perhaps I am embarrassing you?'

'Oh, no, no, no, not at all. It's very kind of you. I'm sure I'd love to have it.'

'Oh, I am glad.' She clapped her hands. 'It will be just right for you, quite the correct thing for a country vet. I'd so much like to think of you wearing it.'

'Right . . . right . . .' I said, still a little bemused. 'Thank you very much.' I laughed. 'Such a nice surprise.'

'Good, good,' she said, laughing too. Then she called across the hall. 'Ruth, Ruth, will you bring one of those big sheets of brown paper to put round this suit, there's a dear.'

As the maid hurried off, Mrs Pumphrey put her head on one side. 'There's just one thing, Mr Herriot. My husband was rather a large man. Some alterations will be necessary.'

'Oh, that's all right,' I said, 'I can see to that.'

As I walked over the gravel to my car weighed down with my parcel, I mused on the upturn in my day. A couple of hours ago I had slunk away like a pariah from a farm after a visit steeped in censure and dislike and with a final tongue-lashing thrown in, and look at me now. Mrs Pumphrey and Ruth were smiling and waving from the doorway. Tricki was back at his window, laughing his head off as he barked his farewell, the curtains moving with the wagging of his tail. My stomach glowed with sherry and savoury biscuits and I had a handsome free suit in my arms.

Not for the first time I thanked providence for the infinite variety of veterinary practice.

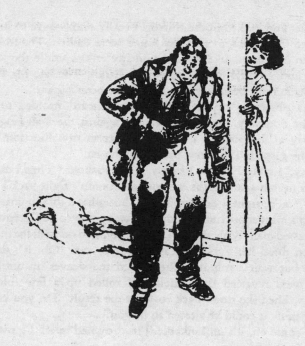

5

'Look at this, Helen!' I cried as I pulled off the brown paper back in Skeldale House. 'Mrs Pumphrey's given me a suit!'

My wife gasped as my new acquisition was unveiled. 'It's beautiful, Jim. So expensive-looking!'

'Isn't it just. I could never afford one like this.'

We looked down at the sumptuous tweed with its faint, scarcely discernible pattern of brownish threads among the Lovat green and Helen held up the jacket to examine it more closely.

'Gosh, it's so thick and heavy, I can hardly lift it! I've never seen such cloth – you'll never feel cold wearing this. Aren't you going to try it on? There's time before lunch – I'll just pop through to the kitchen and see that nothing's boiling over.'

I hurried to our bedroom and, bubbling with anticipation, removed my trousers and pulled on the new ones, then I donned the jacket and looked in the mirror. I really didn't have to look – I realised from the start that my hopes were dashed. The trousers rested in concertina-like folds round my ankles while the jacket sleeves hung several inches below my hands. The late Mr Pumphrey hadn't just been large, he must have been a giant.

I was observing myself sadly when I heard muffled sounds from the doorway. Helen was leaning against the wall laughing helplessly as she pointed a shaking finger in my direction. 'Oh dear,' she gasped. 'I'm sorry, but oh, ha-ha-ha!'

'Okay,' I said. 'I know, I know, it's a washout.' Then I caught sight of myself again in the mirror and couldn't fight back a wry smile. 'You're right, I do look funny, but what a disappointment. It's such a marvellous suit – I thought I was going to be Darrowby's best-dressed man. What the heck are we going to do with the thing?'

Helen dried her eyes and came over to me. 'Oh, it's such a shame, but wait a minute.' She tucked the sleeves up until my hands were revealed then knelt and rolled up a few folds of trousers. Then she stood back to view the result. 'Do you know, I really think it could be altered to fit you.'

'Oh come on, it's unthinkable. I'm drowned in it.' I glowered again at my reflection.

My wife shook her head vigorously. 'I'm not so sure. Looking at you now, I can just imagine how splendid it could be. Anyway, I'm going to take it round to Mr Bendelow and see if I can sweetheart him into doing it quickly.'

I grinned at the thought of our local tailor stirring himself. 'That would be a miracle.'

'You never know,' Helen said. 'I'm going to try, anyway.'

Later that day she came to me with the news that Mr Bendelow had been so dazzled by the quality of the material and the cut that he had promised a rush job.

The excitement over the suit was forgotten as I had an urgent call immediately after lunch.

Ted Newcombe's voice on the phone was strained and shaking. 'It's Clover – she's on calvin' and there's just a head and nowt else. I've had a go, but I can't reach the legs – it's a whopper of a calf. And it's the one I badly want – you remember?'

'Yes, I do remember, of course.'

'Can you get 'ere quick, Mr Herriot?'

'I'm leaving now.'

Clover was his best heifer and had been served by a premium bull. To a hill farmer like Ted, it would be a disaster if he lost the calf. I shouted to Helen and ran out to the car.

Ted's smallholding was a grey smudge high on a hillside near the top of the dale. There was no road to it and my car bumped its way up the grassy slope with my drugs and instruments rattling and clinking behind me. The flagged yard and thick-walled buildings were hundreds of years old; in fact, coupled with its inaccessibility, it was the sort of place where only hard-up people like Ted would dream of trying to make a living. The rent was low and it was all he could afford.

He was coming out of the byre as I drew up, Tall and thin, about my own age, father of a boy and girl who walked down that hill every day and then the two miles to the village school. He looked worried, but managed a grin.

'Nice car, Mr Herriot!' He gave the gleaming bonnet a mock polish with his sleeve but, as was typical of him, that was as far as the mickey-taking went.

I followed him into the little byre and I realised why he didn't feel much like joking. The smile was wiped off my own face immediately I looked at the beautiful heifer groaning and heaving, with an enormous muzzle just peeping from her vulva as she strained.

No vet likes to see that. It wasn't just a case of sorting out a malpresentation, it meant that a huge calf was finding it impossible to find a way out.

'I've 'ad a go,' Ted said as I stripped off and began to wash my arms in the buckets of steaming water. 'But there's no legs – feet are miles away. I remember you tellin' me once to push back the head to reach the feet but I've tried and she's ower strong for me.'

I nodded. The farmer hadn't much flesh on his bones, but he had a stringy power in his arms and I knew what he meant. 'Nobody's as strong as a big beast like that, Ted.'

'And all the time I'm wonderin' if t'calf's still alive. He's been squeezed in there for a hell of a long time.'

That was my worry, too. I soaped my arm and pushed a hand into the vulva alongside the massive head, but as I reached for the shoulder Clover gave another heave and my arm was trapped agonisingly for a few seconds.

'That's no good,' I gasped, 'there's not an inch of room in there. I'll try my luck with the head.'

I put my hand against the muzzle and pushed steadily, leaning hard as the head went back a few inches. That was as far as I got. Another mighty expulsive effort from the heifer sent me back where I started.

I began to wash my hands and arms again. 'It's impossible, Ted. That calf won't come out till we bring the feet round and there's simply no way of reaching those feet. She's a big, powerful heifer and we can't win pushing against her.'

'Oh 'ell!' He looked at me wide-eyed. 'What do we do, then? Caesarean? That's a big job!'

'Maybe not,' I said. 'I've got another trick up my sleeve.'

I was out to the car and back again in a few moments with a syringe and local anaesthetic. 'Grab the tail, Ted,' I said, 'and move it up and down like a pump handle. That's the way.' I felt for the epidural space between the vertebrae and injected 10 ccs, then I stood back and watched.

I hadn't long to wait. In less than a minute Clover began to relax as though her troubles were over. Ted pointed at her. 'Look at that, she's stopped strainin'!'

'She can't strain, now,' I said. 'She's had a spinal anaesthetic and she can't feel a thing back there. In fact, she really doesn't know what's going on.'

'So if she can't push against us we can maybe get the head back inside?'

'That's the idea.' Another soaping of my arm and I pressed my palm against the broad muzzle, and oh, it was lovely to feel the head and neck and the whole calf moving away from me with no sign of resistance. There was room then to pass a noose inside and snare a foot and then another till I had two cloven hooves showing at the vulva. I grasped one in each hand and as I leaned back the calf's muzzle reappeared and, to my great relief, I saw a twitching of the nostrils.

I laughed. 'This calf's alive, Ted.'

'Oh, thank God for that,' the farmer said, blowing out his cheeks. 'We can get on wi' the job now, can't we?'

'Yes, but there's just one snag. Because she's unable to strain she can't help us. We'll have to do everything ourselves.'

It was still a very tight squeeze and we had half an hour of careful pulling on the legs and head and frequent application of lubricating jelly. We soon began to sweat but Clover was totally unconcerned and paid no attention as she picked away happily at the hay in the rack. My big fear was that the calf might stick at the hips but, with a final heave from us, the little creature slid out into the world and I caught the slippery body as it fell.

Ted lifted a hind leg. 'It's a bull. Reckon it had to be when it was as big as that.' He smiled happily. 'Most times I want heifers, but thus 'un will sell well for breedin'. He's got a fine pedigree on both sides.'

He began to rub ribs and head with straw and the calf responded by raising his head and snuffling. Clover looked round quickly at the sound and gave a soft moo of delight and, it seemed to me, surprise, because she had known nothing of the operation and clearly was a little mystified as to how this enchanting newcomer had arrived. We pulled him up to her head and she commenced an enthusiastic end to end licking of the little body.

I smiled. I never got tired of this – the most rewarding thing in my veterinary life. 'Nice to see, isn't it, Ted. I wish all calvings finished up like this.'

'By gaw, you're right, Mr Herriot, and I can't thank ye enough. I really thought I had a dead 'un on me hands this time.' As I bent over the bucket he gave me a friendly thump on the back.

As I dried my arms, I looked round the byre with its row of well-kept cows. Over some months Ted had gutted the place completely, hacking out the ancient wooden partitions and replacing them with tubular metal, plastering the walls, digging up the cobbled floor and laying down concrete. He had done all the work himself.

He followed my gaze. 'What d'you think of me little place now?'

'It's great, you've done wonders, Ted. And you've built a nice little dairy, too.'

'Aye, ah've got to get that TT licence somehow.' He rubbed his chin. 'But there's a few things that don't come up to standard. Like not enough space between the channel and the back wall. There's nowt I can do about that and one or two other points. But if the Ministry'll grant me a licence, I'll get another fourpence on every gallon of milk and it'll make all the difference in the world to me.'

He laughed, as though reading my thoughts. 'Maybe you don't think fourpence is much but, you know, we don't need a lot o' money. We never go out at night – we're quite happy playin' cards and Ludo and dominoes with the kids, and with these cows to milk and feed and muck out twice a day, three hundred and sixty-five days a year, I'm tied to the spot.' He laughed again. 'Ah can't remember when I even went into Darrowby. No, we don't want much money, but right now I'm just hanging on – only keepin' my head above water. Any road, I'll know after next Thursday. They're having a meeting to decide.'

I didn't say anything. I couldn't tell him that I was the one who had to make a confidential report to the Milk Committee on that day about him and his farm and it all rested on whether I could convince them. Ted's fourpence a gallon was in my hands and it frightened me a bit, because if the TT licence didn't go through I dared not think how much longer he could carry on his struggle to make a go of this wind-blown farm with its sparse pastures.

I packed up my gear and we went outside. Breathing in the cold, clean air I looked at the cloud shadows chasing across the tumbled miles of green hills, and at the few acres that were Ted's world. They made a little wall-girt island lapped around by the tufted grass of the moorland which was always trying to flow over and swamp it. Those fields had to be fed and fertilised to keep them from returning to their wild state, and the walls, twisted and bent by the centuries, kept shedding their stones – another job to be done by that one man. I recalled a time when Ted told me that one of his luxuries was to wake up in the middle of the night so that he could turn over and go to sleep again.

As I started the engine, he waved, raising a huge, work-calloused hand. Bumping down the hillside I looked back at the thin, slightly stooping figure standing by the house with its fringe of stunted trees, and an awareness of his situation welled in me as it had done so often before. Compared to his, my life was a picnic.

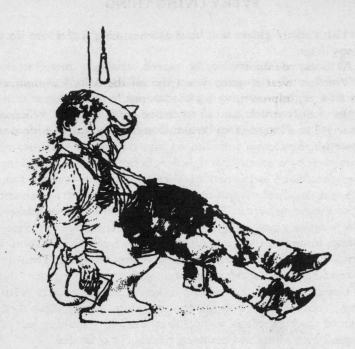

6

The following Thursday I awoke with the words of my appeal for Ted spinning around in my head and I kept mouthing a few phrases in the car as I did a couple of early calls. I was due in the Ministry Office at 11 a.m. and by ten o'clock I was back home ready to change.

I was about to go upstairs when Helen came in.

'You'll never believe this,' she said breathlessly, 'but Mr Bendelow saw me as I passed his window and gave me the suit.'

'Mr Pumphrey's suit?'

'Yes, it's all altered and ready for you to wear.' She stared at me, wide eyed.

I looked at the parcel in amazement. 'Well, that's never happened before. We asked for a miracle and got one.'

'That's right,' Helen said. 'And another thing, I feel sure it's a happy omen.'

'What do you mean?'

'You can wear it when you speak to the Milk Committee. You'll really impress them in a suit like that.'

Her words struck home. As an orator I was no Winston Churchill and I needed any help that was going. In the bedroom I tore off my clothes and climbed into the refurbished trousers. They were now exactly the right length but there was something else, something I hadn't noticed when I had tried them on before. The waistband came right up over my chest until it was almost tucked under my arms. Those were the days of high waistbands which rested comfortably well above the hips, but Mr Pumphrey's stature had vastly accentuated this. I was beaten again. I turned and faced Helen and her mouth began to twitch. Then she lowered her head and her body shook with repressed giggles.

'Don't start that again!' I cried. 'They're nearly as funny as last time. You don't have to tell me. Anyway, I can't wear these damned things, that's all there is to it. I'm just a walking pair of trousers with a head and shoulders poking out at the top.'

I was about to pull off the maddening garment when Helen held up a hand. 'Wait . . . wait . . .' she said. 'Put on the jacket.'

'What good will that do?'

'The lapels are very high, just put it on.'

With a feeling of hopelessness I shrugged myself into the jacket and turned towards her.

Helen was looking at me with something like awe. 'It's wonderful,' she whispered. 'Incredible.'

'What is?'

'Look at yourself.'

I looked into the mirror and Lord Herriot of Darrowby looked out at me. The waistband was quite hidden and the suit was there in all its glory of rich material and superb tailoring, draped on me elegantly as if it had been made for me.

'My God,' I breathed, 'I never knew clothes could make all that difference. I'm like another person.'

'Yes, you are,' agreed Helen eagerly. 'You're like an important,

43

prestigious person. You must wear it for the committee – you'll knock them cold!'

While I washed and combed my hair, I had the warm sense of everything slotting into place when all had seemed lost and as I left after a final admiring glance at myself in the mirror I was filled with an airy confidence.

Outside, a bitter wind swept over the fields but I couldn't feel it. Nothing could penetrate my apparel; in fact, I felt sure that, dressed like this, I could walk in comfort to the North Pole without changing.

In the car, my body heat rose rapidly and I had to open the windows. I was glad when I reached my destination and was able to take a few breaths of the cold air. My relief, however, was short lived because as soon as the swing doors of the Ministry Office closed behind me a stifling heat hit me. On my previous visits I had wondered how people could work in this atmosphere with the central heating going full blast and as I walked along the corridor looking through the glass partitions at the typists and technicians and Ministry officials apparently going about their business quite happily, I marvelled anew. Only this time it was worse. Much, much worse. This time I was cocooned almost up to my chin in two layers of carpet-like material.

It was the waistband, of course, that was the trouble, clamped round my entire rib-cage like a great constricting hand, and I had the silly feeling that the suit itself was carrying me along to the double doors of the Conference Room at the end of the corridor. In the big room it was hotter than ever and I had a moment of panic when I thought I wouldn't be able to breathe, but I settled down as the Committee members welcomed me in their usual friendly way and the chairman ushered me to my seat at the long table.

There were about twenty people on the Milk Committee – big farmers, technical officers of the Ministry, two of the great landowners of the district in Lord Darbrough and Sir Henry Brookly, a physician and one practising veterinary surgeon – me. I had felt honoured when I was invited to join and had tried to fulfil my duties to the best of my ability, but this morning was something special.

Sir Henry was chairman and as he started the proceedings I prayed that it would be a short session. I knew I couldn't stand it for long, tightly muffled in this heat, but as the minutes ticked away with agonising slowness I realised that there was a tremendous amount of business to get through. Long discussions about sterilisation, farm buildings and husbandry, cattle diseases, points of law – it went on and on and I sat there getting hotter and hotter. Quite often I was asked for my opinion and I answered in a breathless way which I hoped went unnoticed, but it seemed that my most important contribution was being kept until the end.

My condition deteriorated steadily until, after an hour, I was sure I was suffocating and it was only a matter of time before I fainted away and had to be carried from the room. I was breathing only with difficulty, I could feel the sweat running down my neck onto my collar and had to fight the impulse to tear open my jacket and let out some of the pent up heat, but the thought of this decorous group of men dissolving into laughter at the sight of my chin-high trousers stayed my hand.

It was after almost two hours that Sir Henry looked around the table and introduced my subject. 'Well, gentlemen,' he said, 'to conclude our business this morning we have to decide on the borderline case of hill-farmer Edward Newcombe's application for a Tuberculin Tested licence and I understand that our young friend, Mr Herriot, has been looking into the matter for us. Mr Herriot . . . ?' He smiled across the table at me.

Somebody began to talk about Ted Newcombe and for a few moments I didn't realise it was myself. The words were familiar but they seemed to be coming from somewhere outside me, panting and hoarse. Through the blur of sweat trickling into my eyes I could see them all looking at me kindly. They had always been kind, these men, maybe because I was the youngest member, but as my utterances tumbled out – 'outstanding stocksman' . . . 'cattle in immaculate condition' . . . 'hard worker' . . . 'meticulous attention to hygiene' . . . 'man of the highest integrity' . . . they kept smiling and nodding encouragingly and as the last phrase emerged – 'Edward Newcombe's buildings may not be perfect but he really is a trier and if he is granted his licence he will never let anybody down,' I seemed to be surrounded by cheerful, friendly faces.

Sir Henry beamed at me, 'Ah, thank you so much, Mr Herriot, that is most helpful and we are grateful to you. I think we can take it, gentlemen, that there will be no difficulty in granting the licence?' Hands went up in agreement all round the table.

I have very little recollection of how I left the room, only of rushing downstairs into the men's lavatory, locking myself into one of the cubicles, throwing off my jacket and collapsing, open-mouthed, onto the seat. As I opened the front of the vast trousers, unbuttoned my shirt and lay back, gasping, waves of heat mingled with relief and triumph rolled from me. I had got it over. Ted had his licence and I was still alive – just.

As I slowly recovered I heard two men come in. From my semi-supine position I could see their feet under the door and I recognised the voices of Sir Henry and Lord Darbrough. The feet disappeared as the men retreated to the opposite wall.

There was a silence, then. 'Tell you what, Henry,' boomed His Lordship, 'it did me good to see that young fella fighting his corner for the hill-farmer.'

'Couldn't agree more, George. Damn good show, I thought.'

'Threw everything into it, by gad. Didn't spare himself. Never seen anything like it – sweat was rolling down his face.'

'Mm, I saw. Dedication, I'd call it.'

'That's it, dedication. Good to see in somebody his age.' There was another pause, then, 'Y'know, Henry, there was something else about that young fella.'

'What was that, George?'

'Knows his clothes. Splendid suit. Rather envy him his tailor.'

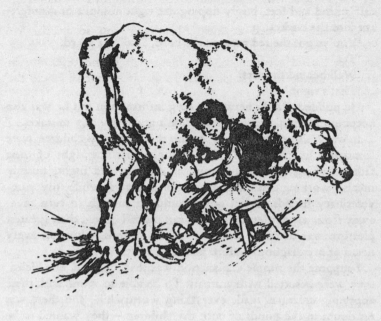

7

'Look at that little lad!'

Farmer Dugdale was amused as he watched Jimmy directing his torch beam as I calved the cow. My son, ten years old, was taking his duty very seriously. It was quite dark in the loose box and he solemnly followed my every movement with his beam, shining on the cow's rear end as I worked, then on the bucket of hot water each time I resoaped my arms or dipped the ropes in the disinfectant.

'Yes,' I said, 'he loves night work.'

Jimmy, in fact, loved all veterinary work, but if I was called out in the evening before his bedtime it was his particular delight to come with me, sitting by me, quite absorbed, as the headlights picked out the twists and turns of the country lanes.

And tonight, when we arrived, he had been into the boot

before me, picking out the different coloured ropes to go on the calf's head and feet, busily tipping the right amount of disinfectant into the bucket.

'You've got the red rope on the head, Dad?' he asked.

'Yes.'

'Well behind the ears?'

'That's right.'

He nodded. Partly he was seeking information but he was also keeping me right, making sure I didn't make any silly mistakes.

It was a source of wonder to me that both my children were fascinated by my job. I often thought that the sight of their father rushing around all hours of the day and night, missing meals, working on Saturdays and Sundays while my non-veterinary friends played golf, would be enough to turn them away from my profession for life, but instead of that their greatest pleasure was to come with me on my rounds, taking in every detail of my diagnostic efforts and treatments.

I suppose the simple explanation was that, like me, like Helen, they were besotted with animals. To be able to work with these appealing creatures made everything worthwhile, and there was no doubt in the minds of both my children – they wanted to be vets.

It struck me now, that Jimmy, at the age of ten was half way there already. As the calf slipped out on to the loose box floor he quickly wiped away the mucus from the little animal's nostrils and mouth, seized a handful of hay and began to administer a brisk rubdown.

'It's a heifer, Dad,' he said, after an expert glance between the hind legs. 'That's good, Mr Dugdale, isn't it?'

The farmer laughed. 'Aye, it is. We want plenty of heifers. That 'un you're rubbing maybe will be a good milk cow one day.'

The following day was a Saturday with no school, and after breakfast, both children were lined up, ready for action. In fact they had already started. They had the lid of the car boot up and were clearing out the empty bottles and cartons, checking up to see that I had everything I might need.

'You're getting a bit short of calcium, Dad,' Rosie said. She was six now and had been doing the rounds since she was two, so she was very familiar with the contents of the big slotted box which a friend had made for me to hold my drugs and instruments.

'Right, my pet,' I replied, 'you'd better go and get some. Calcium is one thing we can't do without.'

Flushed with importance, she ran inside to the stock room, and I wondered, as often before, why it was that, at home and on the farms, she always ran to get things for me while Jimmy invariably walked.

Often, in the middle of a case, I'd say, 'Fetch me another syringe, Jimmy,' and my son would stroll out to the car, often whistling, perfectly relaxed. No matter how interested he was in what was happening he never hurried. And I have often noticed that now, when he is a highly experienced veterinary surgeon, he still doesn't hurry. This is probably a good thing, because ours can be a stressful occupation and going about things calmly must be the best way.

When all was ready we drove out into the hills. It was a bright morning with the bleak outlines of fell and moorland softened by the sunshine. There had been rain in the night and all the scents of the countryside drifted through the open windows.

The first farm was approached by a lane with several gates and Rosie was delighted because this was her job.

As we drew up at the first one she was out of the car in a flash. Red faced and serious, she opened the gate and I drove through.

'Lucky I was with you this morning, Dad,' she said. 'There's two more up ahead. I can see them.'

I nodded. 'It is indeed, sweetheart. If there's one thing I hate, it's gates.'

My little daughter sat back, well pleased. In the days before she started school she used to be really worried. 'What are you going to do without me?' she would say. 'I've got to go to school soon, and Jimmy's there already. You'll be all alone.'

Jimmy always seemed to be reasonably confident that I'd manage to struggle round on my own, but Rosie had grave doubts. Weekends for her were not just a time to play, but a blessed opportunity to look after her father. And for me it was a wonderful time and I marvelled at my luck. So many men with high pressure jobs see very little of their families but I had it both ways with my little son and daughter so often at my side as I worked.

And there was no doubt about it, it was an absolute boon to have the gates opened for me. Rosie stood stiffly to attention as I drove through the last one. Her hand was on the latch and her face registered the satisfaction of a job well done.

A few minutes later I was in the cow byre, scratching my head in puzzlement. My patient had a temperature of 106 but my first confident diagnosis of mastitis was eliminated when I found that the milk was white and clear.

'This is a funny one,' I said to the farmer. 'Her lungs are okay, stomach working well, yet she's got this high fever, and you say she's not eating?'

'Aye, that's right. She hasn't touched her hay or cake this morning. And look how she's shakin'.'

I pulled the cow's head round and was looking for possible symptoms when my son's voice piped up from behind me.

'I think it *is* mastitis, Dad.'

He was squatting by the udder pulling streams of milk on to the palm of his hand. 'The milk's really hot in this quarter.'

I went round the teats again and sure enough, Jimmy was right. The milk in one quarter looked perfect, but it was decidedly warmer than the others and when I pulled a few more jets on to my hand I could feel flakes, still invisible, striking my palm.

I looked up ruefully at the farmer and he burst into a roar of laughter. 'It looks like t'apprentice knows more than the boss. Who taught you that, son?'

'Dad did. He said you could often be caught out that way.'

'And he was, wasn't he!' The farmer slapped his thigh.

'Okay, okay,' I said, and as I went out to the car for the penicillin tubes I wondered how many other little wrinkles my son had absorbed in his journeys with me.

Later, as we drove back along the gated roads, I congratulated him.

'Well done, old lad. You know a lot more than I think!'

Jimmy grinned. 'Yes, and remember when I couldn't even milk a cow?'

I nodded. Milking machines were universal among the bigger farms but many of the smallholders still milked by hand and it fascinated my son to watch them. I remembered the time he stood by the side of old Tim Suggett as he milked one of his six cows. Crouched on the stool, head against the cow's flank, the farmer effortlessly sent the white jets hissing and frothing into the bucket held between his knees.

He looked up and caught the boy's eager gaze.

'Does tha want to 'ave a go, young man?' he asked.

'Oh, yes please!'

'Awright, here's a fresh bucket. See if ye can fill it?'

Jimmy squatted, grasped a teat in each hand and began to pull away lustily. Nothing happened. He tried two other teats with the same result.

'There's nothing coming,' he cried plaintively. 'Not a drop.'

Tim Suggett laughed. 'Aye, it's not as easy as it looks, is it? I reckon it 'ud take you a long time to milk ma six cows.'

My son looked crestfallen, and the old man put a hand on his head. 'Come round sometime and I'll teach ye. I'll soon make a milker out of ye.'

A few weeks later, I returned from my round one afternoon to find Helen standing on the doorstep of Skeldale House, looking very worried.

'Jimmy hasn't come back from school,' she said. 'Did he tell you he was going to any of his friends?'

I thought for a moment. 'No, not that I can remember. But maybe he's just playing somewhere.'

Helen looked out at the gathering dusk. 'It's strange, though. He usually comes home to tell us first.'

We telephoned round his school friends without result, then I began a tour of Darrowby exploring the little winding 'yards', calling in at people we knew and getting the same reply. 'No, I'm sorry, we haven't seen him', and my attempt at a cheerful rejoinder, 'Oh, thanks very much, sorry to trouble you,' as a cold hand began to grip at my heart.

When I got back to Skeldale House, Helen was on the verge

of tears. 'He hasn't come back, Jim. Where on earth can he have got to? It's pitch black out there. He can't be playing.'

'Oh, he'll turn up. There'll be some simple explanation, don't worry.' I hoped I sounded airy but I didn't tell Helen that I had been dredging the water trough at the bottom of the garden.

I was beginning to feel the unmistakable symptoms of panic when I had a thought. 'Wait a minute, didn't he say he'd go round to Tim Suggett's one day after school to learn to milk?'

The smallholding was actually in Darrowby itself and I was there in minutes. A soft light shone above the half door of the little cow house and as I looked inside there was my son, crouched on a stool, bucket between his knees, head against a patient cow.

'Hello, Dad,' he said cheerfully. 'Look in here!' He displayed his bucket which contained a few pints of milk. 'I can do it now! Mr Suggett's been showing me. You don't pull the teats at all. You just make your fingers go like this.'

Glorious relief flooded through me. I wanted to grab Jimmy and kiss him, kiss Mr Suggett, kiss the cow, but I took a couple of deep breaths and restrained myself.

'It's very good of you to have him, Tim. I hope he hasn't been any bother.'

The old man chuckled. 'Nay, lad, nay. We've had a bit o' fun, and t'young man's cottoned on right sharp. I've been tellin' him if he's goin' to be a vitnery he'll have to know how to get the milk out of a cow.'

It is one of my vivid memories, that night when Jimmy learned how to get the milk out of a cow, so that he could diagnose mastitis and put one over on his old man.

To this day I often wonder if I did the right thing in talking Rosie out of her ambition. Maybe I was wrong, but back in the forties and fifties, life in veterinary practice was quite different from now. Our practice was ninety per cent large animal work and although I loved the work I was always being kicked, knocked about and splashed with various kinds of filth. With all its charms and rewards it was a dirty and often dangerous job. On several occasions, I was called to help out in neighbouring practices where the vet had sustained a broken limb, and I had myself been lame for weeks when a huge carthorse whacked my thigh with his iron-shod hoof.

Quite often I didn't smell so good because no amount of bathing in antiseptics could wholly banish the redolence of delivering decomposing calves and the removal of afterbirths. I was used to people wrinkling their noses when I came too near.

Sometimes after prolonged calvings and foalings, often lasting for hours, every muscle in my body ached for days as though I had been beaten with a heavy stick.

It is all so different now. We have long plastic gloves to protect us when we are doing the smelly jobs, there are metal crushes to hold the big beasts instead of having to plunge among them as they were driven into a passage on the farm, and the Caesarean operation has eliminated the rough side of obstetrics. Also, the gentler small animal work has expanded beyond all expectations until it now makes up more than half our work.

When I entered the veterinary college there was only one girl in our class – a tremendous novelty – but now girls make up at least fifty per cent of the students at the veterinary schools and, in fact, excellent girl veterinary surgeons have worked in our practice.

I didn't know all this forty years ago and although I could imagine tough little Jimmy living my life, I couldn't bear the thought of Rosie doing it. Unfairly at times, I used every wile I could think of to put her off veterinary work and to persuade her to become a doctor of humans instead of animals.

She is a happy doctor, too, but, as I say, I still wonder . . .

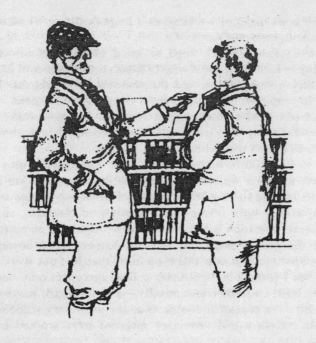

8

'Not to put too fine a point on it, Herriot, I think you are dishonest.'

'What!' I had been called a few things in my time, but never that and it hit me hard, especially coming from a tall, patrician veterinary surgeon, looking down his nose at me. 'What the devil do you mean? How can you possibly say that?'

Hugo Mottram's imperious blue eyes regarded me with distaste. 'I say it only because I am forced to no other conclusion. I consider unethical behaviour to be a type of dishonesty and you have certainly been guilty of that. Also, your attempts to justify your actions seem to me to be sheer prevarication.'

This was really nice, I thought, particularly here in Brawton where I was trying to enjoy my precious half-day. I had been browsing happily in Smith's bookshop, and had spotted Mottram walking along by the shelves and, in fact, had been regarding him with some envy, wishing that I looked a bit like him. He was the perfect picture of my idea of a country vet; check cap, immaculate hacking jacket, knee breeches, stockings and brogues together with a commanding presence and hawk-like, handsome features. He was in his fifties, but as he paced among the books, head high, chin jutting, he had the look of a fit young man.

I took a deep breath and tried to speak calmly. 'Mr Mottram, what you have just said is insulting, and I think you should apologise. Surely you realise that neither my partner nor I have any designs on your clients – it was just an unfortunate combination of events. There was nothing else we could have done in the circumstances and if only you would just think about it . . .'

The tall man stuck out his chin even more. 'I *have* thought about it and I mean what I say. I have no desire to waste any more time in discussing this matter, and my hope is that I shall have no further contact with you in the future.'

He turned quickly and strode from the shop leaving me fuming. I stood there, staring at my boots. Helen would be joining me any minute now – she had been having her hair done – and then our happy programme would start; shopping, tea, then the cinema and a late meal with a lot of good conversation, all with my pal, Gordon Rae, the vet from Boroughbridge and his wife, Jean. It was a simple sequence, but a blessed escape from the hard work and we looked forward to it all week. And now it was in ruins, shattered.

This thing with Mottram had started a few weeks previously. I was examining a spaniel with a skin eruption in our surgery when the lady owner suddenly said, 'Mr Mottram of Scanton has been treating this dog for some time. Says it's eczema, but it's not improving and I think it must be something else. I want a second opinion.'

I looked at the lady. 'I wish you'd mentioned that at the beginning. Really, I should have asked Mr Mottram's permission before I looked at your dog.'

'Oh, I didn't know that.'

'Well, yes, that's how it is, and I'm afraid I'll have to speak to him before I do any more.'

I excused myself and went through to the telephone in the office.

'Mottram here.' The voice was as I remembered. Deep, assured, cool. As a neighbouring veterinary surgeon, I had met him a few times and found I couldn't get very near him. His aristocratic haughtiness was, to me, decidedly off-putting. But I had to try to be friendly.

'Oh, hello, this is Herriot, Darrowby. How are you?'

'I am quite well, Herriot. I trust you are the same.' Damn, he still sounded patronising.

'Well now, I have one of your clients, a Mrs Hickson, here with her dog — I see it has a skin condition. She's asking for a second opinion.'

The voice became suddenly glacial. 'You've seen the animal? I think you might have consulted me first.'

'I'm sorry. I didn't get the chance. Mrs Hickson didn't tell me till I had the dog on the table. I do apologise, and I wonder if I might have your permission to carry on.'

There was a long pause, then again the icy tones. 'Well, I suppose if you must, you must.' The phone went down with a bonk.

My face was hot with embarrassment. What was the matter with the chap? This sort of thing happened all the time in veterinary practice. I'd had to approach other neighbouring practitioners and sometimes they'd had to approach me. The response on both sides had always been 'Oh yes, of course, carry on by all means. I'd be glad to know what you think.' And followed by a description of the treatment to date.

None of that with Mottram, and I wasn't going to phone him again. I'd have to find out the past treatment from the owner if I could.

I told Siegfried later.

'Snooty bugger,' he grunted. 'Remember when I asked him to dinner a long time ago? He said that he felt that vets should have an honourable association with their neighbours in opposition, but he didn't believe in their socialising with each other.'

'Yes, I do remember.'

'Okay, I respect his views, but there's no need for this stupid touchiness.'

A couple of weeks later I had a feeling of impending doom when I was feeling my way over the hind leg of a lame dog and the owner, a nice old man, chirped up. 'Oh, by the way, I should have told you. Mr Mottram over at Scanton has been treating him, but I can see no improvement at all and I'd like your opinion.'

My toes began to curl, but there was nothing else for it. I rang up our neighbour again.

'Mottram here.' That same discouraging voice.

I told him what had happened, and asked his permission.

Again that long pause, then a disdainful 'So you're at it again?'

'At it ...? What do you mean? I'm not at anything, I'm merely asking your permission to do as your client has requested.'

'Oh, do what you damn well like.' And I heard the familiar thud of the phone at the other end.

I began to sense the eerie workings of fate when Siegfried came in a few days later, looking thoughtful.

'You won't believe this, James. I was called to one of Mottram's clients this morning. Bollands by name, and he was in a state. He had a horse with a broken leg and couldn't get hold of Mottram. Phoned me in desperation. I rang the Scanton practice but he was on his rounds and I had to dash out to Bollands' place. It was a ghastly thing – a horrible compound fracture with the poor creature in agony. No possibility of treatment. There was simply nothing for it but to shoot the poor thing immediately. I couldn't let him suffer. But it would be Mottram – I've tried to contact him again now, but he's still not around.'

I had been helping Siegfried to clean out a dog's cankered ears and we were clearing up when, to our complete astonishment, Mottram appeared in the doorway of the operating room. He was immaculate as usual, clearly in a rage, but in cold control of himself.

'Ah, you're both here.' That superior voice again. 'It's just as well, because what I have to say applies to both of you. This latest escapade at Bollands' is really too much, Farnon. I can only conclude that you are conducting a campaign to steal my clients.'

Siegfried flushed. 'Now look here, Mottram, that is ridiculous.

We have absolutely no desire to poach your clients. As to Bollands' horse, I tried in vain to get in touch with you, but . . .'

Mottram held up a hand. 'I don't want to hear any more. You can say what you like, but I believe in *honourable* relations. Now that this has happened I am glad I stuck to my principles about that "out to dinner together" nonsense.' He nodded down to each of us from his great height and left.

Siegfried turned to me ruefully. 'Well, that's finally torn it. I want to be friends with all my neighbours but we're finished there.'

Now in the bookshop in Brawton, recalling the sequence of events, I felt that I hadn't needed this final onslaught from Mottram. Standing there among the wreckage of my half-day, looking at his retreating back, I knew that he had washed his hands of me.

Like my partner, I was unhappy about the situation, but I put it out of my mind until my bedside phone rang at 1 a.m. about a month later. I reached out a sleepy arm.

The voice at the other end was agitated. 'This is Lumsden, Scanton. Mr Mottram's assistant. I'm treating his horse with a bad colic, but I'm beat with it. I need help.'

Suddenly I was wide awake. 'Where's Mottram?'

'He's on holiday in the north of Scotland.' The young man's voice began to quaver. 'Oh, this would happen when he's away. He adores this horse – it's his favourite, he rides it every day. But I've tried everything and it looks like dying. I don't know how I'm going to face him when he gets back.' There was a pause. 'Actually, I was hoping to speak to Mr Farnon. He's good with horses, isn't he?'

'Yes, he is,' I said. In the darkness, I rested the receiver on my chest and looked at the ceiling as Helen stirred uneasily at my side, then I spoke again. 'Look, Lumsden, I'll have a word with my partner. It's his night off, but I'll see what he says. Anyway, I promise you one of us at least will be out to give you a hand.'

I cut short his thanks and dialled Siegfried's home number. I told him the story and could sense him snapping awake at the other end. 'Oh my God! Mottram!'

'Yes. What d'you think?'

I listened to a long sigh, then, 'I've got to go, James.'

'I'll come with you.'

'Really? Are you sure?'

'Of course. It's my night on, anyway, and I might be able to help.'

On the way to Scanton we didn't say much, but Siegfried voiced our thoughts. 'You know, this is uncanny. It sounds as though we're on a hiding to nothing here and Mottram is going to love us even more when he finds we've been in at the death of his beloved horse. Colics are nasty things at any time, always dangerous, even the straightforward ones, and I'd like to bet that this one will have some complications.'

Mottram's house was just outside Scanton and our headlights picked out an avenue of chestnut trees leading to an impressive bulk with a fine pillared doorway. We drove round the back and found Lumsden waving us with his torch into a cobbled court-yard. As we drew up, he turned and ran quickly into a lighted loose box in the corner of the yard. When we followed him, we could see the reason for his haste. And it was a frightening sight. My stomach lurched and I heard a soft 'Oh, dear God!' from Siegfried. A big chestnut horse, head hanging, staring-eyed and lathered in sweat, was stumbling round the box, buckling at the knees, doing his best to throw himself down and roll which, as any vet knows, can cause torsion of the bowel and inevitable death. The young man was hanging on desperately to the halter shank and urging the animal to keep walking round the box.

Lumsden looked about sixteen, but as a qualified veterinarian he had to be nearly ten years older than that. He was slightly built and his naturally boyish face was pale and exhausted.

'Very good of you to come,' he gasped. 'I hate to get you out of bed, but I've been fighting this colic all day yesterday and all day today, and I'm getting nowhere. The horse is worse if anything and I'm about knackered.'

'That's quite all right, old chap,' Siegfried said soothingly. 'James will hold the horse for a minute while you tell me what you've done.'

'Well, I've been giving Istin as a laxative, chloral hydrate to relieve the pain. Largactil, and a few small shots of arecoline, but I'm frightened to give any more arecoline because there's a hell of an impaction in there and I don't want to rupture the bowel. If only he'd pass a bit of muck, but there's been nothing through him for over forty-eight hours.'

'Never mind, my boy, you've done nothing wrong, so don't worry about that.' Siegfried slipped a hand behind the animal's elbow and felt the pulse. Then as the horse staggered around, he reflected the eyelid and examined the conjunctiva. He looked at it thoughtfully before taking the temperature.

'Yes . . . yes . . .' he murmured without changing expression, then he turned to the young man. 'Would you slip into the house now and get us a bucket of hot water, soap and a towel. I want to do a rectal.'

As Lumsden hurried out, Siegfried swung round. 'By God, I don't like this, James. Lousy weak pulse – can hardly detect it – brick red conjunctiva and temperature 103. I don't want to put the wind up this young chap, but I think we're on a loser here.' His eyes widened. 'And Mottram again! Is there such a thing as a jinx?'

I didn't say anything as I hung on to the struggling animal. A weak pulse is a particularly ominous finding in a horse and the other things pointed to a complicating bowel inflammation.

When the young man came back, Siegfried rolled up a sleeve and pushed his arm deep into the rectum. 'Yes . . . yes . . . bad impaction, as you say.' He whistled softly for a few moments. 'Well, first, we've got to relieve his pain.'

He injected the sedative into the jugular vein, speaking gently to the horse all the time. 'That'll make you feel better, old lad. Poor old chap,' and followed this with a long saline infusion intravenously to combat the shock, and antibiotic for the enteritis. 'Now we'll get a gallon of liquid paraffin into him to try to lubricate that lot in there.' Quickly he pushed a stomach tube up the nostril and into the stomach and held it there as I pumped in the oil.

'Next, a muscular relaxant.' Again he gave an intravenous injection.

By the time he had cleaned and rolled up the stomach tube,

the horse looked a lot happier. Colic is a frightful agony and I've always felt that horses seem to suffer pain more deeply than any other animal, a suffering at times almost unbearable to watch. It was a relief to see the big animal calming down, stopping his repeated attempts to collapse, clearly finding a blessed release.

'Well,' said Siegfried quietly, 'now we wait.'

Lumsden looked at him questioningly. 'Are you sure? I feel very guilty about you losing your sleep. It's after two o'clock – maybe I could manage now.'

My partner gave him a wan smile. 'With respect, laddie, it's going to need a combined operation. That horse is only doped for now, and I don't have to tell you that he is in a very serious condition. If we can't get his bowels moving, I'm afraid he'll die. He's going to need more of everything, including the stomach tube. We'll all see it through, one way or another.'

The young man sat down on a pile of hay and gazed dully at his boots. 'Oh God, I hope it's not the other. Mr Mottram's last words to me were, "Now you'll look after Match."'

'Match?'

'Match Box. That's the horse's name. My boss is devoted to him.'

'I'm sorry,' Siegfried said, 'you're in an awkward position. I shouldn't think Mottram would be the easiest man to explain things to.'

Lumsden ran his hands through his hair. 'No . . . no . . .' then he looked up at us. 'Mind you, he's not a bad bloke. He's always treated me right. It's just his personality. When he gives me one of his looks I feel about six inches high.'

'I know the feeling,' I said.

Siegfried gazed at the young man for a moment. 'What's your name? What does your mother call you?'

'Harry.'

'Well, Harry, you're probably right. And I like your loyalty. Maybe it's just his way, but James and I both seem to have caught him at the wrong time. Anyway, can you fetch us a pot of coffee? It could be a long night.'

It was indeed a long night. We took turns at walking the horse when he showed signs of going down. Siegfried repeated his injections, ringing the changes between sedatives and muscular relaxants with another cautious shot of arecoline and at five o'clock used the stomach tube again to give magnesium sulphate. And all the time as we dosed and yawned, slumped on the hay, we looked for a genuine easing of the pain, a raising of the animal's depression and most of all for a movement of the bowels.

For my part, as I watched Match Box's lolling head and trailing steps, my dominating worry was the knowledge that horses die very easily. Cattle and most other species could survive things so much better and the old saying among the farmers that ' 'Osses don't stand much' was so true. As the night wore on and my metabolism slowed down, my spirits drooped with it. At any moment, I expected the horse to halt in his painful circling of the box, pitch forward on to his side and groan his last few breaths away. Then we would drive miserably back to Darrowby.

Over the half-door of the box I could see the gradual disappearance of the stars and a lightening of the eastern sky. At around six o'clock, as the birds began to sing in the chestnut trees and the grey light of dawn crept into the box, Siegfried stood up and stretched.

'The big world has started to turn again out there, chaps, so what are we going to do? We've got to see to both our practices so who's going to stay with Match Box? We can't leave him.'

We were looking at each other, bleary-eyed, when the horse suddenly cocked his tail and deposited a small heap of steaming faeces on the floor.

'Oh, what a lovely sight!' cried Siegfried as our weary faces broke into smiles of relief. 'That makes me feel a lot better, but we mustn't get too cocky yet. He's still got a touch of enteritis, so I'll give him another shot of antibiotic before we go. Harry, I think it's safe to leave him now, so we'll be on our way, but don't hesitate to ring us if he doesn't go on right.'

Out in the yard we shook hands. The young man was blinking with tiredness but he looked happy. 'I don't know what to say,' he mumbled. 'I'm so grateful to both of you. You've got me out of a terrible fix and I can't thank you enough.'

'Not at all, my boy,' Siegfried sang out, 'only too glad to be able to help. Get in touch with us any time – but not about colicky horses for the next day or two, if you don't mind.'

We all laughed and waved goodbye as Siegfried started the engine and drove out of the yard.

There was no word from Lumsden until the following day when I answered the phone. 'Match Box is absolutely fine. Bowels normal, nibbling hay, just great,' he said. 'Thanks – thanks again!'

Three weeks passed and, in the rush of work, the Scanton episode began to recede into all the other memories, but one morning Siegfried looked up from his perusal of the appointments book.

'You know, James, I do think Mottram might have made some acknowledgement of our bit of assistance with his horse. I'm not looking for fulsome thanks, but I think he might have said something.'

With an irritable gesture, he scribbled something in the book. 'I expect the toffee-nosed bugger can't unbend even as far as that.'

'Oh, I don't know, Siegfried. Maybe he's still on holiday. We don't know that.'

'Hmm!' My partner looked at me doubtfully. 'Possibly. Could be I'm doing him an injustice, but anyway, we've got the satisfaction of helping to pull that grand horse round.' His face softened. 'Lovely sort.'

Next day I came in from my morning round and found my partner bending over an open crate from whose depths a row of gold-topped bottles protruded.

'What's that?' I asked.

'Champagne. A dozen.' He pulled out a bottle and looked at the label. 'Bollinger, no less!'

'Gosh, where's that come from?'

'No idea. Delivered this morning while we were out, and there's no message inside. But don't worry, it's for us all right. Look. Messrs Farnon and Herriot, Skeldale House.'

'Wonderful. I wonder . . .'

As I spoke, there was a knock on the office door and Hugo Mottram walked in.

We didn't say anything – just stared at him.

He glanced at the crate. 'Ah, I see you got the champagne.'

We spoke in unison. 'You sent it?'

'Yes . . . yes . . . a small gesture of thanks. I returned from holiday only last night and . . . er . . . Lumsden told me what you did for Match.'

'Oh really there's no need . . . only too pleased . . .' Siegfried for once was almost stammering.

Mottram, too, was finding things difficult. Tall and dignified as always, he was nevertheless acutely uncomfortable; unsmiling, searching desperately for words. 'There is indeed a need . . . a need to express my gratitude which . . . which is deeper than I can . . . can truly say. And there is a need, also . . . to apologise to you gentlemen for my stupid and unforgivable remarks when last we met . . .'

'My dear chap, not another word,' Siegfried burst out. 'We never really –'

Mottram raised a hand. 'Please let me say . . . I am profoundly sorry and ashamed. Why I said such things I do not know . . . I've done it before . . . I just seem to be much too . . . prickly. I'm afraid I can't help it.'

As he spoke, he still pushed his chin out, looking down his nose at us. Maybe he couldn't help that either. But it was obvious that his confession was costing the man dear and I could feel the tension in the room rising.

Siegfried, it was clear, felt the situation needed defusing. He threw his arms wide in an all-embracing bonhomie.

'Mottram, Mottram, my dear fellow. What is all this? Just a simple misunderstanding immediately forgotten. Say no more, I beg of you. I assure you that the only concern of James and myself is that your beautiful horse has fully recovered.'

The big man's face softened. 'He is beautiful, isn't he?'

'I tell you this,' Siegfried said softly, 'I wish I had one like him. I do envy you.'

I could see the flash of rapport as the two horse lovers faced each other.

Mottram nodded. 'Ah well, so glad, so glad,' he murmured.

'And by the way, I have something for you from Lumsden.

He, too, is immensely grateful.' He handed Siegfried a small parcel.

My partner unwrapped it quickly and gave a shout of pleasure. 'A bottle of malt whisky! Good old Harry! This is our lucky day. And I think we ought to celebrate Match Box's recovery – among other things. We have all the ingredients right here.' He lifted a bottle of champagne from the crate. 'What do you say, Mottram, old chap? We have a little time to spare before lunch.'

'You're very kind, Farnon. I'd like that.'

'Splendid, splendid, do sit down and make yourself comfortable. Get the glasses, James!'

Within minutes the champagne had popped and we were seated round the table. Siegfried raised his glass and looked appreciatively at the sparkling contents. 'Here's to Match Box, may he never have belly-ache again!'

We drank, and Mottram cleared his throat. 'There is just one more thing I want to say. I wish we had got to know each other socially long ago. I wonder if both of you would come to dinner next Friday?'

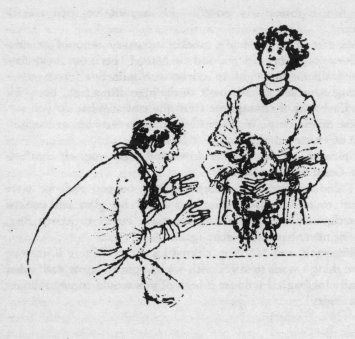

9

I was always apprehensive and ill at ease when I had Mrs Featherstone's problem dog on the table, but this time I felt relaxed and full of confidence. But then I was always like that when I was delirious.

Delirium was only one of the countless peculiar manifestations of Brucellosis. This disease, which causes contagious abortion in cattle, ruined thousands of good farmers of my generation and was also a constant menace to the veterinary surgeons who had to deliver the premature calves and remove the afterbirths.

Thank heaven, the Brucellosis scheme has now just about eradicated the disease but in the fifties such a thing hadn't been dreamed of and I and my contemporaries wallowed almost daily in the horrible infection.

I remember standing stripped to the waist in cow byres –

parturition gowns were still uncommon and the long plastic protective gloves unknown in those days – working away inside infected cows for hours and looking with wry recognition at the leathery placenta and the light-coloured, necrotic cotyledons which told me that I was in contact with millions of the bacteria. And as I swilled myself with disinfectant afterwards, the place was filled with the distinctive acrid odour of abortion.

The effects on many of my fellow vets were wide and varied. One big fat chap faded away to a skeleton with undulant fever and was ill for years, others developed crippling arthritis and some went down with psychiatric conditions. One man wrote in the *Veterinary Record* that as part of his own syndrome he came home one night and decided it would be a good idea to murder his wife. He never got round actually to doing it, but recorded the impulse as an interesting example of what *Brucella abortus* could do to a man.

I used to pat myself on the back and thank God that I was immune. I had been bathing in the infection for years and had never experienced the slightest reaction and as I looked around at some of my suffering friends I was so thankful that I had been spared their ordeal. And after all this time I just knew that such a thing would never happen to me.

That was before I started my funny turns.

This was my family's term for a series of mysterious attacks which came unheralded and then passed off just as quickly. At first I diagnosed them as repeated chills – I was always stripping off in open fields, often in the middle of the night – then I thought I must have a type of flu of short duration. The symptoms were always the same – a feeling of depression, then an ice-cold shiveriness which drove me to my bed where within an hour I shot up a temperature of 105 or 106. Once I had developed this massive fever I felt great: warm and happy, laughing heartily, chattering to myself and finally breaking into song. I couldn't help the singing – I felt so good.

This was a source of great amusement to my children. When I was at the singing stage I could always hear them giggling outside the bedroom door, but I didn't mind – I didn't mind anything.

However, I finally had to find out what was happening to me and a blood test by Dr Allinson dispelled all doubts by showing a nice positive titre to *Brucella abortus*. Reluctantly I had to admit that I had joined the club.

The particular attack when Mrs Featherstone brought her dog to the surgery was on a Saturday. I was driving back from a football match in Sunderland with some of my pals. Our team had won and we were all in high spirits, laughing and joking, and I hardly noticed just when I stopped being the life of the party and went quiet. I did know that when I got to Skeldale House and huddled miserably over the fire, shaking like a man with malaria that another funny turn was on the way.

Helen took one look, chased me upstairs and began to fill the hot water bottles. Feeling like death I crawled between the sheets and lay, cuddling one bottle, feet on another, while the bed vibrated with my terrific rigor. Helen piled another eiderdown on top of me, turned out the light and left me to it. We both knew what was going to happen.

It wasn't long before the familiar pattern started to set in. Quite soon I began to feel a bit better – warmer, more cheerful – then the warmth mounted and increased and spread through every corner of my being until I was floating along in a delicious languor, utterly at peace, all my troubles dissolved and gone. This, I felt, was heaven. I could stay like this forever, but the warmth developed into a fiery heat when I felt even better; no longer languorous, but powerful, dominant, foolishly and riotously happy.

This was the time when I usually extended a burning arm to pick up my bedside thermometer and stick it under my arm. Ah, yes, there it was, 106, exactly as I thought. I chuckled with satisfaction. Everything was just fine.

Lying there, I was so full of the joys of life that I began to talk aloud, discussing interesting matters with myself, and then my bursting high spirits had to find some further outlet and singing was the natural thing. 'Maxwelltown braes are bonny, where early fa's the dew, and t'was there that Annie Laurie gie'd me her promise true.' I let rip at full volume and never had my voice sounded as rich and rounded.

A few hee-hees sounded from behind the door followed by Jimmy's whisper, 'There he goes' and a muffled laugh from Rosie. The little beggars were there again, but what the hell? 'Gie'd me her promise true, which ne'er forgot will be!' I hit the high notes without a trace of self-consciousness, ignoring the further outburst from beyond the door.

I had a further chat with myself, agreeing wholeheartedly with everything I said, then I thought I'd try my John McCormack impression of 'The Rose of Tralee'. I took a long breath. 'The pale moon was shining above the green mountain.'

'Ha-ha-ha-haaa!' My children were having a great time out there. Then I heard the ringing of the front door bell, moments later feet on the stairs, then a knock on the bedroom door.

Jimmy's head poked into the room. 'Hello, Dad.' His face worked in his effort to stifle his laughter. 'Mrs Featherstone's downstairs with her dog. She says it's urgent and Mum's had to go out for a few minutes.'

'Right-oh, old lad.' I swung my legs from the bed. 'I'll be down immediately.'

My son's eyes widened. 'Are you sure?'

'Absolutely. I'll be down in two ticks. Put her in the consulting room.'

With a final startled glance, Jimmy closed the door and left.

As I pulled on shirt and trousers, the blood thundered in my ears and my face was afire. Normally, the very mention of Mrs Featherstone made me shrink. Rich, middle-aged, imperious, she had plagued me for years with the imaginary ailments of her little poodle, Rollo.

Rollo was an outstandingly healthy little dog. In fact, like many poodles, he was a tough little animal with the characteristic of being able to leap six feet in the air from a standing position as though he were operated by springs, but where he was concerned Mrs Featherstone was a raving hypochondriac. From a commercial point of view, it may seem ideal to have a rich client willing to pay for regular visits with her dog which has nothing the matter with it, but I found it increasingly wearing. Endless sessions of 'Really, Mrs Featherstone, the thing you are pointing out is quite normal' or 'I assure you, Mrs Featherstone, you are worrying needlessly' with the lady drawing herself up and sticking out her chin. 'Are you suggesting, Mr Herriot, that I am dreaming these things? That I cannot believe the evidence of my own eyes? My poor Rollo is suffering and I expect you to do something about it.'

Weak-mindedly I invariably submitted and fobbed her off with some form of placebo which would do the little animal no harm, but the sense of shame was deep. I had to admit that I was overawed by the woman, a jellyfish and a wimp in her presence, allowing her to dismiss my wafflings with a wave of her hand. Why couldn't I assert myself?

However, at this moment, knotting my tie, humming a happy tune as the glittering eyes in the vermilion face glared back at me from the mirror, my past diffidence seemed totally incomprehensible. I was really looking forward to seeing the lady again.

I ran downstairs, snatched a white coat from its hook, trotted along the passage and found Mrs Featherstone standing by the consulting-room table.

Damn, she wasn't a bad-looking woman! Very very nice, in fact. Funny I had never noticed that before. Anyway, there was not the slightest doubt in my mind as to what I had to do. I would grab her, give her a big, smacking kiss and a good long squeeze and all our past misunderstandings would melt away like the morning mist in the sun.

I was advancing on her when I noticed something strange. She had vanished. I was quite sure she had been standing there a second ago. I was blinking around me in bewilderment when I saw that she had ducked behind the table. How wonderful that she, too, was feeling skittish and ready for a game of peek-a-boo.

In a moment her head bobbed up and I greeted it with a merry cry. 'Yoo-hoo, I see you!' I trilled, but it seemed she had merely been stooping to lift her dog which she deposited on the table.

She gave me an odd look. 'Have you been on holiday, Mr Herriot? You have such a high colour.'

'No, no, no, no. I just feel extraordinarily well. In fact. I –'

The lady pursed her lips and brushed off the rest of my sentence impatiently. 'I really am most frightfully worried about poor Rollo.'

At the sound of his name, the poodle, aggressively fit, began to caper around on the table and jump up at my face.

'You are? Oh, what a shame. Tell me all about it.' I suppressed a chuckle.

'Well, we had just started on our evening walk when he coughed quite suddenly.'

'Just one cough?'

'No, two, like this. Hock-hock.'

'Hock, hock, eh?' I was having terrible ·trouble keeping a serious face. 'And then what happened?'

'Nothing else happened! Isn't that enough? A nasty cough?'

'Well, tell me, do you mean two hocks or one hock-hock?' I could not suppress a giggle, captivated as I was by my wit.

'I mean, Mr Herriot, one very unpleasant and alarming cough.' A dangerous light glinted in the lady's eye.

'Ah yes.' I took out stethoscope and thermometer and began a thorough examination of the patient. Everything, of course, was normal, and I could swear I detected an apologetic glance from Rollo.

And all the time the giggle was struggling steadily to the surface and finally it burst out into a loud 'Ha-ha!'

Mrs Featherstone's eyebrows shot up and she stared at me. 'Why are you laughing?' she enquired in glacial tones. She made the word seem more portentous by drawing it out into a long 'laawfing'.

'Well, really, ·you see, it's so funny.' I leaned on the table and laughed some more.

'Funny?' Mrs Featherstone's expression was a mixture of horror and disbelief. Her mouth opened soundlessly a few times. 'I fail to see anything *funny* in an animal's suffering.'

Wrapped in my cloak of heat and euphoria, I wagged a finger at her. 'But he's not suffering, that's what's so funny. He never *is* suffering when you bring him in to me.'

'I beg your pardon!'

'It's true, Mrs Featherstone. All Rollo's ailments are imagined by you.' The table shook as another paroxysm seized me.

'How dare you say such a thing!' The lady glared at me down her nose. 'You are being insulting and I really cannot –'

'Hey, just wait a minute. Let me explain.' I wiped a few tears away and took a few gasping breaths. 'Do you remember being worried to death by that habit of Rollo's where he lifts up a hind leg for a few steps, then puts it down again? I told you it was nothing, just a mannerism, but you insisted on my treating him for arthritis?'

'Well, yes, but I was worried.'

'I know, but you wouldn't believe me and he's still doing it. There's nothing wrong with him. Lots of little dogs do it.'

'Well, possibly, but . . .'

'And another thing,' I said between my chuckles, 'there was the time you made me give him sleeping pills because of his terrible nightmares.'

'Yes, and rightly so. He made the most pathetic whimpering sound while he was sleeping and his paws kept working as though he was running away from something terrible.'

'He was dreaming, Mrs Featherstone! Probably a nice dream about chasing his ball. All dogs have these dreams.'

I took hold of Rollo's head. 'And look here, ha-ha! You must recall your insistence that there were things growing over his eyes. You would never believe me that they were his normal third eyelids, ha-ha-ha! And see, they're still there, aren't they? You can see them now and he's quite happy with them, ha-ha-ha-ha!' I abandoned myself completely and bent over to dig her in the ribs, but she drew back and evaded my finger.

She put her hand over her mouth and continued to stare at me. Her eyebrows had taken up permanent residence high on her forehead. 'You . . . you cannot really mean all this!'

'Oh, but I do, I do. I could go on and on.'

'Well, I don't know what to say. And about his cough tonight?'

'You can take him away,' I said, 'And if there are any more hock-hocks, bring him back tomorrow, but there won't be.' I wiped my streaming face and lifted Rollo from the table.

The lady seemed in a daze as I steered her along the passage to the front door. She kept putting a hand over her mouth and giving me an incredulous sidelong glance, but she remained silent as though stunned.

After I had shown her out I retired to bed and drifted to sleep with the satisfied feeling of having cleared up a problem happily and effortlessly. I had handled the whole thing beautifully.

I didn't feel like that next morning. My latest funny turn was following its usual course. After the elation of the night before, a devastating deflation, lethargy, gloom, despondency and, in this case, the horrid spectre of remorse. As I lay in bed, pulling the sheets round my chin, my recollection of the previous evening was a frightening jumble. I couldn't get any of it sorted out in my mind.

I had been awake only a few moments before the memory hit me. Mrs Featherstone! Oh, my God! What had I said to her? What had I done? Desperately I tried to bring back the details without success, but the main indisputable fact was that I had laughed, even jeered at her, possibly even pawed at her person. Had I really attempted to embrace her? Had I given her a little cuddle as I walked her down the passage? My mouth opened in a series of soft moans.

Of one thing I could be sure – I had been guilty of the most ghastly impropriety and I had a searing conviction that I would have to pay dearly for it. Certainly she would never set foot in my surgery again. The whole shameful story would get around. She might even report me to the Royal College. I could see the headlines in the *Darrowby and Houlton Times*. VETERINARY SURGEON ON SERIOUS CHARGE, HERRIOT TO APPEAR BEFORE DISCIPLINARY BODY.

Groaning, I huddled deeper, gazing sightlessly at the cup of tea which Helen had placed by my bedside. After my funny turns I always had a day's rest and after that I made a remarkably quick recovery. But this time the mental scars would take a long time to heal. And how about the dire consequences?

I couldn't stand the self-torture any longer. I swallowed my tea, pulled on my clothes and trailed downstairs.

'Feeling better, Jim?' my wife asked brightly as she washed the dishes. 'You'll soon be okay again, you always are. What a strange business it is, but anyway, the kids enjoyed it. I understand you were in excellent voice last night.' She giggled as she reached for the towel.

I thought a gentle stroll in the fresh air would make me feel better, so I set off to walk around the town. I could hardly believe it when I saw Mrs Featherstone approaching a mere hundred yards away. Panic-stricken I scuttled over to the other side of the street, but the lady had spotted me and she crossed over too. And as the expensively tweeded figure bore down on me with purposeful strides I knew there was no escape.

Ah well, I told myself, here it comes. 'Mr Herriot, I thought you might be interested to know that I have placed the matter of Saturday night in the hands of my solicitors. Your behaviour was quite outrageous and I feel it my duty to ensure that defenceless women are protected from you in future. I can scarcely believe that a professional man would act as you did – taking advantage of your situation, betraying the trust placed in you. And as for your incredible callousness in the face of my poor dog's suffering – well, I cannot bear to think of it.'

But it wasn't like that at all. When Mrs Featherstone came up to me she put a hand on my arm. 'Now, Mr Herriot, you did me a service last night.'

'Eh?'

'Yes, you were so understanding. I realise now that I have been foolish about Rollo. I must have been such a nuisance to you.'

'Oh, no, no, no . . .'

'You are kind, but I know I have been unreasonable, troubling you over nothing at inconvenient times and here again I was at your door on a Saturday night.'

'I assure you . . .'

'But instead of being upset, you laughed, and it was so wonderful how you made me see the funny side of my silliness. I feel so ashamed that I always refused to listen to you when you so rightly tried to explain that I was worrying needlessly, and I do hope you can forgive me. From now on, I intend to be a sensible dog owner. And Rollo really is quite healthy, isn't he?'

Waves of relief rolled over me as I looked at the little dog, bright eyed, laughing-faced, leaping almost head high at the sound of his name. 'Well, I'm not too sure. He doesn't look very lively to me.'

'Oh, now you are trying to make me laugh again.' She put her hand over her mouth with the same embarrassed gesture I remembered, then gave me a quizzical look. 'I feel I'm going to laugh a lot more in future.'

I haven't had a funny turn for thirty years. They just gradually disappeared from my life. But when I think of that Saturday night with Mrs Featherstone, I still get an attack of the shivers.

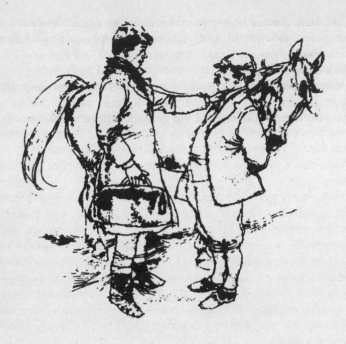

IO

I couldn't believe I was going to launch this boy on his own into the jungle of veterinary practice. Young John Crooks, so familiar a face after the months he had spent seeing practice with us during his university vacations, watching us work, picking up the practical hints and knowledge, doing the odd job himself, but always under our wings, was standing there by my desk, cheerful and smiling as always, but oh, so youthful. He looked about seventeen. It didn't seem fair to send him out there unprotected.

However, there was no doubt that it was J. L. Crooks Esq., MRCVS standing there, suitcase by his side, bright eyed and eager to go, and I had to adjust to the fact.

I cleared my throat. 'Well, John,' I said, smiling up at him, 'congratulations on qualifying. You're a fully fledged veterinary surgeon now, all your examinations behind you, and it's good to see you here. And, you know, this is quite an occasion. You are the very first assistant to be employed in the practice of Farnon and Herriot.'

He laughed. 'Really? That makes me sound very important. But when I was here as a student you had people working for you?'

'Yes, that's right. Tristan, of course, but he's one of the family and we never thought of him as an assistant. And there were one or two temporary people, but you are the first *official* man.'

'Well, that's nice. And now I'm here I'd better start earning my keep.'

'Okay, we'll get your car kitted out and then you'd better report to your digs. You're lodging with Mrs Barrie, aren't you?'

As the young man filled the car boot with the drugs and instruments he was going to need I could see that he was keen to pitch into the unpredictable world of practice, but I wondered just how nervous he was at the prospect of confronting the tough Yorkshire farmers on his own. Would he make the grade? Some new graduates just couldn't do it, and as he drove away in his Ford 8 with his bag of tricks rattling behind him I found myself crossing my fingers.

I have a big streak of old hen in me as my family will testify and throughout the day I was almost wringing my hands. How was the poor lad getting on? We were so busy that I didn't see him to talk to, and I kept hoping he hadn't come up against any awkward situations. Although our farmers were nearly all no-nonsense but kindly men, there was the odd very difficult client.

I recalled my session with Major Sykes a few days ago. That fierce little man barking at me as I treated his horse. 'Herriot, good God, man! Can't you do better than this? You don't seem to have much idea how to treat this blasted animal!' Then shouting at his groom, 'No, don't put the bucket down there, you bloody fool!' He was impossible to please and verbally steam-rollered people into the ground, treating everybody, especially it seemed, vets, like the more dim-witted private soldiers of his army days. In fact, despite myself, I often found my thumbs edging into line with the seams of my trousers, taking me back to my days in the RAF.

It was late afternoon when I came into the surgery and looked at the appointments book, and the words jumped out at me. 'Major Sykes, Hunting horse, laminitis.' John had ticked it – he'd be there now.

My eyes popped. One of those adored and valuable hunters – and laminitis, a condition with so many nasty possibilities. No job for a newly qualified young chap. The Major would eat him alive. I had to check up and I hurried out to Roova Grange.

As I got out of the car I could hear the Major's aggressive tones coming from a loose box and I feared John was already going through it.

I peeped over the half door of the box. A fine bay mare was standing there in the painful, crouching position of laminitis, her hind feet drawn under her body. A foal, obviously only a few days old, was close by her side. The Major, hands on hips, was almost shouting up into John's face.

'Now look here, er . . . er . . . what d'ye say your name is? Crooks, yes, now look here dammit, Crooks, you say this mare has a bad laminitis. Bloody great temperature, all crippled up, and you're trying to tell me that she'll be all right. Well, I bought her in foal and I bought her in good faith, is she always going to be subject to this, eh, eh? I've heard about horses which are always getting it. Have I been sold a pup, d'ye think? D'you know enough about the job to tell me that, eh, eh?'

The young man, however, did not seem at all put out. He spoke soothingly. 'Now, Major Sykes, I've told you the cause of the trouble. Your mare retained her afterbirth when she foaled and she developed metritis. Laminitis is a common complication of this, and what you have here is an isolated case. I've given her a shot of antibiotic and I'll repeat it over the next day or two. That will clear the metritis.'

Still bristling, the little man stuck out his chin. 'And how about the bloody laminitis, what're you going to do about that, eh, eh?'

'Well, as you saw, she's had an injection for that, too.' John gave him a serene smile. 'And if you'll keep her on bran for a few days and stand her in your pond to cool the feet as I directed I'm sure she'll soon be back to normal.'

'And d'you think she's had it before?'

'No, no, no.'

'How the hell d'ye know that?'

'Well, now, she's got no lines round her hooves, and look here,' he lifted one of the mare's fore feet, 'a lovely concave sole. She's never had laminitis before.'

'And it won't come back, eh?'

'No likelihood of a recurrence.'

'Just hope you're right,' the Major grunted.

'I'm sure I am. You'll see. You worry too much, you know.'

I shuddered and closed my eyes as John reached out and gave the little man a comforting pat on the shoulder. For a moment I thought the Major would erupt, then, to my amazement his face broke into something like a shy smile. 'You think so, eh?'

'I do indeed. You really oughtn't let things upset you so much.'

This was something new in the little man's experience and for a few seconds he looked up into John's face, then he took off his cap and scratched his head. 'Well, maybe you're right. Maybe you're right, young man. Heh–heh–heh!'

I couldn't believe it. He was laughing. John threw back his head and laughed too. It was like a reunion between two old college chums. And suddenly I realised that that wasn't little John Crooks, our student, in there; it was a tall, good–looking, self–assured veterinary surgeon with a fine big voice which lent authority to everything he said. I slunk away to my car and drove off with a resolution already formed in my mind. I wasn't going to worry about John any more.

He had been with us for a few weeks when I answered the phone one morning. 'Hello, is that Mr Herriot?' a cheerful voice enquired. I recognised one of our farmer clients.

'Yes, Mr Gates,' I replied. 'What can I do for you?'

'Nay, it's awright. Ah want to speak to t'yoong man.'

A pang, unexpectedly deep and piercing, shot through me. What was this? I was the 'yoong man', always had been. That was how the clients had invariably referred to me even though I was only six years younger than Siegfried. There was some mistake here.

'Who did you say you wanted?' I asked.

'T'yoong man – Mr Crooks.'

Ah well, there it was. I hadn't realised that I had become so attached to my title and, walking along the passage to fetch John, I felt strangely wistful as I faced the fact that, although I was still in my early thirties I wasn't the 'yoong man' any more.

From then on, I had to live with an ever-increasing flood of requests for the services of a yoong man who wasn't me. However, it was only depressing for a short time, because the compensations were enormous. As John settled in to the practice, I found a miraculous easing of my life. It was rather wonderful to have an assistant, especially a good one like him. I had always liked him, but when I got a call to a calving heifer at three o'clock in the morning and was able to pass it on to him and turn over and go back to sleep, I could feel the liking deepening into a warm affection.

John had his own ideas about treatment and wasn't afraid to express them. One day Siegfried found the two of us in the operating room.

'I've been reading about this Inductotherm. Revolutionary new treatment for strained tendons in horses. You just wrap this electric cable round the leg for a certain time every day and the heat clears up the strain.'

I gave a non-committal grunt. I seldom had any ideas and, in fact, was constitutionally opposed to any change, any innovation. This trait, I knew, irritated my partner intensely so I remained silent.

John, however, spoke up. 'I've read about it, too, but I don't fancy it.'

'Why not?' Siegfried's eyebrows went up.

'Smacks of witchcraft to me,' John said.

'Oh, rubbish!' Siegfried frowned at him. 'I think it sounds perfectly rational. Anyway, I've ordered one of the things and I'd like to bet it'll be a big help to us.'

Siegfried was the horse specialist so I didn't argue, but I was very interested to see how the thing worked and we soon had the opportunity to find out. The Lord of the Manor of Darrowby, usually called the Squire, kept his horses in some stables at the foot of our street, a mere hundred yards away, and it seemed like fate when he reported a case of strained tendons.

Siegfried rubbed his hands. 'Just what we wanted. I've got to go over to Whitby to inspect a stallion, so I'll leave it to you to handle this case, John. I've got a feeling you'll think the treatment is a great advance.'

I know my partner was looking forward to saying 'I told you so' to the young man, but after a week of the treatment, John still wasn't impressed.

'I've been winding this thing round the horse's leg every day and hanging about for the required time, but I can't see any difference. I'm having another session this afternoon, but if it still isn't any better I'm going to suggest a return to the old treatment.'

Around five o'clock that afternoon, with heavy rain sweeping along on the wind, I was drawing up outside the surgery when I froze in my seat. I was looking out at something terrible. Several of the Squire's men were carrying a body down the street. It was John. As I got out of the car they bore him into the house and deposited him at the foot of the stairs. He seemed to be unconscious.

'What on earth's happened?' I gasped, looking down in horror at the form of my colleague draped over the lower steps.

'T'yoong man's electrocuted 'isself,' one of the men said.

'What!'

'Aye, it's right. He were soaked wi' rain and when 'e went to connect up the machine to the plug, 'e must have got his fingers on the live metal. He started to yell, but 'e couldn't let go. He went on yellin', but I were hangin' on to the horse's head and I couldn't help 'im. He sort of staggered about, like, and at t'finish he fell over the horse's hind leg and that broke 'is grip on the thing or I think he'd have been a goner!'

'My God! What can we do?' I turned to Helen who had appeared from the kitchen. 'Could you phone the doctor,' I cried. 'But wait a minute, I think he's coming round.'

John, stretched out on the stairs, had begun to stir, and as he peered up at us through half-closed eyes, an amazing flow of colourful language began to pour from him. He went on and on and on.

Helen stared at me, open-mouthed. 'Just listen to that! And he's such a nice young man, too!'

I could understand her astonishment, because John was an upright, very correct lad who, unlike most vets, did not swear. However, he had a wonderful store within him because some of the words were new even to me, which was surprising considering that I grew up in Glasgow.

After a while the torrent slowed down to an unintelligible mumble, and Siegfried, who had just come in from his round, began to ply him with neat gin which, I believe, is contra-indicated in these cases.

There is no doubt that John could have lost his life but, mercifully, as the minutes passed he recovered steadily until he was able to sit up on the stairs. At last, as we adjured him to take it easy and stay where he was, he shook himself, got up, drew himself up to his considerable height and faced Siegfried.

'Mr Farnon,' he said with great dignity, 'if you ask me to operate that bloody apparatus again I shall tender my resignation.'

And so that was the end of the short career of the Inducto-therm.

It was a few days later and as always, I felt a little wary when I saw the formidable figure of Sep Craggs bearing down on me in the passage at Skeldale House.

'Hey, 'erriot,' he barked, 'I want a word wi' you!'

He was a rude man but I was used to his mode of address and put up with it because he was a valuable client with a large farm which he ran with four grown sons whom he bullied and terrorised.

'Well, Mr Craggs, what's the trouble?' I asked peaceably.

He glared down at me from his six foot four bulk and pushed his face close to mine. 'Ah'll tell ye what the trouble is! You've been wastin' ma time!'

'Oh, really? In what way?'

'Remember them mastitis powders you were goin' to put out for me?'

Oh God, those sulphanilamide powders. I'd forgotten about them. 'I'm terribly sorry, I . . .'

'You forgot 'em, didn't you! "Come down this afternoon," you said. "They'll be in the box at the door for you." Well, I came down at three o'clock, but there was nowt in the box and nobody knew a thing about it. Ah'm bloody cross, I tell ye!'

'Well, as I say, Mr Craggs, I'm very sorry . . .'

'Aye, it's awright bein' sorry, but that doesn't help *me*. It's a bloody long way to Darrowby from ma place and I had to leave ma haymakin'. And all for nowt. I'm a busy feller tha knows, and I can't afford to have ma time wasted like this!'

Oh hell, he was rubbing it in, but he had me cold. I picked up the powders from the dispensary and handed them to him.

He was still grumbling. 'I don't want any more of this in the future, so think on. If ye ask me to come here for anything, just think on and 'ave it ready for me.'

I nodded dumbly, but he wasn't finished yet.

'It's you that needs powders,' he grunted. 'Thinkin' on powders!' He gave me a final glare and left.

I took a few deep breaths and hoped fervently that I would never transgress again in that quarter.

The incident was still fresh in my mind the following week when I again found Sep Craggs waiting for me at the surgery when I returned from a round.

His face was inscrutable but I felt a twinge of apprehension as he again towered over me.

'Ah came this mornin' to pick up a bottle of liniment, but it wasn't in the box,' he muttered.

Oh no! Please not again! Was I losing my mind? I dug my nails into my palms. 'I'm so sorry . . . I . . . I really can't remember arranging this.'

But there was no outburst this time. The man was strangely subdued. 'It wasn't you, it was t'yoong man.'

So it was poor John's turn to fall under the lash. How could I divert the wrath from him? I gave a light laugh. 'Oh . . . I see . . . well, Mr Crooks is a splendid chap but he hasn't the best of memories.'

'Nay, nay – don't criticise t'yoong man! He's got enough on 'is mind without botherin' about a little thing like a bottle of liniment.'

'Eh?'

'Aye, don't start blamin' him! I'm not havin' that!' He gave me a disapproving scowl. 'With all he's got to think about, you can't expect 'im to remember everything.'

I opened my mouth, but no words came.

I had never seen Mr Craggs smile, but his granite features relaxed a little and an almost dreamy look came into his eyes. 'By gaw, he does know a lot, does that lad – ah've never met anybody with such learnin'. Ah'll tell tha' summat, 'erriot. He came to a bullock wi' foul in the foot and 'e didn't mess about wi' tar and salt for a week like you do. Never touched the flippin' foot. All 'e did was inject into the *shoulder*, and t'beast was better in two days. What d'ye make of that, eh?' He tapped me on the chest.

I knew he wouldn't believe me if I told him that I, too, was using the new sulphadimidine injection now, so I didn't say anything.

'And ah'll tell tha summat else,' he went on. 'It was the *right* leg that was lame, but 'e injected into the *left* shoulder.' His eyes widened. 'It was like magic!'

'Good ... good ...' I croaked. 'Well, I'll get you that liniment.'

I brought the bottle from the dispensary and handed it to him. 'Well, here it is, Mr Craggs. I'm sorry you've had an extra journey.'

The big man shook his head. 'Nay, that makes no matter. It only takes a few minutes to get 'ere.'

As in a dream, I saw him out of the door and as I watched him walk down the street one thought was uppermost. If John could touch the heart of Sep Craggs his future was assured.

In fact, I think it was then that I realised that John was destined for something big. I had from the start begun to detect the seeds of greatness in him because of his uncanny ability to get through to people of all stations in life. It wasn't just his appearance, his confident approach, his rich voice, there was something else and I couldn't quite identify it, but whatever it was, everything about him stamped him as the 'young man most likely to succeed'.

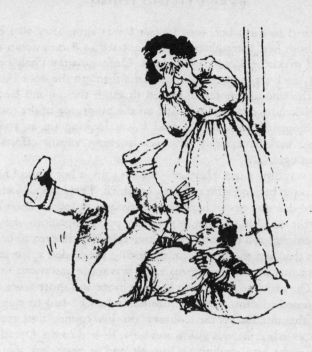

I I

John's home town was Beverley with its glorious Minster; this
was fifty miles from Darrowby, and on his half days he usually
went home for a few hours. Over the next year as he talked to
me about these visits, a girl's name began to crop up more and
more frequently. She was called Heather and whenever he mentioned her his eyes were inclined to take on a faraway look and
his features to fall into an ethereal smile. These symptoms became
more and more marked over the months until one day he
confided to me that he was engaged and that he and Heather
hoped to marry soon.

One wintry day I was kicking the snow off my boots in the
porch at Skeldale House when John appeared in the doorway.

'Heather's inside,' he said a little breathlessly. 'She's in the
office – I'd like you to meet her.'

I wanted to meet her, too. In fact I was agog after all I had heard about her. I straightened my tie, tried to flatten down my hair and strode briskly into the room. Unfortunately I had a ball of snow stuck on my heel and as I came through the door I took off on the smooth linoleum, soared through the air and landed with a sickening crash on my back on the other side of the room. When I opened my eyes I found I was looking up at a very attractive dark-haired girl who was making valiant efforts to keep a straight face.

That was how I met Heather – looking up at her – and I have looked up to her and admired her ever since. There are all sorts of words to describe her in her future marriage to John – cherished partner through life, staunch helpmeet, happy companion – she was all those things and the mother of three splendid children to boot.

After that first meeting, John's courting proceeded apace and I could see that his impending marriage was more and more on his mind. The previous symptoms became more and more acute and he confessed to short bouts of amnesia when he had to stop his car in the middle of the country on his rounds and try to remember where he was going and what he had to do. Occasionally I caught him smiling to himself and it was clear that his thoughts were on something rather wonderful ahead.

Just how much his future was preoccupying him became clear one wet afternoon. One of our farmers phoned me.

'I've had a message passed on to say that Mr Crooks's fiancée has been taken ill. He'd just left my place and I thought I'd missed 'im, but then I saw that his car had got stuck in the ford just beyond our gate.'

'Oh dear, I'd better come and get him.'

'Nay, there's no need. I slipped down in my car and gave him the message and he jumped out and asked me to run 'im to Darrowby station. He caught a train and he was off.'

'Gosh, that was quick.'

'Aye, by gaw, he didn't mess about!'

'And where's the car now?'

'Still stuck in t'water.'

'Right. Thanks for letting me know. I'll come out with Mr Farnon and we'll fetch it back.'

The scene which met Siegfried and me when we got to the ford is one of the vivid memories of John's time with us. There was a dip in the narrow, hill-girt road where the beck flowed over the tarmac and John's little Ford 8 was standing there, axle deep in the water. There were signs of a hasty exit – the driver's door was hanging open and the windscreen wipers were still in motion, flip-flopping lazily across the glass. John hadn't delayed his departure for a second.

Happily, Heather's illness was not serious and life in our busy practice went on with John doing his share of the routine calvings, foalings, lambings, castrations of colts and proving himself daily as the right man in the right job.

The young couple were married on a fine day in May and they settled in part of Siegfried's house. Heather was a teacher and she taught Siegfried's two children throughout her stay in our practice.

It was a jolt when the inevitable day came when John decided to branch out on his own. He left to set up a practice in Beverley and I felt the loss not only of a great assistant but a friend. I was only about ten years older than John – close enough to have interests and pursuits in common. I suppose as the years passed and other 'yoong men' came and went in our practice, I progressed through the status of ageing colleague, elder statesman and, finally, quaint old fossil, but with the first few assistants I was still in their world, and John and I had a lot of fun together.

Skeldale House had always been a place of laughter and, thank heaven, John brought a vivid brand of humour of his own to the practice. He had his failures and disasters like all of us and used a wonderful gift of mimicry to describe them. He was sensitive and totally lacking in vanity despite his forceful personality.

Above all, I still think of him as a typical Englishman of an almost old-fashioned sort with a passion for cricket, an unshakable belief in the old values and a reverence for the beautiful county in which we worked.

After he had left to set up his own practice in Beverley, we were absorbed in our own busy lives and inevitably saw less and less of each other. There were special occasions, of course. Helen and I were honoured to become Godparents to Annette, the first born of the Crooks family, then we had happy notice of the arrival of James and then Elizabeth. We managed to meet Heather and John occasionally in Scarborough and I saw John at veterinary meetings but the old chapter was closed.

However, with my conviction that he would rise high in the profession, I followed his progress over the years, and noted the rapid growth of his practice until he was employing several assistants. He was being increasingly recognised for his drive and organising ability and was involved in the growth and administration of the profession. I was right in my prognostication; the only thing that at last stopped John's rising was that he couldn't go any higher. In 1983, thirty years after he left Darrowby, he was elected President of the British Veterinary Association.

It touched me then that after all that time he reached back to his first boss and asked me to make the induction speech at his inauguration.

'Those years in Darrowby were the happiest time of our lives for Heather and me,' he said. 'I want you to do it.'

So there it was. The great day came with me sitting in the conference hall of Lancaster University among hundreds of vets from all over the world. All the notables were there – distinguished names everywhere – but as I looked up at the august company on the platform after I had said my piece, it gave me a tremendous kick to realise that right in the middle and the most important of them all was t'yoong man from Darrowby.

My speech over, the ceremony proceeded and John stood tall as he was arrayed in the regalia of President. The Association Secretary helped him into the handsome black gown with green watered silk facings, then the President of the previous year placed the chain of office around his neck. As I saw this chain being fastened from behind, the whole thing suddenly reminded me of dressing up in an obstetric gown before a calving with the farmer tying the tapes from the rear. It seemed that John felt exactly the same because at that very solemn moment he said, 'Could I have a bucket of hot water, soap and a towel please.' A roar of laughter went up from the audience – so many of us had uttered those words a thousand times.

Finally, in full raiment, he turned and faced the assembly. He was bulkier than in his Darrowby days and his hair was a silver thatch, but he was profoundly imposing. I looked towards the front row of the auditorium where Heather and all the family sat, gazing up proudly. Among them I saw baby Emily, first of the grandchildren, perched on James's knee and the years rolled away. Ah well, John wasn't t'yoong man any more, but he was a famous and happy one.

In my speech, I had tried to bring out John's unique ability to influence people and when I had still been stuck for the right words, I had paraphrased a lager advertisement by saying he could reach the parts other veterinary surgeons couldn't reach.

As I sat there watching the ceremony on the platform, the memory of that lonely road among the hills and the stranded car in the water with the door hanging open and the windscreen wipers going flip-flop, flip-flop swam up into my mind. It occurred to me that there could be a clue there. Maybe that epitomised two of the aspects of John's character which had taken him to the top of the profession – devotion to his wife and the power of instant decision.

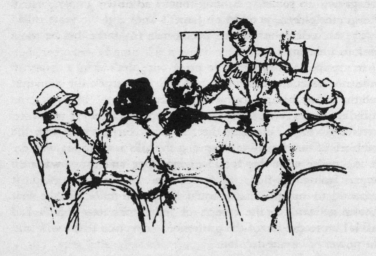

12

'This house is a woman killer, Mr Herriot.'

I was seeing a farmer out and he was looking down at Helen scrubbing the front door steps. His words went through me like a knife. He was stating baldly something which had been eating away at my mind for a long time.

'Aye,' he said again, 'it's a grand old house, but it's a woman killer.'

That was the moment when I decided that somehow, some way, I had to get Helen out of Skeldale House. We loved the old place but it had vast disadvantages for a young couple of moderate means. It was charming, graceful and undoubtedly a happy house in its atmosphere, but it was far too big and a veritable ice box in cold weather.

I looked up over the ivy covered frontage at the big bedroom windows, then further to the next storey where there was a suite of rooms where, in the early days, we had had our bed-sitter. There was another storey if you counted the tiny rooms under the tiles; here there was a big bell mounted on the end of a spring which used to summon a little housemaid down to the ground floor in the early days of the century.

The old doctor who lived in Skeldale House before we took over had had six servants including a full-time housekeeper, but Helen looked after the whole place with the aid of a series of transient maids, most of whom soon grew tired of the hard work and the impossible inconvenience of the house.

Before going back inside I looked down again at my wife scrubbing away. This was crazy, and the words 'Please stop it!' bubbled up in my mind. But I didn't speak them. It was no good. I had tried to stop her again and again but it was a waste of time. That was the way she was made. She was domestically minded and she just couldn't sit back and admit defeat. She was absolutely determined to keep inside and outside clean and tidy.

This was something which worried and exasperated me. I was married to a beautiful, intelligent, warm-hearted girl, but I wished with all my heart that she would be kinder to herself and take more time to rest. When we were first married, I tried by pleading, and at times by making angry scenes which I wasn't much good at, to make her alter her ways but it was like talking to a wall – she slogged on regardless. Cooking, too. I had never met anybody who could work such magic with food, and as a dedicated eater I realised my good luck, but I wished fervently that she would spend less time over the oven. However, when all my entreaties were in vain and she went her own way, I consoled myself that I could hear her singing as she went round the house with her Hoover and duster. At this moment, she was actually humming softly to herself as she scrubbed that accursed step.

Even now, fifty years later and when we are coming up to the supreme accolade of getting our Golden Wedding pictures in the *Darrowby and Houlton Times*, she still sings as she potters busily around in another, mercifully much smaller house. It dawned on me long ago that she's happy that way.

From the front door, I went along the tiled passage which

would have been full of sunlight and character in the summer but on this cold spring day was just as cold and shivery as the street outside; on and on past dining room and sitting room, then turned left down to the dispensary, then right and left again and to another stretch of passage past consulting room, breakfast room and finally to the kitchen and scullery at the end of the long offshoot at the back of the house. I seemed to have travelled about fifty yards and who could blame Tristan in the old days for riding his bicycle to get to the front door?

On the way, I passed little Rosie, clattering over the tiles in her strong shoes, her legs muffled in thick pantaloons as Jimmy's used to be. I sometimes wondered how we had brought the children up in this relentless cold and I was grateful that they didn't seem to suffer from more coughs and sneezes than other children. The main casualty was Helen who was plagued with terrible chilblains round her ankles.

Next morning as soon as I awoke, my decision welled strongly in my mind. We had to get out. Skeldale would be fine as the practice quarters but we had to find something smaller to live in.

It was the beginning of a kind of obsession and I could think of nothing else that morning as I jumped out of bed, tried in vain to see out of the frosted windows and then dressed quickly in the icy atmosphere. I threw open the bedroom door and, at full gallop, began my morning routine. Down the stairs two at a time, full tilt along the freezing passage – the secret was to keep running – to the kitchen where I put the kettle on. Back along to the dining room at top speed where the bloody-minded anthracite stove was out again. It was the only source of warmth in the whole house but I hadn't time to relight it now.

Back over the long stretch to the kitchen where I made the tea and took up a cup to Helen. Then, blowing on my hands and jumping around to stop the blood freezing, I started a fire in the kitchen. I was never much of a boy scout at fire-lighting – unlike Helen who could have a fine blaze going in no time – and by the time the family came downstairs I had my usual fitful flame peeping out among the coals.

Breakfast was a cheerless affair with a little one-bar electric fire fighting an unequal battle and all of us trying to stop our teeth from chattering. I was silent over the meal, my mind wholly occupied with my fierce resolve, and I kept thinking back over previous festive seasons, remembering how we huddled round the fire in the big sitting room while our backs froze and the Christmas decorations swayed in the assorted draughts.

It was still uppermost in my mind when I called at Mrs Dryden's little semi-detached house on the outskirts of Darrowby. I had been treating her cat for a very bad attack of otodectic mange in the ears.

'Come on, Sooty,' I said, as I lifted him on to the table. 'You look a lot better today.'

His mistress smiled. 'Oh, he is. He's stopped shaking his head and scratching. He was goin' nearly mad before you cleaned his ears out.'

I did some more swabbing then trickled some lotion into the ears as the black cat purred happily. 'Yes. He won't need any more attention from me. Just keep putting the drops in the ears night and morning for another few days and I'm sure he'll be fine.'

I went over to the kitchen sink to wash my hands and looked out of the window at the neat garden. 'This is a nice little house, Mrs Dryden.'

'Aye, it is, Mr Herriot, but I'm leaving it soon.'

'Really, why is that?'

'Well, I need the money. That's the top and bottom of it. When Robert died, he didn't leave much.'

I could believe her. She was a retired farmer's widow, and I knew what a struggle they had had to scrape a living on their smallholding. Bob Dryden and I had shared some hard experiences up there on the hills. Tough calvings and lambings, and I could remember a disastrous spring when many of their calves had died of scour. He was a fine man and I remembered him as a friend.

'But where will you live?' I asked.

'Oh, I'm going to live with me sister in Houlton. I'll be all right there, but I'll be sorry to part with this nice little house. Robert and I were that pleased to be able to buy it when he retired. Still, I'm hopin' to get two thousand pounds for it and that'll be a godsend to me in my old age.'

I had one of my blinding flashes then. This was just the place for us. It was perfect, and I felt sure I'd be able to get a mortgage to buy it.

'Would you sell it to me?' I asked eagerly.

She smiled. 'I would if I could, Mr Herriot, but the arrangements are all made. It goes up for auction at the Drovers' Arms on Wednesday.'

My heart started to thump. 'Well, I'll be there bidding, Mrs Dryden.'

I was positive I would get the house, and as I looked round the kitchen all my worries seemed to dissolve. What a piece of luck! I could just see Helen at that window, looking out on the little garden which gave on to green fields, with the church tower rising from the trees on the other side of the river. And everything was so compact. There was a hatch into the living room – no hiking fifty yards with the food. A little hall with the stairs leading to three bedrooms, almost at arm's length away. You could reach out and touch everything, and I loved the thought. In my frame of mind at that time, small was beautiful. Nothing else mattered.

I saw the man at the Building Society and there was no problem. They would grant me a mortgage. It was a house which would probably fetch around fifty to sixty thousand pounds at the present day but, in the early fifties, two thousand was about right.

I was walking on air until the Wednesday when I rolled up with Helen to the Drovers for the auction. The room was full and as Helen and I took our seats a farmer client nudged me. 'There's old Seth Bootland,' he murmured. 'He wants this house for his son who's just got married. Reckon he'll get it, too. He's rollin' in brass, but he's a hard businessman.'

I looked over at the rich grain merchant. He was impressive with his high-coloured, beaky face and camel coat, and his face wore an expression of grim confidence. I felt a qualm, then came a return of my steely resolve. I was going to buy that house.

The bidding started at fifteen hundred and went rapidly – more rapidly than I had expected – up to my top figure of two thousand. Bootland made it two thousand one hundred. He clearly was used to this sort of thing and just twitched a bored forefinger. I stabbed the air eagerly to put on another hundred – I was quite sure my mortgage could be stretched another little bit – but Bootland flicked the finger again and it was up to me.

Soon there was just the two of us. All other bidders had fallen out and I felt cruelly exposed. The bids were down to fifty now and as the price crept up and up toward three thousand my heart began to pound and I could feel my palms sweating.

Helen was clutching my knee and with each new bid, she whispered desperately, 'No, Jim, no! We haven't any money!' But I was seized by a kind of madness. The money meant nothing. All I could see was Helen in that trim little house looking out on her garden from the pretty kitchen. That was the vision which wouldn't go away and I ploughed on doggedly.

When the price got above three thousand, the audience in the packed room had begun to emit an excited 'Ahh!' at each new bid. It had got down to raises of twenty-five pounds.

'Mr Bootland bids three thousand two hundred and twenty-five.' My mouth was dry as the auctioneer gazed at me enquiringly.

Helen's grip on my knee was like a vice. She was shaking it with her entreaties. 'No, Jim, *no!*'

I raised my hand.

'And fifty. Thank you,' and then the glance at Bootland. 'And seventy-five.' The auctioneer's and everybody's eyes were on me. As in a dream, I raised my hand.

'We have three thousand three hundred pounds.'

Bootland waggled his finger.

'And twenty-five.'

Once again, in the vibrating silence, all the eyes were on me. I felt utterly drained, parched, exhausted. I was trembling and only slightly aware of Helen punching my leg and almost sobbing. 'Stop it! Please stop it!' I thought she was going to cry. I shook my head at the auctioneer and the thing was over.

There was an excited hum of conversation in the room, but I stayed slumped in my seat, only dimly aware of Bootland going up and talking to the auctioneer and of Helen sitting very still beside me. Finally, I rose and looked at her.

'Good heavens, Jim, you're as white as a sheet!' she gasped.

I nodded wordlessly. I did feel extremely white. On the way out I received a savage glance from Mr Bootland. Thanks to me, he had had to pay one thousand three hundred and twenty-five pounds – around thirty thousand at present day prices – more than the house was probably worth. I certainly wasn't his favourite man.

But I didn't care. All I felt was the sense of abject failure. My happy vision of Helen looking out of that window onto the fields beyond was shattered and I was right back where I started. I had accomplished nothing.

Outside in the market place I stood for a moment, drawing in the cool air. I took Helen's arm and was about to move on when I felt a hand on my shoulder. I looked down at the sweet face of Mrs Dryden. She was smiling at me.

'Eee, Mr Herriot, I'm right sorry you didn't get the house, but you've done a lot for me – you'll never know how much. I've got all that extra money to put by me, thanks to you. Believe me, it'll make all the difference in the world. I really cannot thank you enough.'

As she walked away, I looked at her thin, bent figure and her white hair. There was the wife of good old Bob Dryden and he would have been pleased. I had done something after all.

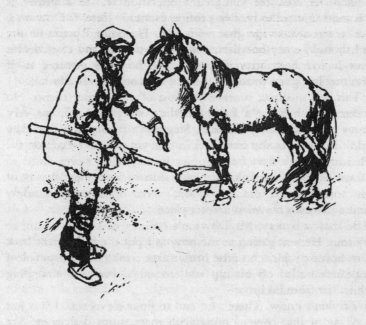

13

I unwound the spiral Hudson's instrument from the cow's teat and drew forth a strong jet of milk.

'Eee, that's wonderful, marvellous,' breathed Mr Dowson reverently. 'I don't know 'ow you do it – you've saved me again. You're a great man, Mr Herriot.'

We were still doing a lot of these teat operations, because milking machines had not come into general use and the farmers' horny-handed pulling at the cows' teats often resulted in damage to the lining and blockage. It wasn't a particularly popular procedure with the vets because there was an excellent chance of having your head kicked off as you crouched down there by the udder, but it was undeniably satisfying to bring a useless teat back to life. A lot of a cow's value was lost when she became a 'three-titted 'un'.

However, valuable though the operation was to a farmer, it was most unusual to receive profuse gratitude like Mr Dowson's. But it was always like that with him. He poured praise on me and though, over the years, I was sure that all my cases on his farm hadn't been triumphs, that was how he pictured it. If anything had gone wrong in the past he would never admit it.

This was in direct contrast to most of our farmer clients. No matter how brilliant a feat of healing we pulled off, we very rarely heard anything about it. Siegfried's theory was that they didn't like to mention our cures in case we put a bit extra on the bill and he may have had a point because they never failed to inform us about our failures. Comments such as 'Hey, that beast you treated never did any good,' were often embarrassingly shouted across a crowded market place.

Be that as it may, Mr Dowson's attitude was always balm to my soul. He was gazing at me now as I put the instrument back in its bottle of spirit, his little brown face crinkled in a benevolent smile. He pulled off his cap and smoothed back the straggling white hair from his brow.

'Ah don't know. There's no end to your cleverness. I was just thinking of that cow of mine with magnesium deficiency. She was laid there like a dead thing – ah was sure she'd stopped breathin' – but you put a bottle into 'er vein, then you looked at your watch. "Mr Dowson," you said, "this beast will get up on her legs in exactly twelve and a half minutes."'

'I did?'

'Ah'm not jokin' nor jestin', that's what you said, and you can believe me or believe me not, just the very second the hands on your watch got round to twelve and a half minutes that cow jumped up and walked away.'

'Good heavens! Did she really?'

'She did that, and I'll tell you summat else, she's never looked back since.'

'Well, that's great.' I had the same feeling of bewilderment as I always felt at Mr Dowson's panegyrics. I could never remember the magical things I had done, but it was very pleasant all the same. Was I really that brilliant or did he make it all up? His habitual phrase of 'believe me or believe me not' suggested that he may have had doubts about it himself, but that didn't alter the fact that his eulogies were always delivered with the greatest certainty and emphasis.

Even the surroundings of his farm were idyllic, and as I walked to my car with a gentle breeze, full of the scents of summer, eddying around me, I looked back at the little farmhouse tucked into the green hillside which dipped down over rig and furrow to the river, sparkling in the sunshine.

As always, I drove away in a rosy glow with Mr Dowson waving until I was out of sight.

I was back there again within a week to deal with a calving heifer. Mr Dowson was worried because she was overdue, but the delivery was uneventful and I soon had a large bull calf snuffling and snorting among the straw in the byre.

'Well, that's fine,' I said. 'Sometimes these big calves are a bit late. It was a tight squeeze, but all's well.'

'Aye, aye,' said the farmer. 'There was no need to worry. I should've known. You told me more than a month ago that that heifer would be exactly five days late, and you were right as usual.'

'Did I really say that? I don't see how I would know . . .'

He shrugged his shoulders. 'Well, Mr Herriot, them was your words. I ought to remember them.'

As we left the byre, Mr Dowson stopped to pat a little Dales pony which was happily cropping the grass by the side of the house. 'Remember this little feller? Remember that bad stoppage he had?'

'Ah yes, of course I do. He looks fine now.'

'He does that, and by gaw 'e was ill! Thought ah was going to lose 'im. Right bunged up and groanin' in pain he was. I'd given him all sorts o' medicines to try to move 'is bowels but they did no good – nothing came through 'im for two whole days. Then I got you in and I'll never forget what you did.'

'What did I do?'

'Ah tell ye, it were like a miracle. You came in the morning and you gave him two injections and you said to me, "Mr Dowson, his bowels will move at two o'clock this afternoon."'

'I said that?'

'You did an' all, and then you said, "At first he'll pass exactly a handful, just like this."' He cupped his hands to illustrate. 'And right on two o'clock, that's what 'e did. No more, no less.'

'Gosh!'

'Aye, and then you said, "At half past two he'll pass just enough to fill that small shovel."' Mr Dowson hurried busily over to the house and picked up a little shovel which stood by the coal bunker. He held it out to me. 'There's the very thing. And right on the dot by my watch he passed just the amount you said. I measured it.'

'Never! Are you sure?'

'You can believe me or believe me not. Then you said, "At three o'clock he'll have a good clear out," and that's just what happened. I was lookin' at my watch when he cocked his tail and got rid of everything that was troubling 'im. And he's been right as ninepence ever since.'

'Well, that's wonderful, Mr Dowson. I'm so pleased to hear it.' I shook my head to dispel the mists of fantasy which had begun to billow around me. I am a run of the mill veterinary surgeon, hard working and conscientious, but that's all, and it knocks me out of my stride to be hailed as a genius, but as always, listening to Mr Dowson was like soothing oil being poured on my oft-bruised ego. I had to admit I enjoyed it, and I didn't demur when he went on.

'And while you're 'ere, just have a look at this pig.' He took my arm and led me into an outbuilding. 'There she is,' he said, leaning over a pen and pointing to a fine big sow stretched on the straw with a litter of piglets sucking busily at her teats. 'That's the one that had that nasty great swelling on her foot. Dead lame she was, and I was right worried about 'er. You gave her a jab and left me some salve to rub on the lump and next morning it was gone!'

'You mean . . . it vanished overnight? All of it?'

'Aye, that's right, ah'm not jokin' nor jestin'. It was gone!'

'Well . . . that's quite amazing.'

'Not to me, it isn't, Mr Herriot. Everything you do for me turns out right. Ah don't know what I'd do without you.'

Even through my confusion I found his faith touching. I hoped it would never be shattered.

I thought that moment had arrived when Mr Dowson called me to his farm a few weeks later.

'What's the trouble this time?' I asked.

The old man rubbed his chin. 'Well, it's a funny one, I tell you. It's this calf.' He pointed to a sturdy young animal about a month old. 'He won't drink 'is milk properly. Look. I'll show ye.' He tipped some milk into a big bucket and set it down in front of the little creature, but the calf, instead of drinking, put his head down and with a fierce butt, sent the bucket flying, spilling the milk in all directions.

'Does he do this every time?'

'Aye, knocks it over every time. It's a dang nuisance. Wastes me good milk, too.'

I examined the calf, then turned to the farmer. 'He seems perfectly healthy to me.'

'Oh aye, he is. Fit as a flea and full o' life. It's just this one thing wi' the bucket. I thought you'd maybe be able to give 'im one of your magic injections to stop him doin' it.'

'Well, really, Mr Dowson,' I said, laughing, 'this isn't a medical problem, it's psychological. He just doesn't like buckets. I'm afraid I can't do anything for you this time. Can't you hold the bucket while he drinks?'

'Yes, that's what I have to do, but even then 'e keeps bashin' at it with his head.' He dug his hands into his pockets and gave me a crestfallen look. 'Ah'm sure you could do something. You say it's not a medical problem, but it's an animal problem and everythin' you've done for me wi' animals has been successful. I wish you'd have a try. Go on, give 'im an injection.'

I looked at the old man's doleful face. I had a feeling that if I walked off the farm without doing something, he would be truly upset. How could I please him without being an absolute charlatan? If I didn't inject something it was going to break his heart, but what . . . what . . . ? Mentally I searched the contents of my car boot and was beginning to despair when in my mind's eye I saw the bottle of Thiamin – Vitamin B injection. We used it for a brain disease called cerebrocortical necrosis and while, of course, the calf wasn't suffering from that or anything like it, at least it had to do with the head. Anyway, I stilled my conscience with the thought that I wouldn't charge the old man anything.

I hurried to the car. 'I'll give him a shot of this,' I said and was rewarded by a radiant smile lighting up Mr Dowson's face. I injected a few ccs with the knowledge that I wasn't doing any harm. The injection would be useless, but it was serving its purpose. The old man was happy and, really, when I thought about it, it would be no bad thing if, for once, my treatment was ineffective. My mantle of infallibility would be stripped from me and I wouldn't be expected to do the impossible any more.

It was more than a month before I saw Mr Dowson again. He was leaning over a rail at the cattle market and he waved and came over to me. I was intrigued at the prospect that for the first time ever he would have to report a failure. What words would he employ? He had never had to do it before. And I was pretty sure that he would hate telling me.

He looked up at me with wide eyes. 'Well, you've done it again, Mr Herriot!'

'Done it again?' I looked at him blankly.

'Aye, that calf. Your injection worked.'

'What!'

'It did an' all.' The familiar happy smile flooded over his face. 'He's never butted a bucket since that day!'

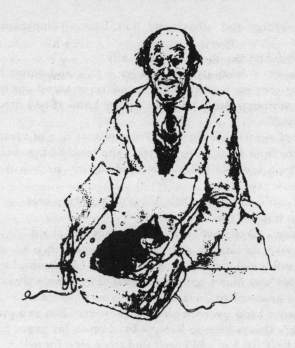

14

Sometimes, when our dog and cat patients died, the owners brought them in for us to dispose of them. It was always a sad occasion and I had a sense of foreboding when I saw old Dick Fawcett's face.

He put the improvised cat box on the surgery table and looked at me with unhappy eyes.

'It's Frisk,' he said. His lips trembled as though he was unable to say more.

I didn't ask any questions, but began to undo the strings on the cardboard container. Dick couldn't afford a proper cat box, but he had used this one before, a home-made affair with holes punched in the sides.

I untied the last knot and looked inside at the motionless body. Frisk. The glossy black, playful little creature I knew so well, always purring and affectionate and Dick's companion and friend.

'When did he die, Dick?' I asked gently.

He passed a hand over his haggard face and through the straggling grey hairs. 'Well, I just found 'im stretched out by my bed this morning. But . . . I don't rightly know if he's dead yet, Mr Herriot.'

I looked again inside the box. There was no sign of breathing. I lifted the limp form on to the table and touched the cornea of the unseeing eye. No reflex. I reached for my stethoscope and placed it over the chest.

'The heart's still going, Dick, but it's a very faint beat.'

'Might stop any time, you mean?'

I hesitated. 'Well, that's the way it sounds, I'm afraid.'

As I spoke, the little cat's rib cage lifted slightly then subsided.

'He's still breathing,' I said, 'but only just.' I examined the cat thoroughly and found nothing unusual. The conjunctiva of the eye was a good colour. In fact, there was no abnormality.

I passed a hand over the sleek little body. 'This is a puzzler, Dick. He's always been so lively – lived up to his name, in fact, yet here he is, flat out, and I can't find any reason for it.'

'Could he have 'ad a stroke or summat?'

'I suppose it's just possible, but I wouldn't expect him to be totally unconscious. I'm wondering if he might have had a blow on the head.'

'I don't think so. He was as right as rain when I went to bed, and he was never out during t'night.' The old man shrugged his shoulders. 'Any road, it's a poor look out for 'im?'

'Afraid so, Dick. He's only just alive. But I'll give him a stimulant injection and then you must take him home and keep him warm. If he's still around tomorrow morning, bring him in and I'll see how he's going on.'

I was trying to strike an optimistic note, but I was pretty sure that I would never see Frisk again and I knew the old man felt the same.

His hands shook as he tied up the box and he didn't speak until we reached the front door. He turned briefly to me and nodded. 'Thank ye, Mr Herriot.'

I watched him as he walked with shuffling steps down the

street. He was going back to an empty little house with his dying pet. He had lost his wife many years ago – I had never known a Mrs Fawcett – and he lived alone on his old age pension. It wasn't much of a life. He was a quiet, kindly man who didn't go out much and seemed to have few friends, but he had Frisk. The little cat had walked in on him six years ago and had transformed his life, bringing a boisterous, happy presence into the silent house making the old man laugh with his tricks and playfulness, following him around, rubbing against his legs. Dick wasn't lonely any more, and I had watched a warm bond of friendship growing stronger over the years. In fact, it was something more – the old man seemed to depend on Frisk. And now this.

Well, I thought, as I walked back down the passage, it was the sort of thing that happened in veterinary practice. Pets didn't live long enough. But I felt worse this time because I had no idea what ailed my patient. I was in a total fog.

On the following morning I was surprised to see Dick Fawcett sitting in the waiting room, the cardboard box on his knee.

I stared at him. 'What's happened?'

He didn't answer and his face was inscrutable as we went through to the consulting room and he undid the knots. When he opened the box I prepared for the worst, but to my astonishment the little cat leaped out onto the table and rubbed his face against my hand, purring like a motor cycle.

The old man laughed, his thin face transfigured. 'Well, what d'ye think of that?'

'I don't know what to think, Dick.' I examined the little animal carefully. He was completely normal. 'All I know is that I'm delighted. It's like a miracle.'

'No, it isn't,' he said. 'It was that injection you gave 'im. It's worked wonders. I'm right grateful.'

Well, it was kind of him, but it wasn't as simple as that. There was something here I didn't understand, but never mind. Thank heaven it had ended happily.

The incident had receded into a comfortable memory when, three days later, Dick Fawcett reappeared at the surgery with his box. Inside was Frisk, motionless, unconscious, just as before.

Totally bewildered, I repeated the examination and then the injection and on the following day the cat was normal. From then on, I was in the situation which every veterinary surgeon knows so well – being involved in a baffling case and waiting with a feeling of impending doom for something tragic to happen.

Nothing did happen for nearly a week, then Mrs Duggan, Dick's neighbour, telephoned.

'I'm ringin' on behalf of Mr Fawcett. His cat's ill.'

'In what way?'

'Oh, just lyin' stretched out, unconscious, like.'

I suppressed a scream. 'When did this happen?'

'Just found 'im this morning. And Mr Fawcett can't bring him to you – he's poorly himself. He's in bed.'

'I'm sorry to hear that. I'll come round straight away.'

And it was just the same as before. An almost lifeless little creature lying prone on Dick's bed. Dick himself looked terrible – ghastly white and thinner than ever – but he still managed a smile.

'Looks like 'e needs another of your magic injections, Mr Herriot.'

As I filled my syringe, my mind seethed with the thought that there was indeed some kind of magic at work here, but it wasn't my injection.

'I'll drop in tomorrow, Dick,' I said. 'And I hope you'll be feeling better yourself.'

'Oh, I'll be awright as long as t'little feller's better.' The old man stretched out a hand and stroked the cat's shining fur. The arm was emaciated and the eyes in the skull-like face were desperately worried.

I looked around the comfortless little room and hoped for another miracle.

I wasn't really surprised when I came back next morning and saw Frisk darting about on the bed, pawing at a piece of string which the old man was holding up for him. The relief was great but I felt enveloped more suffocatingly than ever in my fog of ignorance. What the hell was it? The whole thing just didn't make sense. There was no known disease with symptoms like these. I had a strong conviction that reading a whole library of veterinary books wouldn't help me.

Anyway, the sight of the little cat arching and purring round my hand was reward enough, and for Dick it was everything. He was relaxed and smiling.

'You keep gettin' him right, Mr Herriot. I can't thank you enough.' Then the worry flickered again in his eyes. 'But is he goin' to keep doin' it? I'm frightened he won't come round one of these times.'

Well, that was the question. I was frightened too, but I had to try to be cheerful. 'Maybe it's just a passing phase, Dick. I hope we'll have no more trouble now.' But I couldn't promise anything and the frail man in the bed knew it.

Mrs Duggan was showing me out when I saw the district nurse getting out of her car at the front door.

'Hello, Nurse,' I said, 'you've come to have a look at Mr Fawcett? I'm sorry he's ill.'

She nodded. 'Yes, poor old chap. It's a great shame.'

'What do you mean? Is it something serious?'

'Afraid so.' Her mouth tightened and she looked away from me. 'He's dying. It's cancer. Getting rapidly worse.'

'My God! Poor Dick. And a few days ago he was bringing his cat to my surgery. He never said a word. Does he know?'

'Oh yes, he knows, but that's him all over, Mr Herriot. He's as game as a pebble. He shouldn't have been out, really.'

'Is he . . . is he . . . suffering?'

She shrugged. 'Getting a bit of pain now, but we're keeping him as comfortable as we can with medication. I give him a shot when necessary and he has some stuff he can take himself if I'm not around. He's very shaky and can't pour from the bottle into the spoon. Mrs Duggan would gladly do it for him, but he's so independent.' She smiled for a moment. 'He pours the mixture into a saucer and spoons it up that way.'

'A saucer . . . ?' Somewhere in the fog a little light glimmered. 'What's in the mixture?'

'Oh, heroin and pethidene. It's the usual thing Dr Allinson prescribes.'

I seized her arm. 'I'm coming back in with you, Nurse.'

The old man was surprised when I reappeared. 'What's matter, Mr Herriot? Have you left summat?'

'No, Dick, I want to ask you something. Is your medicine pleasant tasting?'

'Aye, it's nice and sweet. It isn't bad to take at all.'

'And you put it in a saucer?'

'That's right. Me hand's a bit dothery.'

'And when you take it last thing at night there's sometimes a bit left in the saucer?'

'Aye, there is, why?'

'Because you leave that saucer by your bedside, don't you, and Frisk sleeps on your bed . . .'

The old man lay very still as he stared at me. 'You mean the little beggar licks it out?'

'I'll bet my boots he does.'

Dick threw back his head and laughed. A long, joyous laugh. 'And that sends 'im to sleep! No wonder! It makes me right dozy, too!'

I laughed with him. 'Anyway, we know now, Dick. You'll put that saucer in the cupboard when you've taken your dose, won't you?'

'I will that, Mr Herriot. And Frisk will never pass out like that again?'

'No, never again.'

'Eee, that's grand!' He sat up in bed, lifted the little cat and held him against his face. He gave a sigh of utter content and smiled at me.

'Mr Herriot,' he said, 'I've got nowt to worry about now.'

Out in the street, as I bade Mrs Duggan goodbye for the second time, I looked back at the little house. ' "Nowt to worry about," eh? That's rather wonderful, coming from him.'

'Oh aye, and he means it, too. He's not bothered about himself.'

I didn't see Dick again for two weeks. I was visiting a friend in Darrowby's little cottage hospital when I saw the old man in a bed in a corner of the ward.

I went over and sat down by his side. His face was desperately thin, but serene.

'Hello, Dick,' I said.

He looked at me sleepily and spoke in a whisper. 'Now then, Mr Herriot.' He closed his eyes for a few moments, then he looked up again with the ghost of a smile. 'I'm glad we found out what was wrong with t'little cat.'

'So am I, Dick.'

Again a pause. 'Mrs Duggan's got 'im.'

'Yes. I know. He has a good home there.'

'Aye . . . aye . . .' The voice was fainter. 'But oftens I wish I had 'im here.' The bony hand stroked the counterpane and his lips moved again. I bent closer to hear.

'Frisk . . .' he was saying, 'Frisk . . .' Then his eyes closed and I saw that he was sleeping.

I heard next day that Dick Fawcett had died, and it was possible that I was the last person to hear him speak. And it was strange, yet fitting, that those last words were about his cat.

'Frisk . . . Frisk . . .'

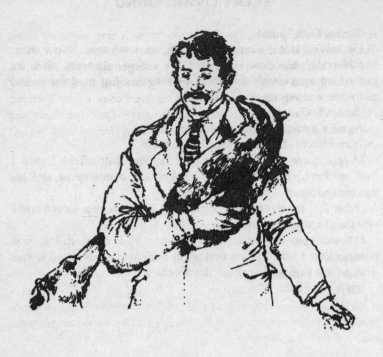

15

I have to go back now to those early days when John Crooks departed from the practice and it was difficult to adjust my mind to the fact that he had gone for good. I couldn't believe that I would never hear that booming voice on the other end of the phone saying, okay, I could stay in my bed and he'd go out into the cold darkness to calve that heifer. And it wasn't just that. As I have said, I was young enough then to be a friend to an assistant and I was losing a friend now – two, in fact, when John and Heather set off to build their own life in Beverley – and it left me with an empty feeling.

However, it was no use brooding. We had to have another assistant and since our advertisement in *The Veterinary Record* had been successful, there was one on his way to us at this moment. I looked at my watch. It was nearly two thirty. Calum Buchanan's train would be pulling in to Darrowby in a few minutes. I ran out to the car and drove to the station.

When the train drew in, only one passenger alighted. He was a tall young man with a huge lurcher dog trotting by his side, and as he came along the platform towards me I took in the battered suitcase, flowing black moustache and very dark eyes, but the most striking feature was a large hairy animal draped over his left shoulder.

He put out his hand and grinned. 'Mr Herriot?'

'Yes ... yes ...' I shook his hand. 'You'll be Calum Buchanan.'

'That's right.'

'Good ... good ... but what's that on your shoulder?'

'That's Marilyn.'

'*Marilyn?*'

'Yes, my badger.'

'Badger!'

He laughed – a carefree laugh. 'Sorry, maybe I should have warned you in my letter. She's my pet. Goes everywhere with me.'

'Everywhere?'

'Absolutely.'

All kinds of apprehensions boiled up in my mind. How did a veterinary assistant carry out his duties with a wild animal hanging from his shoulder at all times? And what sort of man would roll up to a new job not only with a badger but with a giant dog?

Anyway, I knew I would soon find out, so I pushed my misgivings to one side and led him out to the car, running a gauntlet of pop-eyed stares from a booking-clerk, two ladies sitting on the platform seat and from a porter who nearly wheeled a load of packing cases into a wall.

'I see you've got a dog, too,' I said.

'Yes, that's Storm. Lovely, good-natured animal.'

The lurcher waved his tail and gazed up at me with kind eyes. I patted the shaggy head. 'He looks it.'

'Incidentally,' I said, 'with a name like yours, I was expecting a Scottish accent and you haven't got one.'

He smiled. 'No, I grew up in Yorkshire, but my ancestry is Scottish.' His eyes gleamed and his chin went up.

'You're proud of that, eh?'

He nodded gravely. 'I am indeed. Very proud.'

At Skeldale House, I showed him his car and helped to kit him out with the essential equipment we all carried – the drugs, instruments, obstetric gown and protective clothing – then I took him up to the flat where his main interest seemed to be directed not at the interior but at the birds and flowers he could see through the window overlooking the long garden.

'By the way,' I said, 'I should have asked you earlier. Have you had lunch?'

'Lunch?'

'Yes, have you had something to eat?'

'Eat . . . eat . . . ?' The black button eyes took on a thoughtful expression. 'Yes, I'm sure I had something yesterday.'

'Yesterday! My God, it's nearly four o'clock in the afternoon. You must be starved!'

'Oh no, not at all, not in the least.'

'You mean you're not hungry?'

He seemed to find the question unusual, even irrelevant, and replied with a non-committal shrug of the shoulders.

'Anyway,' I said, 'I'll slip downstairs and see what I can find for you.'

In the office cupboard was a large uncut fruit cake which Helen had just baked to go with the cups of coffee we snatched between visits. I put it on a plate with a knife and took it up to the flat.

'Here you are,' I said, placing the cake on the table. 'Help yourself and then you can get a proper meal later.'

As I spoke I heard footsteps on the stairs and Siegfried burst into the room.

'Calum Buchanan, Siegfried Farnon,' I said.

They shook hands then Siegfried pointed a trembling finger at the young man's shoulder. 'What the devil is that?'

Calum smiled his engaging smile. 'Marilyn, my badger.'

'And you're going to keep that animal here?'

'That's right.'

Siegfried took a long breath and let it out slowly through his nose, but he didn't say anything. Instead, he continued to look fixedly at our new assistant.

The young man was talking easily about his experience in practice, his pleasure at coming to a charming town like Darrowby, and about the things he could see in the garden.

He had started on the cake, but didn't bother to use the knife. Instead, he crumbled pieces off absently as he spoke. 'What a beautiful wisteria! Finest I've ever seen. There's a pretty little bullfinch, and surely that's a tree creeper on your apple tree – not many of them about.' And, popping a large chunk of sultana-laden comestible into his mouth, 'My word, I can see an albino blackbird over there – what a beauty!'

Siegfried was a keen naturalist and ornithologist and normally this conversation would have been right up his street, but he remained silent, his eyes straying unbelievingly from the badger to the dog and to the steadily disappearing cake.

Finally, Calum swept up the last few crumbs with his fingers – I had the impression that he had no interest in what he had eaten – and turned away from the window.

'Well, thank you very much. I'll get unpacked now, if I may.'

I swallowed. 'Right, see you later.'

We went downstairs and Siegfried led me rapidly into the empty office. 'What the hell have we got here, James? An assistant with a blasted badger round his neck! And a dog as big as a donkey!'

'Well, yes . . . but he seems to be a nice bloke.'

'Maybe so, but *very* strange. Did you see – he ate that whole bloody cake!'

'Yes, I saw. But he was very hungry – he hadn't eaten since yesterday.'

Siegfried stared at me. 'Not since yesterday! Are you sure?'

'Sure as I can be. He didn't seem to know himself.'

My partner groaned and slapped a hand against his forehead. 'Oh, God, we should have had an interview before we took this chap on. But he had such glowing references from the university. They said he was outstanding. I thought we couldn't go wrong.'

'You never know. He may be good at the job, that's what really counts.'

'Well, we'll have to hope so, but he's a bloody odd ball and I sense trouble.'

I didn't say anything, but I had my own misgivings. John Crooks with all his great qualities was, at bottom, just an ordinary nice guy, but there was nothing ordinary about that dark-eyed young man upstairs.

The telephone interrupted my musings. I took the call and turned to Siegfried. 'That's Miles Horsley. He's got a heifer calving.'

My partner nodded, then pursed his lips thoughtfully. After a few moments he raised a decisive finger. 'Right, we'll send the new man. We've been wondering if he can do the job. This is our chance to find out.'

'Wait a minute, Siegfried,' I said. 'The young chap's newly qualified and this is Miles Horsley. He's an expert – you never get an easy calving there, and it's a heifer, too. It could be very tough. Maybe I'd better go.'

Siegfried shook his head vigorously. 'No, I want to find out what this fellow's made of and the sooner the better. Shout him down will you.'

Calum received the instructions calmly, whistling softly as we pointed out the farm on the map. As he turned to go, Siegfried fired a parting shot. 'This could be a difficult job, but don't come back till you have calved that heifer. Do you understand?'

My blood froze but Calum didn't seem in the least put out. He nodded, gave us a casual wave of the hand and went out to his car.

After he had left, Siegfried turned to me with a grim smile. 'You may think I'm hard, James, but I don't want him coming back here in half an hour with the story that it's an unusual presentation and would we take over. No, in at the deep end, I say. It's the best way.'

I shrugged. I just hoped the new young man could swim.

That was around five thirty and by half past seven I was suffering from almost unbearable tension. Pictures of the hapless rookie rolling around on a byre floor, covered in blood and muck, passed through my mind and I found myself looking at my watch every five minutes. I had almost reached the stage of pacing the floor when Siegfried came in, carrying a little dog which had torn its flank and needed stitching. 'How did Buchanan get on?' he asked.

'I don't know. He's not back yet.'

'Not back!' My partner gave me a level stare. 'Something's wrong, then. Let's get this dog stitched, then one of us had better get out there and see what's going on.'

We were both silent as I anaesthetised the little animal and Siegfried began to clean out the wound. I knew we were thinking the same thing – it had been a mistake to send the new man to the Horsley farm. As Siegfried inserted the sutures I noticed that he, too, kept glancing at his watch.

It was just after eight o'clock when the operating room door opened and Calum Buchanan walked in.

My partner, needle poised, looked at him. 'Well . . . ?'

'I'm afraid it was an impossible presentation,' Calum replied. 'Small heifer, huge calf with lateral deviation of the head. Right away back, out of reach. No way I could possibly calve her.'

Siegfried flushed and a dangerous light glinted in his eyes.

'So . . . ?'

'So I did a Caesarean.'

'You did what?'

Calum smiled calmly. 'A Caesarean. It was the only thing to do. The calf was alive, so embryotomy was out of the question.'

Siegfried looked at him open-mouthed. 'And tell me . . . what . . . what happened?'

'Oh, pretty straightforward, really. The heifer was up and looking fine when I left, and we got a lovely live calf.'

'Well . . . well . . .' My partner seemed lost for words – the Caesarean operation on cows was a rare undertaking in the fifties – but finally his natural sense of justice reasserted itself. 'Well, my boy, you've obviously done a splendid job and I do congratulate you. It was your very first call as a qualified man, too. Well done indeed.'

The young man flashed his dark-eyed smile. 'Thank you very much.' He looked down at his hands, 'I could do with a bath now if you don't mind.'

'My dear chap, by all means. And get something to eat, too.'

As the door closed behind our new assistant, my partner gave me a wide-eyed look. 'Well, what do you make of that?'

'Absolutely great!' I said. 'Anybody who can tackle a job like that when he's only just arrived must be good. My God, he's hardly had time to get his instruments sorted out in his car!'

'Yes . . . yes . . .' Siegfried's expression was preoccupied as he finished his stitching and he didn't say anything as he put down his needle and went over to the basin against the wall to wash his hands. Then he turned to me suddenly. 'You know, I still can't quite believe it, James! Do you think he's having us on?'

I laughed. 'Oh no, of course not. He wouldn't dare.'

'I don't know,' grunted Siegfried. 'There's something very odd about that chap. I don't know where I am with him somehow.' He finished drying his hands and then his face broke into a slow smile. 'Tell you what. When we've cleared up here, we'll slip out to Miles Horsley's place. It's only ten minutes' drive and we can have a beer in the village pub. It's nearly opposite the farm. I won't be satisfied till I've had a look for myself.'

Miles Horsley was a rangy, six foot Dalesman — a decent man but not one to cross. An advanced dairy farmer, a perfectionist. His granite features relaxed as he answered the door.

'Now then, gentlemen, we're seeing a lot o' vets this evening. What's up?'

'Ah yes, Miles,' Siegfried said airily. 'James and I were having a drink over at the Blacksmith's Arms and we thought we'd just check on your heifer.'

The farmer nodded. 'Aye, right. Come and see.' He led the way over the dark yard, opened a loose box at the far end and switched on the light.

A fine roan heifer was nibbling casually at a rackful of hay while a strapping calf sucked at her udder. On the heifer's left flank an almost perfect rectangle of hair had been shaved away and running down the middle of it was as neat a row of stitches as I had ever seen.

'That's a good young feller you've got,' said the farmer. 'But, mind you, I wondered who was comin' when I saw that badger on his shoulder!'

Siegfried was still staring bemusedly at the operation site. 'Yes . . . yes, indeed.'

'Aye, very confident was t'lad,' continued the farmer. 'And I liked the way he went about the job. Careful and very clean. Brought all 'is instruments into the house and boiled them up thoroughly before he started work. There'll be no infection after this job, I'll warrant. And I've got a real smashin' calf into the bargain.'

Siegfried ran his hand over the heifer's back and rubbed the calf's head. 'I'm so pleased things have turned out well. Many thanks, Miles, for letting us have a look.'

In the Blacksmith's Arms my partner took a thoughtful pull at his glass. 'Beautifully tidy work, James, but it's a funny thing – I can't help feeling there's a catch somewhere.'

'Why, whatever do you mean? We've got a first class vet in the practice, that's obvious.'

'Oh yes, so it seems. But he's very peculiar – and I keep thinking about that damn badger. And that funny big walrus moustache. And that cake! I've never seen anybody demolish an enormous bloody fruit cake at one go – and he didn't seem to notice what he was doing.'

I laughed. 'Oh yes, I know. There's no doubt he's a very unusual young man. But he looks to me like a nice fellow – there's something very likable about him – and he's good at the job. That's the main thing.'

'I agree, I agree.' Siegfried ran his hand through his hair and churned it about a bit. 'I'm probably worrying needlessly, but . . . time will tell . . .'

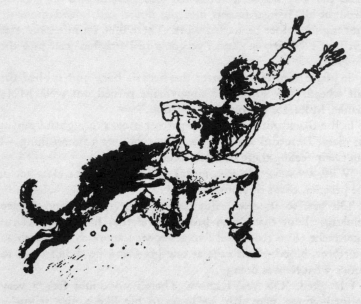

16

'Nice dog,' I said, as I evacuated the anal glands of the big animal on the table. He was making a grumbling sound up front, but it was good to see the waving, friendly tail even though he couldn't have been enjoying my squeezing at his bottom. 'I'm glad his tail is wagging.'

'Aye, but –' old Mrs Coates began, but she was too late. As I moved forward to take a look at his eyes, the dog, to my astonishment, turned on me, all teeth and snarling lips, and made a ferocious grab at my face. My evasive technique has become polished over the years, but I only just avoided a nasty wound.

'Stop it, Wolfie! You naughty bad dog!' screamed the old lady. 'Just behave, or I'll give you such a smackin', that I will!'

The big animal subsided under his mistress's scolding and I took a step back out of harm's way. 'You know, Wolfie is remarkable,' I said, looking at him, wide-eyed. 'His tail is still wagging like mad and yet he's growling and showing his teeth as if he'd like to tear me to bits.'

'Aye, that's t'trouble, Mr Herriot. He's allus givin' people the wrong impression. They think he's that good-natured when they see 'im waggin', then they get a shock.'

'Well, he certainly had me fooled, Mrs Coates. He's the only dog I've ever seen that wags and growls at the same time. Depends which end you look at, doesn't it?'

Mrs Coates lived in a row of council bungalows for old people. Some time after my visit I called on an elderly couple, Mr and Mrs Hart, further along the same row.

Their cat which was, like themselves, quite old was losing its hair and going bald in places. As I parted the hair and examined the skin I could see the obvious signs of miliary eczema.

'This is a condition which often affects neutered toms like your Peter. I'll be able to clear it up with a hormone injection and a course of tablets.'

Peter didn't stop purring as I inserted the needle under his skin – he was a cat who appreciated any kind of attention – but I noticed that his owners looked a little uneasy. They seemed even more unhappy when I tipped some tablets into a box and began to write the instructions.

'We're a bit worried, Mr Herriot,' the old man said suddenly. 'This treatment will cost a bit and we can't pay you. Not today, any road.'

'That's right,' his wife broke in. 'We allus like to pay on the dot, but we 'aven't any money right now. We've been robbed.'

'Robbed?'

'Aye, unfortunately. My husband hasn't been well lately and the garden's got a bit untidy. Two men came in and said they'd do the garden up for us, but when we were talkin' to one of them here in the parlour, the other 'un was in the kitchen stealin' our pension money and a bit o' ready cash we kept on the mantelpiece.'

'Well, what a dirty trick!' I said. 'But please don't worry about paying me. Any time will do. I'm really very sorry – this must have upset you terribly.'

As I left the house it was difficult to believe that there were such people – who would come into the homes of decent old folks and rob them of their precious few pounds. But sadly I had heard this story before. These two men had been going around Darrowby lately, getting into houses on any pretext and carrying out their despicable actions. They specialised in robbing elderly people. They weren't very brave.

A few days later I happened to be passing Mrs Coates's bungalow so I thought I might as well check on Wolfie. The old lady let me in and I looked at the big dog lashing his tail vigorously and snarling at the same time.

'He's champion,' Mrs Coates said. 'Never shuffles round on 'is bottom now.'

'Oh, that's good,' I said. 'It's an unpleasant thing for a dog.'

She caught my arm. 'Ah've got summat else to tell you. Ah've had the thieves in!'

'Oh no, those two men? Not you, too! I'm so sorry.'

'Aye, but listen!' she said excitedly. 'One of them fellers was talkin' to me and t'other was in the kitchen with Wolfie. I heard 'im sayin' "Nice doggie, nice doggie," then there was a terrible yell and a scuffle and the feller went past the parlour door screamin', with Wolfie hangin' on to 'is backside. The other 'un ran off, too, but Wolfie caught 'im just as he was goin' through the door and he didn't half holler out! Last thing I saw was the two of them runnin' for their lives down t'street with Wolfie after them.'

She reached into the corner of the fireplace and handed me a jagged piece of blood-stained cloth, obviously from the seat of a man's trousers. 'Wolfie brought that back with 'im.'

I laughed so much that I had to lean against the mantelpiece. 'Oh, what a lovely story. I bet we'll never see those two around here again.'

'Nay, nay, that we won't.' The old lady put her head in her hands and giggled. 'Eee, I can't help laughin' when I think of that feller saying, "Nice doggie, nice doggie."'

'Yes, it's very funny,' I said. 'He must have been looking at the wrong end.'

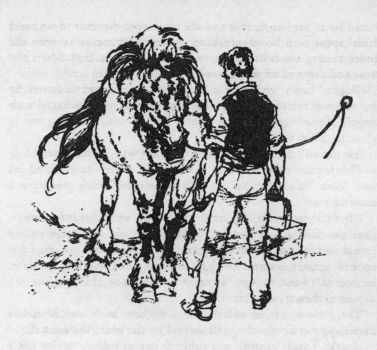

17

Ninety per cent of horses' lamenesses are in the feet. So the old saying goes and I could see it was true here.

The big Clydesdale was lifting his near hind leg, holding the foot, quivering, a few inches from the ground, then putting it down carefully. I had seen this sort of thing a hundred times before and it was diagnostic.

'He's got gravel,' I said to the farmer. This was the local term for an infection of the foot. It happened when the horse bruised or cracked its sole, allowing the entrance of bacteria. An abscess formed and the only cure was to pare down the horn and evacuate the pus.

This involved lifting the hoof and either resting it on your knee in the case of a hind foot or between your legs in a fore and cutting through the sole with a hoof knife. Sometimes the horn could be as hard as marble and the exact spot difficult to find and I had spent many back-breaking sessions hacking away with the horse resting his full weight on me as the sweat ran down my nose and dripped on to the hoof.

'Right,' I said, 'let's have a look at it.' I ran my hand down the leg and was reaching for the foot when the horse whickered with anger, turned quickly and lashed out at me, catching me a glancing blow on the thigh.

'He can still kick with that bad foot, anyway,' I murmured.

The farmer took a firmer grip on the halter and braced his feet. 'Aye, he's a cheeky sod. Watch yourself. He's given me a clout or two.'

I tried again with the same result and, at the third attempt, after the flailing foot had narrowly missed me, the horse swung round and sent me crashing against the side of the box. As I got up and, grimly determined, had another go at reaching the foot, he reared round at me, brought a fore foot crashing on my shoulder, then tried to bite me.

The farmer was an elderly man, slightly built and he didn't look happy as he was dragged around by the plunging animal.

'Look,' I said, panting and rubbing my shoulder, 'we've got a bit of a problem. I have to bring Denny Boynton out to another gravelled horse near here this afternoon. We'll call in about two o'clock and treat this chap. He's got a shoe on, anyway, and it's a lot easier to do the job with a blacksmith.'

Farmer Hickson looked relieved. 'Aye, that'll be best. I could see we were goin' to have a bit of a rodeo!'

As I drove away, I mused on my relationship with Denny. He and I were old friends. He was a bit younger than I and accompanied me regularly on horse visits. In the fifties, the tractor had more or less taken over on the farms but some farmers still liked to keep a cart horse and took a pride in them. Most of them were big, docile animals and I had always had a strong empathy with them as they plodded patiently through their daily tasks, but that one back there was an exception.

Normally I would have taken the shoe off without much trouble before exploring the foot. All vets did courses in shoeing early in their education and I carried the tools with me, but I would have had some fun trying to do that with Hickson's animal. It was a job for Denny.

The Boynton smithy stood right at the end of Rolford village and as I drove up to the squat building with its clustering trees and backdrop of green hillside I felt, as I often did, that I was looking at one of the last relics of the past. When I first came to Yorkshire, every village had its blacksmith's shop and Darrowby itself had several. But with the disappearance of the draught horse they had just melted away. The men who had spent their lives in them for generations had gone and their work places which had echoed to the clatter of horses' feet and the clang of iron were deserted and silent.

Denny's shop was one of the few which had survived, mainly because he was an expert farrier, skilled in the often specialised shoeing which riding horses required. As I walked in, he was bent over the foot of a strapping hunter, laughing and joking with the attractive young owner who stood nearby.

'Now then, Mr Herriot,' he cried as he saw me. 'Be with you in a few minutes.' He was holding the hot shoe against the foot and the smell of the smoke rising from the seared horn, the glow of the forge and the ringing bang-bang as his still sprightly father hammered the glowing metal on the anvil evoked a hundred memories of a richer past.

Denny wasn't very big but he was lean and hard, the muscles on his forearms bulging and tensing as he worked. He had the broad strong back essential to his trade but, apart from that, he projected the same image of stringy durability as the Dales farmers who worked alongside me every day.

Now he was tapping the nails into the shoe and after a couple of minutes he straightened up and slapped the horse's rump. 'Right, Angela, you can take this awd screw away, now,' he said, flashing the girl a white-toothed grin.

She giggled and it struck me that it was a typical scene. Denny with his impish eyes and the hint of recklessness in his craggy features was undoubtedly attractive to the many county young ladies who brought their horses to him and I had never seen him working without a running badinage. A visit to the Boynton smith was in some ways a social event.

As horse and rider left, he reached for his bag of tools. 'Right, Mr Herriot. At your service!'

'Will you have time to do another gravel job on the way, Denny?' I asked.

He laughed. 'We'll mek time. Anything to oblige a gentleman!'

As we drove away I felt I ought to put him in the picture about Hickson's horse. I knew he had been dealing with skittish, often dangerous horses since childhood, and I had seen him again and again pushing big, explosive animals around effortlessly as though they were kittens, but it was only right to warn him.

'Denny,' I said, 'this horse at Hickson's could be difficult. He's a wild beggar and I could hardly get near him.'

'Oh aye?' Tool bag on knee, cigarette dangling from his lips, the young man was lazily observing the passing countryside. He didn't seem to be listening.

I tried again. 'He had a few goes at me with his hind foot, then started to wave his fore feet about . . .'

He dragged his eyes unwillingly from the window. 'It'll be right, Mr Herriot, it'll be right,' he murmured absently, stifling a yawn.

'He's a biter, too. Damn nearly got me on the shoulder just as I was trying to get away from –'

'Hey, wait a minute!' Denny shouted as we passed a roadside farmhouse. 'That's George Harrison in the yard. Just slow down a second, will you, Mr Herriot?' He wound down the window quickly. 'Nah then, George, how ista?' he yelled at the young farmer who was shouldering a straw bale. 'Have ye sobered up yet? Ha-ha-ha-ha!'

The two men exchanged a few shouted pleasantries before we took off. Denny turned to me. 'By gaw, George had a skinful last night at the Licensed Victuallers' Ball. Still looks a bit green – heh-heh!'

I decided to give up my attempts at warning him. He clearly wasn't interested.

He chatted away, filling me in with some uproarious details of the previous evening, but as we drew up in Hickson's yard he fell silent. His face was suddenly drawn and serious as he peered this way and that through the car windows. I knew what was coming next.

'Any savage dogs here, Mr Herriot?'

I suppressed a smile. Through all the years I had known him, he had always said this.

'No, none at all, Denny,' I replied.

He stared suspiciously at an elderly sheep dog enjoying a drink of milk at the kitchen door. 'How about that 'un?'

'That's old Zak. He's twelve! Quiet as a sheep.'

'Aye, mebbe, but that doesn't mean you can trust 'im. Get 'im inside, any road.'

I walked across the yard, waited until the old dog had licked out his bowl then ushered him, white muzzle upturned and tail waving at the attention, into the house. I had done this so many times, but still Denny wasn't keen to leave the car. After a final inspection in all directions he got out and stood warily on the cobbles for a few moments, then he hurried to the loose box where Farmer Hickson and horse were waiting.

The farmer gripped the halter tightly and smiled uncertainly at Denny as he came in. 'Watch 'im, lad. He's a funny sod.'

'Funny, is he?' The young man, hammer dangling from his hand, grinned and stepped close to the horse, and the animal, as though determined to prove the words, laid back his ears and lashed out.

Denny avoided the flying foot with practised ease and gave a demon king's laugh, throwing back his head. 'Aha! You're like that, are ye? Right, ya bugger, we'll see!' Then he moved in again. I don't know how he kept clear of the horse's repeated attempts to injure him, but within a minute he caught the claw of his hammer in the iron shoe in full flight and pulled it toward him. 'Okay, ya big bugger, I've got ye now, haven't I, eh?'

The horse, on three legs, made a few half-hearted attempts to pull his foot away as Denny hung on and chattered at him but it was clear that he realised that this new man was an entirely different proposition. Denny, with the foot on his knee, reached for his tools, muttering threats all the time and as I watched unbelievingly, he knocked up the clenches, drew out the nails with his pincers and removed the shoe. The horse, motionless except for a quivering of the flanks, was totally subjugated.

Denny displayed the sole for my inspection. 'Now, where d'you want me, Mr Herriot?' he asked.

I tapped along the sole until I found a place which seemed tender. To make sure, I squeezed at the place with the pincers and the animal flinched.

'That's the spot, Denny,' I said. 'There's a crack there.'

The young farrier began to cut away the horn with expert sweeps of his sharp knife. This was a job I had done so often by myself, but it was a joy to see an expert doing it. In no time at all he had followed the crack down and there was a hiss then a trickle of pus as he reached the site of the infection. It was one of the most satisfactory things in veterinary practice because, if the abscess is not evacuated, it causes the most acute agony for the animal. Sometimes the pus can work up under the wall of the hoof until it bursts out at the coronet after a long period of pain, and in other cases I have seen horses having to be put down when all attempts to relieve the infection have failed and the poor animal was laid groaning with a hugely swollen foot. Such memories from the old carthorse days always haunted me.

Nothing of that was going to happen this time and my relief was as strong as always. 'Thanks, Denny, that's great.' I administered antibiotic and antitetanus injections and said to the farmer, 'He'll soon be sound now, Mr Hickson.'

Then Denny and I set off for our next appointment. As we drove out of the yard I looked at the young blacksmith. 'Well, you certainly dealt with that wild horse. It was amazing how you quietened him.'

He leaned back in his seat, lit another cigarette and spoke lazily. 'Nobbut a bit daft, 'e was. It was nowt. There's lots like 'im – silly big bugger.'

He resumed his account of the previous evening, chuckling softly at times, and as I glanced round at him, totally relaxed, cap on the back of his head, smiling his carefree smile, he looked as though nothing could ever upset him. However, as I stopped the car at the farm where we had to see the other horse, his insouciant air fell away from him as though snatched by an unseen hand. Clutching his tool bag, he anxiously scanned every corner of the farmyard. I waited confidently for his next words.

'Any savage dogs here, Mr Herriot?'

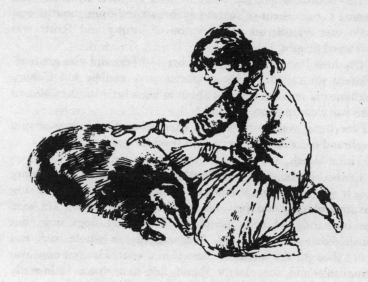

18

'What is it?' 'What the devil is that?' 'A badger? Never!'

Pandemonium broke out in the Drovers' Arms. Calum and I had just returned from a communal visit and when I suggested a beer he got out of the car, slung Marilyn over his shoulder and strode into the bar.

The eyes of the regulars popped, they spluttered into their glasses and in a few seconds we were the centre of an excited crowd. I detached myself and sat quietly with my beer as the young man held court, answering the volleys of questions calmly and with a quiet satisfaction. It was clear that he loved to display his adored pet to anybody who was interested, and with most people it wasn't just a case of interest, he created a sensation wherever he went.

It was the same when I introduced him to my family in the

sitting room at Skeldale House. My children were making music, Rosie at the piano and Jimmy with his harmonica, when the tall, walrus-moustached figure came in with his wild animal. I had become a connoisseur of soaring eyebrows and open mouths, and Helen was typical, but the reaction of Jimmy and Rosie was wide-eyed delight.

'Oh, how lovely!' 'Can I stroke her?' 'Where did you get her?' 'What is she called?' Their questions were endless and Calum, laughing and teasing, was just about as big a hit with the children as his hairy companion.

Everything was going with a bang when Dinah, our second beagle and successor to Sam, ran in from the garden.

'This is Dinah,' I said.

'Oh-ho, oh-ho, little fat Dinah,' said Calum in a rumbling bass. It was not a complimentary remark, because my little dog was undoubtedly too fat, and an embarrassment to a vet who was constantly adjuring people to keep their dogs slim, but Dinah didn't seem to mind. She wagged her whole back end until I thought she would tie herself in a knot. Her response was remarkable and she clearly found this new voice immensely attractive. Calum bent down and she rolled on her back in ecstasy as he rubbed her tummy.

Helen laughed. 'Gosh, she really likes you!'

We didn't know it then, but her words were setting a scene which would be a familiar and intriguing one in the future. I was to find that all animals were attracted to Calum and that he had a rapport with them which was unique. They loved the very sound, sight and scent of him – a heaven-sent asset for a veterinary surgeon.

When the civilities were over with Marilyn scuttling merrily round the floor, happily accepting the petting of the children, Calum sat down on the piano stool and began to play. He was no Rubinstein, but he could knock out a rollicking tune with no trouble at all and the children clapped their hands and stamped their feet in delight.

Jimmy held out his harmonica. 'Can you play this, too?'

Calum took the instrument and held it to his mouth with his hands in a Larry Adler-like attitude, and after the first few notes you could see that he was in a different league from my son whose concert piece was 'God save the Queen'. After a couple of minutes of Mozart my new assistant handed back the harmonica and roared with laughter.

The young people were enchanted. 'I'm going for the concertina,' cried Jimmy.

He ran from the room and came back with one of the relics from my visits to house sales when Helen and I were first married. In those days I was often despatched to house sales to bring back essentials like tables and chairs and usually returned with quite impractical objects, ornamental ink stands and such like. In this case it was the concertina. It was an ancient little instrument, six-sided, with carved wooden ends and leather straps worn and frayed with age. It raised images of a mariner playing sea shanties on the deck of an old-time sailing ship and I had found it irresistible, but unfortunately nobody had been able to extract a tune from it and it had rested for years in the attic with many of my other useless purchases.

Calum lifted it from its wooden box and turned it over tenderly. 'Oh nice, very nice.' He slipped his hands through the straps, his fingers felt their way over the little ivory buttons and in a moment the room was filled with melody of a piercing sweetness. It was 'Shenandoah' and as we listened, suddenly hushed, to the totally unexpected richness which came from the instrument I was back on the deck of the sailing ship which I had dreamed of all those years ago.

I have many memories of Calum, but the one which lingers most hauntingly in my mind is that one of him sitting among my family, his dark eyes, unfathomable as they often were, fixed somewhere high on the wall, while his fingers coaxed that plaintive music from our little squeeze-box.

When he finished there was a spontaneous burst of applause and the children jumped about, clapping their hands. Calum was fixed in their minds for ever as a wonder man. He had a badger, he could play anything, he could do anything.

Just then, we began to wonder about Marilyn. She had been wandering quietly around the room but now there was no sign of her. We peered under the sofa and tipped up the arm chairs without success and were looking at each other in bewilderment when there was a rattling from the fireplace and the badger, abundantly clothed in soot, shot out from the chimney. She didn't want to be caught and raced a few times round the room before Calum grabbed her and carried her outside.

Jimmy and Rosie were almost hysterical. They hadn't had such fun for a long time, but Helen and I, looking at the devastation to our carpet and furniture, were not so amused.

It was a sudden comedown from inspirational heights to chaos, and in an intuitive moment a thought came to me. Was this the way it was always going to be with Calum?

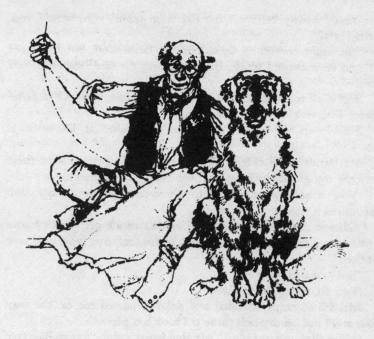

19

I have heard it said that all tailors used to sit cross-legged on a
table to ply their trade, but the only one I ever saw in this
position was Mr Bendelow.

The cottage door opened straight from the street into the
kitchen and the scene was so familiar. The cluttered little room
with a thousand cloth clippings littering the floor, the sewing
machine in the corner; Blanco, his enormous white dog, giving
me a welcoming wag as he lay by the fire and Mr Bendelow,
cross-legged on the table, talking to a customer, his needle poised
above some garment or other.

It struck me, not for the first time, that Mr Bendelow's needle
always seemed to be poised. I don't think I had ever seen it actually
dig into any fabric, because he was always too busy talking. He was at
it now, chattering into the slightly bemused face of a farmer's wife.

'You'd hardly believe what I've been tellin' you, would you, Mrs Haw?'

'No, right enough, I wouldn't, Mr Bendelow, but I wonder if you've managed to do that waistcoat for me husband. You said –'

'But it all really happened all them years ago, sure as I'm sittin' here. You wouldn't credit the things –'

'I'd like to tek it with me if you've finished it. He wants it for a –'

Mr Bendelow cackled. 'Ah'm not an old man, nobbut fifty, but the things that went on in them days . . . I remember . . .'

'You've had that waistcoat for three months, you know, you promised it for –'

'Oh aye, ah knaw, ah knaw. I've that much on. Don't know where to turn. But come back in a fortnight, love, you shall 'ave it then.'

'But 'e wants it for –'

'Best ah can do, love. Ta-ra.'

Mrs Haw, empty-handed and doleful, passed me on the way out and I put on my best smile as I took her place.

'Now then, young man.' Mr Bendelow's thin, gypsy-like face did not change expression but his eyes shot a sidelong glance of sheer hatred at the trousers I carried on my arm.

'Now what's this you've got for me?' he grunted.

'Well, it's these trouser bottoms, Mr Bendelow. They've got a bit frayed and I thought . . .'

'Aye, ye thought I'd just mek 'em like new for you. No trouble at all. You'll kill me, you know, you'll kill me. I'm goin' like 'ell with Christmas comin' on. At it night and day – never a minute.'

'Well, it's just the bottoms, Mr Bendelow . . .'

'And then there's me bad leg. How long have I had it? Oh, years. I went to Dr Allinson. He said, "Have you had this before?" I said, "Yes." He said, "Well, you've got it again." He gave me sixty tablets and when I'd had 'alf I was a lot better and when I'd 'ad the lot I was nearly cured. But the doctor 'ad planned that. "Mr Bendelow," he said, "when you've had half of these tablets you'll be much better and when you've had the other half you'll think you're cured. But you won't be, you know, you won't be. I know what you're like and you won't want to come back to me. But when you've had your sixty tablets I want to see you. On that very day."

'So I goes back to 'im on the very day he said, and he says, "Now then, Mr Bendelow, you're here then." And I said, "Yes, Doctor, right on the day you said." "And you've finished your sixty tablets?" he says. And I says, "Yes, I've 'ad the lot." And 'e gives me another 'undred.'

'Well, that's fine, Mr Bendelow. My wife says if you would just take a look at these frayed bottoms –'

'And he says, "You've got to stop runnin' up and down them stairs." And I says, "I can't, Doctor. I can't stop. I'm always workin'. I never cease." But listen to this, Mr Herriot. I'm goin' to tell you something now. I've never made a penny. And I'll tell you something else. If you've never made a fortune before you're forty you'll never make one.'

'These bottoms are just a little bit frayed as you can see . . .'

'Ah yes, you can talk about makin' a fortune on the football pools if you like, Mr Herriot. I can tell you about Littlewoods. Just listen to this, now.'

As he leaned forward from the table, his face intent, the street door opened and a big man came in. I recognised Jeremy Boothby, son of one of the big landowners and a person of considerable presence.

'You'll excuse me,' he boomed as he brushed past me. 'I've called for my suit, Bendelow. I was in last week.'

The tailor didn't even look at him. 'Do you know that I used to win regular on Littlewoods? But allus on the four aways and the most I won was six bob. So I says to myself if you go for the big money then you'll win the big money.'

'Do you hear me, Bendelow?' The great voice filled the room. 'I've been in every week since October and –'

'So I fills up a perm on the treble chance and I had twenty-four points straight away. I was waitin' for the big cheque for seventy-five thousand comin', but it never came. Oh no, I got a letter from one of the head men at Littlewoods.'

'Now look here, Bendelow!' Mr Boothby's shout made the windows rattle. 'You've had that suit for a year now and –'

He stopped in mid flow. Blanco had strolled round from the fireside and was standing by the table, looking up at him. He didn't have all that far to look, because he must have been just about the biggest dog I had ever seen. Mr Bendelow had described him to me as a Swedish Mountain Dog and I could remember his smug smile of superiority when I told him I had never heard of that breed. I was pretty sure Blanco was a cross but whatever he was he was magnificent — snow-white and vast. And now as he stood close to Mr Boothby, quite motionless, the lion head poised, there was a menacing fixity in his gaze and a faint growl rolled from deep in his rib cage.

As man and dog eyed each other the growl became louder and for a second Blanco's lips fluttered upwards giving a glimpse of a row of crocodilian teeth.

Boothby stepped back, then spoke in a softer tone. 'Will you let me have my suit . . . ? I . . .'

Mr Bendelow, clearly irritated by the interruption, gestured with his needle. 'Not ready yet — call next week.'

With a final glance at Blanco, the big man turned and left.

'A lovely letter of apology, it was,' continued the tailor. 'He told me I had got the twenty-four points all right but he couldn't give me the seventy-five thousand because of one little detail. Yes, I'm tellin' you, one little detail. I'd put down sixteen matches instead of eight. It was a lovely letter and 'e sounded real sorry, but there was nothing he could do about it.'

'Well, well, what a shame. Could you possibly do these trousers for some time next week. I would be very —'

'But all that money would be no good to me. I could tell you something about moneyed people . . .'

I dropped the garment on the table, gave him a hurried farewell wave and fled.

As I walked slowly down the street, my head spinning with the barmy torrent of words which, thanks to contemporary note-taking, I have reproduced here verbatim, I ruminated on the phenomenon of Mr Bendelow. In time, he did disgorge the work brought to him, so presumably he did most of his sewing and cutting at night. He was, in fact, a fine tailor and I had seen suits of such perfect fit and neat hand-stitching that I realised why people like Boothby continued to patronise him. It was all a question of luck – occasionally he had surprised me by coming up with a repair or an alteration in reasonable time.

He had supreme confidence in his own ability and intellectual gifts. In fact, convinced as he was that he knew everything about everything, particularly in the realm of domestic finance, he considered it his bounden duty to impart his knowledge to anybody who crossed his path, and since he had never married, he had no other outlet than his customers.

I had only once seen him at a loss. It was some years earlier when he measured Helen for a skirt and didn't give her a fitting until several months later. When that day finally came, the skirt waist didn't meet by a couple of inches. He stared in disbelief and tugged and pulled at the cloth a few times but it made no difference. Quickly he passed a tape measure round her middle, then consulted his notebook and measured again. From his kneeling position he looked up at us, totally baffled.

Helen smiled and relieved his agony. 'I should have told you,' she said, 'I'm pregnant.'

He looked at her narrowly, but since he was responsible for the long delay he was in no position to complain. However, the unheard of loss of face might have put a strain on our relations but for my long-standing rapport with Blanco, to whom he was devoted.

Blanco was around five years old and although he had been mainly healthy he had required my attention a few times, usually to extract pins embedded in his pads. He was the only tailor's dog I knew and I had often thought that it was an occupational hazard, lying daily as he did among the debris of his master's trade. There was no doubt that those pins often got right in and had to be extracted by digging deep with forceps. Blanco always appeared to be grateful; in fact, he was one of those dogs who actually enjoyed coming to my surgery. Some dogs crossed to the other side of the road when they entered Trengate and slunk past the surgery with their tails down, but Blanco nearly tugged Mr Bendelow off his feet as he fought to drag him through our door.

He had been in for his annual distemper booster the previous week and he had come prancing along the passage, wagging his tail furiously and poking his head sociably round the office door on his way to the consulting room. So different from a big yellow labrador bitch who followed him and had to be sledged along on her bottom the entire length of the passage tiles, her face a mask of misery even though she was only going to have her paw bandaged.

Blanco was the soul of good nature and the only time he showed a gleam of anger was if he thought Mr Bendelow was being threatened. This protectiveness was invaluable to the tailor because the set-up in that house was conducive to exasperation and I had heard a few blustering men and screeching women driven to distraction by the interminable delays. But the great white head and cold eyes appearing round the corner of the table had a wonderfully calming effect. Sometimes a little growl or a pointed sniffing round the customer's ankles was required but I had never seen a failure.

In my musings, I had often thought that Blanco was a vindication of my long-held theory that big dogs came from little houses and little dogs from big ones. In fact, it seemed to me to be the ultimate corroboration because in the greatest of battle-mented, multi-acred mansions you got down to Border Terriers and Jack Russells while in tiny, one-up, one-down dwellings you found something like Blanco.

A week later, ever optimistic, I returned to Mr Bendelow's establishment. He was in his usual place, cross-legged like a little gnome on his table.

Another customer, a disgruntled-looking farmer, was just about to leave, but he was giving the tailor a few parting words.

'Ah'm about fed up comin' here every week after you've promised.' His voice took on an angry tone. 'You don't seem bothered, but it's not good enough, you know.'

Mr Bendelow gave the familiar gesture with his needle. 'Next week . . . next week.'

'Aye, that's what you always say,' barked the farmer, and I looked over the table at Blanco, stretched by the fire. This was the sort of thing that always brought him to his feet, but he showed no interest and didn't move as the farmer, with a final snort, turned and left, banging the door behind him.

'Good morning, Mr Bendelow,' I said briskly. 'I've just dropped in for –'

'Now then, Mr Herriot!' The little man stabbed his needle at me. 'I was just goin' to tell you summat about moneyed people when you left. Old Crowther, down Applegate. Left eighty thousand and when I patched his trousers for 'im he had to stay in bed. I'm not jokin' nor jestin', he had to stay in bed.'

'Talking about trousers, Mr Bendelow –'

'He 'ad a housekeeper – Maud something was her name – she did everything for 'im. Got 'im in and out of bed, cooked for 'im, slaved for 'im for thirty years. But, do you know, he never left her a penny. She contested the will, you know, but she only got five hundred pounds. Money all went to some distant relatives.'

'Are my trousers ready? I do need them for –'

'And I could tell you a worse case than that, Mr Herriot. When I was a lad, I worked for a farmer. That man was worth thousands, but he never went into a pub, never went to the pictures, never went anywhere. Saved every penny. Don't know what 'e did with it all. Maybe kept it about the house. Oh, that reminds me of a story.'

I was about to utter another plea when a stout lady behind me burst out. 'Now look 'ere, I don't want to butt in, but I'm in a hurry. I want my dress now – you promised it for today.'

The tailor waved his needle. 'Not ready. Been too busy. Come next week.'

'Too busy! Too busy chatterin' is more like it.' She had a high, piercing delivery and she gave the tailor the full blast. I looked at Blanco, still motionless by the fire. His lack of interest was unusual.

Mr Bendelow, too, seemed to miss his dog's support because he was untypically abashed by the lady's attack.

'Aye, well,' he mumbled, 'you shall 'ave it next week, definite.' He gave me a sidelong glance. 'You, too, Mr Herriot.'

When I called the following week, I stopped in the doorway, transfixed by the amazing sight. Mr Bendelow was actually stitching. Up on his table, his head bent low over a jacket, his hand flashing over a lapel with wonderful deftness. And he wasn't talking.

The talking was being done by a man and his wife who were submitting him to an aggressive barrage of complaints. The tailor, silent and unhappy, made no reply. And Blanco was still asleep by the fire.

In the quest for my trousers, I called in a few times during my rounds but there was always a queue and I didn't have time to wait. I did notice, however, that on each occasion Mr Bendelow on his table was working, silent and subdued, while his dog was motionless by the fire. The picture saddened me. Talking was the little man's life, his hobby and solace in his bachelor existence. Something was very wrong.

I called round one evening and found Mr Bendelow alone, still stitching.

I didn't mention my trousers. 'What's wrong with Blanco?' I said.

He looked at me in surprise. 'Nowt, as far as I know.'

'Is he eating all right?'

'Aye, he is.'

'Getting plenty of exercise?'

'Yes, a good walk night and mornin'. You know I look after me dog, Mr Herriot.'

'Yes, of course you do. But . . . he's not up round your table like he used to be. Not . . . er . . . interested in the customers.'

He nodded miserably. 'Aye, that's t'only thing. But he isn't ill.'

'Let's have a look at him,' I said. I went over to the fire and bent over the dog. 'Come on, Blanco, old lad, let's see you on your feet.'

I tapped him on the rump and he got up slowly. I looked at the tailor. 'He seems a bit stiff.'

'Aye, maybe, but 'e soon works it off when I take him out.'

'Not really lame, though? No pins?'

'Nay, nay, ah can allus tell when he's picked one up.'

'Hmm. Still, I'd better check on his paws.'

Whenever I lifted one of Blanco's feet I had the same feeling as when I examined a horse's hoof and, indeed, had to stop myself from saying 'Whoa, there, boy' and tucking the paw between my knees.

I carefully inspected each foot, squeezing the pads which were the usual sites for the dangerous pins, but all seemed normal. I took his temperature, auscultated his chest and palpated his abdomen without finding any clues. But as I looked down at the big animal I could not rid myself of the nagging certainty that there was something amiss.

Blanco, tiring of my attention, sat down, and he did so gingerly, lowering himself carefully on to the fireside rug.

That wasn't right at all. 'Get up, lad,' I said quickly.

There had to be some trouble at his rear end. Impacted anal glands, perhaps? No, they were all right. I passed my hands down the massive thighs and on the left side, as I felt my way down the musculature, the dog winced suddenly. There was a painful swelling there and as I clipped away the hair all became clear. Deeply embedded in the flesh was one of his old enemies, a pin.

It was a moment's work to extract it with my forceps and I turned to Mr Bendelow. 'Well, there it is. He must have sat on this when it got onto the rug. It's a wonder he hasn't been lame, but there's a little abscess which has been upsetting him. An abscess is a depressing thing.'

'Aye . . . aye . . . but what can you do?' He looked at me with worried eyes.

'I'll have to get him round to the surgery and drain the pus away. Then he'll be fine.'

Blanco's visit to Skeldale House passed off smoothly. I evacuated the abscess and filled up the cavity by squeezing a few of the ever-useful penicillin intramammary tubes into it.

I didn't visit Mr Bendelow for another week. I clung to the hope that he might have repaired my working trousers. My wardrobe was very limited and I sorely needed them.

The scene was as always. The tailor on his table and Blanco stretched by the fire. And strangely, Mrs Haw, the farmer's wife I had seen at my first visit was there.

She was having a kind of tug-of-war with her husband's waistcoat which Mr Bendelow had apparently mended at last but was reluctant to release. His lips were moving rapidly with his quick-fire delivery. 'And that's what the feller said to me. You wouldn't believe it would you, and that's not all . . .'

With a quick tug, the lady managed to win possession of the waistcoat. 'Thank ye very much, Mr Bendelow. I'll 'ave to go now.' She nodded, waved and scurried past me, looking exhausted but triumphant.

The tailor turned to me. 'Ah, it's you, Mr Herriot.'

'Yes, Mr Bendelow, I was wondering . . .'

'You'll remember I was just goin' to tell you that story about the rich man.'

'About my trousers . . .'

'He was an old farmer, he kept his brass in the house in buckets. His missus brought up a bucket and she said, "There's fifteen hundred pounds in this bucket," and the old chap said, "There's summat wrong somewhere. There should be two thousand in that 'un." And do you know, that man and his wife used to pay separately for their own food. It's true what I'm tellin' you – she went out and bought hers and 'e did the same. And I'll tell you summat else, Mr Herriot . . .'

'Have you, by any chance managed to –'

'Just listen to this, Mr Herriot –'

'Hey, Bendy!' A big man had just come in and was roaring at the tailor over my shoulder. 'I can 'ear you and ah'm not listenin'! I want my bloody jacket!'

It was Gobber Newhouse, hugely fat, notorious drunk and a bully. Stale beer fumes billowed around him as he bellowed again. 'Don't give me any of your bloody excuses, Bendy, ah know you!'

Like a surfacing white whale, Blanco rose from the fireside and surged to the table. He seemed to know the kind of man he was dealing with and didn't waste any frills on him. Stretching up his mighty head, he opened his mouth wide and bayed with tremendous force into the red sweating face. 'Whaaa! Whaaa!'

Gobber backed away. 'Bloody dog . . . siddown . . . gerrim away, Bendy.'

'Whaaa! Whaaa! Whaaa!' went Blanco.

The big man was half out of the door when Mr Bendelow signalled with his needle. 'Come next week.' Then he turned

his full attention to me. 'As I was sayin', Mr Herriot . . .' he
continued.

'I really do need –'

'Next week, definite, but let me tell you . . .'

'Must go, I'm afraid,' I muttered, and escaped into the street.

Out there my feelings were mixed but, on the whole, happy. I
still hadn't got my trousers, but Blanco was right back on form.

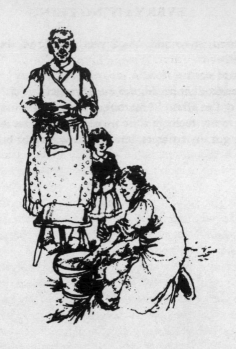

20

Five o'clock in the morning and the telephone jangling in my ear. Ewe lambing at Walton's, a lonely farm on the high moorland, and as I crawled from the haven of bed into the icy air of the bedroom and began to pull on my clothes, I tried not to think of the comfortless hour or two ahead.

Pushing my arms through my shirt sleeves I gritted my teeth as the cloth chafed the flesh. In the pale dawn light, I could see the little red fissures which covered my hands and ran up to my elbows. In lambing time I hardly ever seemed to have my jacket on and the constant washing in the open pens or in windy fields had turned my skin to raw meat. I could detect the faint scent of Helen's glycerine and rose water which she applied to my arms every night and made them bearable.

Helen stirred under the blankets and I went over and kissed her cheek. 'Off to Walton's,' I whispered.

Eyes closed, she nodded against the pillow, and I could just hear her sleepy murmur. 'Yes . . . I heard.'

Going out of the door I looked back at my wife's huddled bulk. When this happened, she, too, was jerked into the world of work and duty. That phone could blast off again at any time and she would have to get in touch with me. And on top of this, she would have to get the fires lit, the tea made and the children started with their breakfast – the little tasks I tried to help her with and which weren't easy in our big, beautiful ice box of a house.

Through the tight-shut, sleeping little town, then on to the narrow road winding between its walls until the trees dwindled and disappeared, leaving the wide windswept fells bare and unwelcoming at this hour.

I wondered if there was any chance of the ewe being under cover. In the early fifties, it didn't seem to occur to many of the farmers to bring their lambing ewes into the buildings and I attended to the great majority out in the open fields. There were happy times when I almost chuckled in relief at the sight of a row of hurdles in a warm fold yard or sometimes the farmers would build pens from stacked-up straw bales, but on this occasion my spirits plummeted when I drew up at the farm and met Mr Walton who came out of the house carrying a bucket of water and headed for the gate.

'Outside, is she?' I asked, trying to sound airy.

'Aye, just ower there.' He pointed over the long, bracken-splashed pasture to a prone woolly form in the distance which looked a hell of a long way 'ower there'. As I trailed across the frosty grass, my medical bag and obstetric overall dangling, a merciless wind tore at me, picking up an extra Siberian cold from the long drifts of snow which still lay behind the walls in this late Yorkshire spring.

As I stripped off and knelt behind the ewe I looked around. We were right on top of the world and the panorama of hills and valleys with grey farmhouses and pebbled rivers in their depths was beautiful but would have been more inviting if it had been a warm summer afternoon and me preparing for a picnic with my family.

I held out my hand and the farmer deposited a tiny sliver of soap on my palm. I always felt that farmers kept special pieces of soap for the vet – minute portions of scrubbing soap which were too small and hard to be of any use. I rubbed this piece frantically with my hands, dipping frequently into the water, but I could work up only the most meagre film of lather. Not enough to protect my tender arm as I inserted it into the ewe, and the farmer looked at me enquiringly as I softly ooh'd and aah'd my way towards the cervix.

I found just what I didn't want to find. A big single lamb, jammed tight. Two lambs are the norm and three quite common, but a big single lamb often spells trouble. It was one of my joys in practice to sort out the tangles of twins and triplets but with the singles it was a case of not enough room and the big lamb had to be eased and pulled out as gently as possible – a long and tedious business. Also, often the single lamb was dead through pressure and had to be removed by embryotomy or a Caesarean operation.

Resigning myself to the fact that I was going to spend a long time crouched on that windy hilltop, I reached as far as possible and poked a finger into the lamb's mouth, feeling a surge of relief as the little tongue stirred against my hand. He was alive, anyway, and with a lifting of my spirits I began the familiar ritual of introducing lubricating jelly, locating the tiny legs and fastening them with snares and, finally, as I sat back on my heels for a breather I knew that all I had to do now was to bring the head through the pelvis. That was the tricky bit. If it came through I was home and dry; if it didn't I was in trouble. Mr Walton, holding back the wool from the vulva, watched me in silence. Despite his lifetime experience with sheep he was helpless in a case like this because, like most farmers, he had huge, work-roughened hands with fingers like bananas and could not possibly have got inside a ewe. My small 'lady's hand' as they called it was a blessing.

I hooked my forefinger into the eye socket – my favourite trick, there was nothing else to get hold of except the lower jaw which was dangerously fragile – and began to pull with infinite care. The ewe strained, crushing my hand against the pelvic bones – not as bad as in a cow but painful, and my mouth opened wide as I eased and twisted and pulled until, with a blessed surge, the head slipped through the bony pelvic opening.

It wasn't long, then, until feet, legs and nose appeared at the vulva and I brought the little creature out onto the grass. He lay still for a moment, snuffling at the cold world he had entered, then he shook his head vigorously. I smiled. That was the best sign of all.

I had another wrestle with the morsel of soap, then the farmer wordlessly handed me a piece of sacking to dry my arms. This was quite common in those days. Towels were scarce commodities on the farms and I couldn't blame the farmers' wives for hesitating to send out a clean towel to a man who had just had his arms up the back end of an animal. An old soiled one was the usual and, if not, the hessian sack was always at hand. I couldn't rub my painful arms with the coarse material and contented myself with a careful patting, before pushing them, still damp, into the sleeves of my jacket.

The ewe, hearing a high-pitched call from her lamb began to talk back with the soft deep baa I knew so well, and as she got up and began an intensive licking of the little creature I stood there, forgetful of the cold, listening to their conversation, enthralled as ever by the miracle of birth. When the lamb, apparently feeling he was wasting time, struggled to his feet and tottered unsteadily round to the milk bar I grinned in satisfaction and made my way back to the car.

After breakfast, my next call was to a 'cleansing', the removal of the afterbirth from a cow and again, after a struggle with a rock-hard marble of soap, I was offered a sack to dry myself, only this time it had recently contained potatoes and I found I was powdering my chapped arms with soil. Later that morning, after a rectal examination for pregnancy diagnosis, I had the choice of a truly filthy 'cow house towel' which must have had an astronomical bacterial count and declined it in favour of yet another piece of hessian.

My arms were red hot inside my sleeves when I drove into the Birrell farmyard, but I knew better things awaited me here. Wonderful things, in fact.

I never knew what George Birrell's attitude to towels might be or that of his wife, but his mother, old Grandma Birrell, had very clear views on the matter. When I had finished stitching a tear on the cow's udder I stood on the cobbles, blood-spattered and expectant, waiting for the old lady. Right on cue, she came into the byre, hand in hand with four-year-old Lucy, the youngest of her grandchildren. She set down a milking stool and laid out in a perfectly folded oblong a newly laundered towel of snowy whiteness and on top of this she placed a tablet of expensive lavender toilet soap in its wrappings, virgin and unopened. A brightly scoured aluminium bucket of steaming water completed the picture, as pretty a one as ever I had seen.

Reverently I peeled the paper from the soap – it was always a new tablet – and as I dipped into the water and spread the rich lather on my burning arms, inhaling the fragrance of the lavender, I almost crooned with ecstasy. The farmer stood by impassively with perhaps the faintest twitch of amusement round his mouth, but Grandma Birrell and Lucy watched my ablutions with rapt enjoyment.

It was always like this at the Birrells and I loved it but I could never quite understand why it happened. Maybe Siegfried had a point when he said that old ladies liked me, and he was always pulling my leg about my 'harem' of over-seventies who insisted on my services for their dogs. Anyway, whatever the cause, I revelled in the patronage of Grandma Birrell. In her eyes, everything had to be right for me. Nothing was too good for Mr Herriot.

It was a Saturday morning when Siegfried pushed the *Darrowby and Houlton Times* across the office desk to me.

'Bit of sad news for you, I'm afraid, James,' he murmured, pointing to an entry.

It was in the deaths column. 'Mrs Marjorie Birrell, aged 78, dearly beloved wife of the late Herbert Birrell ...' I read it through with a growing sense of loss, a rising wistfulness at the feeling of something good coming to an end.

Siegfried gave me a lop-sided smile. 'Your old clean-towel friend, eh?'

'That's right.' Her clean towels were her expression of friendship and it was as a friend I would always remember her. In my mind's eye, I could see her plainly in her flowered apron standing by the milking stool with Lucy. She was of the farming generation which had come through the tough times before the war and her gaunt, slightly bowed frame and lined face bore testimony to the hard years. It was the kind of face I had seen on so many of the old Yorkshire folk – grim, but kindly. I knew I was going to miss her.

Just how much I would miss her came to me forcibly on my next visit to the Birrell farm. As I finished my job I looked at my soiled hands with the renewed pang of realisation that the old lady wouldn't be coming through that door. I knew George Birrell wouldn't offer me a sack, but what was going to happen?

As I pondered, the half-door was pushed open and little Lucy came into the byre, staggering slightly as she carried the familiar shining bucket of hot water. Then from under her arm she produced a towel and soap and laid them on a milking stool. And it was the same spotless, geometrically folded towel and the same pristine toilet soap as before.

Slightly flushed, the little girl looked up at me. 'Gran said I had to look after you,' she said breathlessly. 'She told me what to do.'

I swallowed a big lump. 'Well, Lucy . . . that's wonderful. And you've done everything just right.'

She nodded, well pleased, and I stole a look at her father, standing there, leaning on a cow. But George's face was inscrutable.

I peeled the wrapper from the soap and began to wash and as the scent of the lavender rose around me I was carried back to all the other days.

I lathered my hands in silence, then the little girl spoke again. 'Mr Herriot, the only thing is, I'm five now and I'll soon be goin' to school. I don't know how you're goin' to manage.'

An overwhelming flood of déjà vu washed over me. My own daughter, Rosie, at that same age, had been consumed with worry at how I was going to carry on my life without her and had consoled me with the reassurance that she'd still be available at weekends.

I didn't know what to say, but her father broke in.

'Don't worry, luv,' he said, 'I'll do me best if you'll teach me how, and anyway, from now on I'm goin' to try to call Mr Herriot out only on Saturdays.'

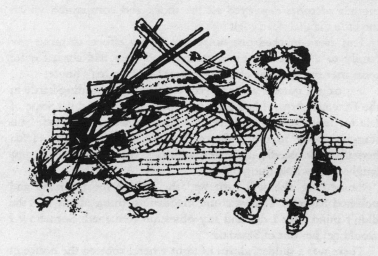

21

I felt a little breathless as I lifted the phone.

'I'm sorry, Lord Hulton,' I said, 'I'm afraid I'll be a little late in visiting your horse this morning. My house blew down last night.'

There was a silence at the other end and I could sense the amiable peer having some difficulty in absorbing my announcement. I felt I should explain further.

'As you know, there was a gale during the night – ninety miles per hour, I understand – and the house I am having built had just got to roof height. I've been along to have a look as I usually do each morning and, as I say, it's blown down. Piles of bricks everywhere and masses of twisted scaffolding. I have a few arrangements I must make.'

There was another silence, quite a long one, then just two words.

'Oh, crumbs.'

It was a traumatic moment in my life and I have never forgotten that brief riposte from the eccentric but endearing Marquis of Hulton. Those two words in his habitual exquisitely modulated tones conveyed all the shock and compassion which the little man so clearly felt.

This event marked one more step in my efforts to move my family to a more suitable dwelling, and they had started quite soon after my abortive attempt to buy Mrs Dryden's house.

It took me quite a while to recover from that bidding battle in the Drovers' Arms. I had built my hopes so high and the sense of failure hung heavily on me as I had to watch my wife still slogging away in the wide reaches of Skeldale House. Helen herself, undoubtedly a better adjusted character than I, just laughed the whole thing off.

'Something else will turn up,' she said as she scrubbed and polished happily. That was the maddening thing about it – she didn't mind. But I did and my obsession remained. Somehow I would get her out of Skeldale.

There was a sudden gleam of light when I spotted the notice in the *Darrowby and Houlton Times*.

'Look at this, Helen!' I said eagerly, pointing to a picture among the estate agents' advertisements on the front page. 'I know that house. It's a very nice place.'

She peered over my shoulder. 'Oh yes, along the Dennaby road. I've seen it – very attractive.' Then she gave me a questioning glance. 'But it's a detached house, not too big, I know, but not like Mrs Dryden's little semi. It will make a lot of money.'

'No, old Bootland and I between us pushed up the price of Mrs Dryden's. That little place was only worth about two thousand pounds. This one will go for its right price – around three thousand. I think the building society would lend me that much.'

I came in for lunch that day, flushed with success. The man at the society had been very accommodating – the mortgage would be possible.

'Things are looking up, Helen,' I said. 'Really it's a good job we didn't get the other house. This one is just right. A bit bigger, but compact and a nice sized garden with an orchard and a lovely view down the dale. The auction is next Friday so we haven't long to wait. This is it, Helen – I know it is!'

My wife gazed at me thoughtfully. 'Jim, I'll only agree to this if you promise to keep calm at the sale.'

'Calm? What do you mean?'

'Well, you know very well that you got all worked up and bid way past the price we could afford. All I'm asking is for you to keep calm and not get yourself into a state like last time.'

'Calm . . . ? State . . . ? I don't understand you,' I said haughtily.

Her smile was patient. 'Oh, you must remember. You were white, like a ghost, and shaking all over at the end of it. I wondered if you'd ever be able to get up and walk out.'

'You're exaggerating,' I replied with dignity. 'I was under a certain amount of pressure, that's all.'

Helen's smile suddenly turned to a grin. 'Oh, I know, but I'm not going with you unless you promise to go as far as that three thousand and not a penny more. I mean it, Jim.'

'Right . . . right . . . I promise, of course. I wouldn't do anything so silly, anyway.'

This little contretemps vanished quickly from my mind and I was soon back in my old fantasy – imagining Helen floating around effortlessly in the new house, the children climbing the trees and picking the fruit in the orchard. On my rounds I kept changing my route so that I could go along the Dennaby road and feast my eyes on the place. Helen and I had had a look round and it was perfect. And soon, very soon, it would be mine.

I didn't come off my cloud until the Friday afternoon when we walked across the market place to the Drovers. When we went into the crowded room where the auction was to be held I felt a sudden lurch at my stomach. It was all horribly reminiscent of last time. Same room, same rows of heads, same auctioneer on the platform drumming his fingers on the table in front of him and looking over the throng with a pleased smile. By the time we had squeezed into a place and sat down, my heart was thumping.

Soon the auctioneer started his preamble, telling us all the nice things I already knew about the house. As he went on, Helen, squashed tightly against me and possibly sensing some slight quivering in my limbs, gripped my hand, interlacing her fingers with mine.

'Just relax, Jim,' she whispered.

I sniffed. 'I'm perfectly relaxed, I assure you,' I mumbled, trying to ignore the thudding in my ears as the bidding started. I did feel, however, that a few deep breaths would help in a situation like this.

It was at about the third deep breath that I heard the words 'And now I have two thousand nine hundred' from the auctioneer. He seemed to have arrived at the figure unexpectedly quickly and I shot up my hand. Other hands rose all around me and I heard 'I have three thousand.'

At that moment Helen's grip on my hand tightened fiercely. She was a big strong girl and it came to me with certainty that if I pursued this matter further she would reduce my fingers to a pulp.

It would have made no difference anyway because the whole business was raging away out of my control. 'Three thousand one hundred, two hundred, three hundred, three thousand four hundred . . .' Then, in no time at all, as I sat mute, he was over four thousand with forests of bids going in. There was a slight slowing down in the late four thousands but before I had finished my deep breathing exercise I heard the hammer going down on the table – sold to Mr Somebody-or-other for five thousand pounds. It was all over – and I hadn't even had a look in.

As we rose and began to shuffle out with the crowd, I saw a grey-haired man shaking hands with the auctioneer and laughing in what I thought was an insufferably smug manner, then we were outside, walking over the cobbles of the market place.

The deflated feeling was the same as before. Helen was still holding my hand and I managed to work up a smile.

'Well, it's happened again,' I murmured. 'But maybe I'm not as white this time?'

My wife studied my face for a moment. 'No . . . a bit pale perhaps, but nothing like last time.' Then she laughed. 'Poor old lad, you never had the chance to go really white. It was over in a flash. Anyway, never mind – I often think that so many things happen for the best.'

'Still, it's another disappointment,' I said. 'Last time we had Mrs Dryden to console us a bit, but there's nobody today.'

As I spoke, I felt a tug at my sleeve. I turned and saw Bert Rawlings, whose smallholding's fields bordered the house which had just been sold.

'Hullo, Bert,' I said. 'Been to the sale?'

'Aye, I 'ave, Mr Herriot, and I'm right glad you didn't get that 'ouse.'

'Eh?'

'I say it was a lucky thing you didn't get it, because I've been in that place many a time and I can tell ye it's not all it appears.'

'Really?'

'Aye, it's a good-lookin' house, but the roof leaks like 'ell.'

'Never!'

'I'm not jokin'. I've been up in the attic and seen rows of buckets and pots and pans set out to try to catch the watter. They've been tryin' to mend that roof for years but they've never managed it.'

'Heavens!'

'And the timbers up there are rotten with all the damp.'

'My God!'

He patted my arm and laughed 'So you see, you 'ad a lucky escape. Just thought I'd tell ye.'

'Well, thanks, Bert. That does make us feel better.' I waved to him as he hurried away across the market place, then I turned to Helen.

'Well, isn't that strange. We have had somebody to cheer us up after all. Maybe next time will be third time lucky.'

Despite our latest defeat our determination was as strong as ever, or rather mine was, because, as I say, Helen didn't seem all that worried. But my mind was set in a groove. I scanned all the advertisements in the local newspapers, stopped eagerly at every For Sale board in the gardens of the district, but nothing really got moving until we were introduced at a party to Bob and Elizabeth Mollison. They were young architects, about our own age, who had opened an office in a nearby market town.

'You know', said Elizabeth, 'you're going through the mill

trying to find a suitable house, but we could build you a really nice house for £3,000 – planned by yourselves with all the features you want. It would be a far better prospect for you, and in fact, probably cheaper in the long run.'

Helen and I looked at each other. We had never thought of that.

'If you can find a plot of land, Bob and I could have a place built for you in a few months,' Elizabeth went on. 'Think it over, anyway.'

I really didn't need to think it over. The whole horizon seemed filled with blinding light. 'This is the right idea,' I said eagerly, and Helen nodded, too. 'Why didn't we think of this before? We'll do it!'

The Mollisons regarded us uncertainly. 'Are you quite sure? Why don't you think about it for a few days.'

I shook my head decisively. 'No, no, we'll go right ahead. You draw up some plans and I'll find a plot somewhere as I go round the country.'

Bob smiled. 'Fine, but hold on – we'd have to have a proper conference to know just what you want. We'd need a lot of details.'

'We want a hatch,' I said.

'A hatch? That's all . . . ? How about you, Helen?'

'A hatch,' replied my wife firmly. In both our minds there floated the heavenly image of our meals being handed through that little hole in the wall from kitchen to dining room. After the years of tramping the long passage at Skeldale House that had to be number one on the list.

The Mollisons had a good laugh at this, but then they hadn't seen the Skeldale passages.

'Right,' Elizabeth said between giggles, 'so we design this house round the hatch, eh?'

'Absolutely.' More laughter, but for Helen and me there was a very serious core to our jollity.

Later, we did have our conference and worked out the less important aspects like bedrooms and bathrooms and it wasn't long before the young couple produced a most attractive plan.

'It's a lovely house,' Helen murmured as she studied it. 'Such a nice little hall and staircase and all those useful cupboards and wardrobes built in. You've thought of everything.'

'Especially the hatch!' said the Mollisons together, and the laughter started again.

Meanwhile I was scouring the countryside for a plot and this was proving very difficult. Something called Town and Country Planning had come into being so it was no good asking one of my farmer friends to sell me a bit of land in one of their fields where there was a nice view.

Nice chaps as they were, they wanted to help, but couldn't.

'I'd be delighted, Jim,' one of them said, 'but it's not allowed. I can't even build a house in my fields for me own son!'

That was the story everywhere and finally I realised that I had to find a bit of ground somewhere inside the tight building line which had been drawn around Darrowby. My search became more and more desperate until, one day, I ended up with a plot between two houses on the edge of the town. It was a pleasant situation but very narrow.

'There's only one thing for it,' Bob Mollison said. 'If you buy this plot we'll have to put the house in long ways on.'

This worried us. 'But what a shame,' Helen said. 'It's such a pretty house – I just love that frontage.'

Bob shrugged. 'I'm afraid it's that or nothing. Lots of people are trying to find land to build on. You might have to wait ages for anything else to turn up. And we can make modifications. We can make it look very attractive the other way round.'

Elizabeth came to us with a modified design and indeed it was an acceptable compromise. We bought the land and prepared for action.

Almost immediately we came up against other unexpected snags. In the early fifties, Britain was still recovering from the austerities of the war. Many things were still in short supply – including builders. We tried everywhere but couldn't find anybody to take on the contract. Finally we decided that the only way to get started was to employ the various tradesmen – joiners, bricklayers, plumbers etc. – ourselves. This was done and before long we had the foundations laid.

It was exciting from then on, but frustrating, too, because time after time I would call at the site to find the bricklayers sitting about smoking and drinking tea. The explanation was always the same: 'We can't get on. The joiners haven't turned up.' Or it was the joiners drinking tea because the bricklayers hadn't arrived. 'We can't get on' was a phrase I grew to dread.

Because of this, progress was slow. After several weeks, the walls were only knee high. We went off for a fortnight's summer holiday and as we drove past the site on our return, expecting to see a big advance, our hopes were dashed when we found that the house had not grown at all.

However, the troubles began to sort themselves out at last and there was a rush of activity over several weeks when the place began to rise at magical speed. The big day arrived when the bricklayers, honest lads and keen to please me, had the gable end nearly up to roof height.

'We'll have t'roof on tomorrow, Mr Herriot,' one of them said cheerfully. 'Only thing is the joiners should've been here to put the ridge and last spars in, but we'll build up the gable to full height and the joiners will be here this afternoon to support it. Then we'll all be happy – we'll put up the flag. You'll be glad to see that!'

He spoke the truth. I would be more than glad, in fact ecstatic and fulfilled, to see the roof on our new house with the traditional flag flying. I couldn't wait to get along first thing next morning to see it.

It had been a windy night with a ninety mile an hour gale according to the radio, but I didn't think anything about it until I drew up my car and looked out at the devastation. The joiners had not arrived when expected and the unsupported gable which fronted the road lay in a tumbled heap of bricks in the front garden. Twisted scaffolding hung around everywhere. I cannot quite describe my emotions.

Yes, on that one fateful night, the gale came and blew the whole thing down. It was just bad luck, nobody's fault, and that was how I came to be apologising to Lord Hulton for my delayed visit to his horse.

Like most of the little disasters of life, this was overcome. The gable was rebuilt and the house triumphantly completed within weeks. And a fine house it was; a brilliant success and a lasting testimony to the skills of Bob and Elizabeth with its many innovative features and modern ideas.

The whole concept of building for ourselves was vindicated and in the end we had what we wanted – a happy home for our family for many years. But at times my mind goes back to that morning when I drove along the Brawton road and looked from my car as the wind still howled over the heap of bricks and mangled scaffolding.

That was a really bad moment. Oh crumbs, it was.

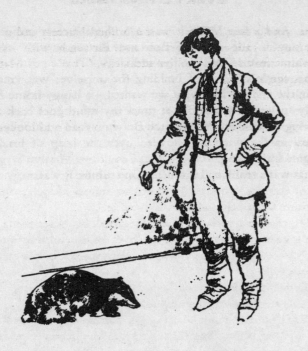

22

There was one time during Calum's reign when I was sure I was hallucinating. I came in through the front door of Skeldale House one morning and there, in the passage, I saw Calum's badger, Marilyn, waddling unhurriedly towards me. She had the run of the house now and I had grown fond of the amiable little animal.

'Hello, old girl,' I said, patting the attractive striped head. 'You really are friendly, aren't you? I'm beginning to understand your master's passion for your breed.'

I turned into the office and stood in shock for a moment. Calum was sitting at the desk with Marilyn on his shoulder.

'What . . . what . . .' I stammered.

Calum looked up and was about to reply when Siegfried strode into the room. For a few seconds he stared unbelievingly at the young man. 'What the hell's this? I nearly tripped over your bloody badger out there and now she's in here.'

Calum smiled. 'Ah yes,' he said airily. 'That's not Marilyn in the passage, it's Kelly.'

'Kelly?'

'Yes, my other badger.'

Siegfried flushed. '*Other* badger . . . I didn't know you had *another* one.'

'Oh well, I just had to get him. I could see Marilyn was lonely – I know the signs. You see,' he said earnestly, 'I know she has me for company, but really, when an animal's lonely, there's no substitute for another of the same species.'

'Yes, that's all very fine,' said Siegfried, his voice rising, 'but I wasn't keen on having one of those things around and now there's two. What d'you think this place is – a lonely-heart home for badgers?'

'Oh no, no. But you must admit that they're nice, friendly little things – they're no trouble at all.'

'That's not the point – I . . .' My partner was stopped in mid flow by the phone ringing. He lifted the receiver and, as he listened, Kelly shuffled into the room. After a few moments Siegfried put down the phone and jumped to his feet. 'Damn! That good horse at Lord Hulton's isn't any better, in fact, it's worse. I've got to go.' With a final incredulous glance at the two badgers, playing now on the office floor, he hurried from the room.

'He isn't upset, is he?' Calum enquired.

'Well, just a bit, but he'll forget about it. I'd leave Kelly in your flat for a few days if I were you.'

He nodded, then pointed out of the window. 'There's Rod Milburn's van just arrived. He's brought a ewe. Thinks it's ringwomb.'

We were in the thick of lambing, and this was the year when the Caesarean operation on sheep, previously uncommon, soared into popularity. The reasons were several. Farmers and vets were unanimous that in many protracted lambing cases it was better to operate on the ewe and 'tek 'em out of t'side' as the saying went. It was absolutely fatal to be the slightest bit rough with a ewe –

forcing open a cervix to pull out an oversized lamb could easily tear the tissues – and for some reason the condition of ringwomb had become very common.

Ringwomb was when the cervix didn't present its usual corrugated feel but was simply a smooth band of tissue which just would not yield, even after the usual injections for undilated cervix. In these cases it was best to operate without delay to avoid suffering for the ewe and to obtain one or more live lambs.

Vets were also doing the Caesarean for bad cases of pregnancy toxaemia because, once delivered of her lambs, the ewe had a better chance of recovery. The upshot was that we were doing the operation so frequently that often the farmers would bring their ewes into the surgery to save us a journey.

We ushered Rod Milburn round to the yard where Calum scrubbed up an arm and explored inside the ewe.

'Typical ringwomb, Rod,' he said, 'so we'd better not mess about. We'll boil up while you do your clipping.'

The farmer produced his clippers from the van, tipped up the ewe and expertly cut away the thick fleece from the flank. I shaved, disinfected and infiltrated the site with local anaesthetic before Calum reappeared with the sterilised instruments on a tray. I have never known a vet more meticulous about asepsis – wherever he went on his rounds, he carried a metal container with freshly boiled knives, forceps and needles and he hadn't been with us very long before his high rate of success became apparent. When Calum operated, his patients lived.

I was letting him have a go now and it was impressive to see his big, strong-fingered hands at work, quickly incising skin, muscles and peritoneum before opening the uterus and drawing out two wriggling black-faced lambs. In no time at all, he was stitching up, grinning at the two tiny creatures determinedly tottering towards the udder.

Rod was delighted. 'That's great! A good job I came down right away. We've got live twins and a healthy mother.' He lifted the lambs into the straw in the back of his van and the ewe hopped in after them as though nothing had happened to her.

I had done a lot of these operations, but I never ceased to be amazed at how little the ewe seemed to be affected. On one occasion I had just finished stitching after a Caesarean in a loose box on the farm when the ewe jerked her head from the farmer's grasp, jumped from the straw-bale operating table where she had been lying and, with a mighty leap, cleared the half-door and galloped off across the field.

When I saw the farmer a few days later and enquired about her, he said, 'Aye, she came back for 'er lambs, otherwise God knows when I'd 'ave seen her again!'

After Rod Milburn had driven away with the new family, we started on our work in the surgery. I did a laparotomy on a labrador which had swallowed his favourite ball and Calum removed a mammary tumour from a springer spaniel with his customary aplomb.

We were cleaning up when he pointed to three cat cages standing by the door. 'What's happening to those cats?'

'Oh, they're spays. I'm taking them through to Granville Bennett.'

'Don't you ever do those jobs yourself?'

'No. All cat and bitch spays go to Granville.'

Calum stared at me. 'Why on earth do you do that?'

'Oh, he's a top man – brilliant. Makes a great job and they all come back in good shape.'

'I'll bet they do. I've heard all about Granville Bennett, but Jim, you're perfectly capable of doing these yourself.'

'Oh, I know, but we've always done it this way. We're a large animal practice. This is only a side line.'

He laughed. 'Since I came here I've seen you do laparotomies, enterotomies, pyometras. What's the difference?'

'Well, I really don't know, Calum. These other things are emergencies. Maybe it's because when you're doing a spay you're starting on a healthy animal. Silly, I suppose.'

'I know what you mean. You can't bear the thought of a client bringing in his fit little animal and then the operation goes wrong.'

'Something like that. Maybe it all stems from a lack of confidence. I can't help thinking of myself as a farm animal doctor who shouldn't be doing such things.'

Calum raised a finger. 'Well, with respect, Jim, you've got to change your ideas. Small animal work is the thing of the future and the day has gone when country vets can turn their backs on routine things like spays just because they think they haven't the time.'

'Maybe you're right. I suppose we ought to start some time.'

'Why not now?'

'Eh?'

'Let's have a crack at these three. Spays are easy – I did quite a few at the college clinic.'

I was beginning to raise objections, but Calum hoisted a cage onto the table and lifted out a pretty twelve-week-old kitten. 'Here we go,' he cried, 'spay number one – the beginning of a new era in Skeldale House.'

I was carried along by his enthusiasm and we soon had the little creature anaesthetised and the site prepared. Calum poised his knife and made a tiny incision in the flank. 'Key-hole surgery is the order here. It's so easy that you don't need a lot of room to work. You just fish out the uterus like this.' He probed through the incision with forceps. 'It's no trouble at all.'

He fished out a slender strand of tissue on the end of the forceps. 'There it is, you see. Child's play.' Then he paused. 'No, that's not it.' He pushed the thing back and searched further within. But when he withdrew the forceps it still wasn't the uterus he had hold of but the same mysterious pink-white thread.

'Damn! I've never had this trouble,' he grunted, and began another exploration in the small abdomen. He had just pulled the wrong thing out again when the phone rang.

'Milk fever, flat out. Urgent. Afraid I've got to go, Calum. Can you manage?'

'Of course, I'm okay. But where the hell is this uterus?'

I left him staring down at the little cat in exasperation.

When we met later in the day, he gave me a rueful grin. 'I'm sorry I made a hash of my demonstration, Jim. You'd hardly got through the door before I found the uterus and finished the job in a few minutes. I did the other two cats after that on my own – no problem.'

I believed him. If ever there was a naturally gifted surgeon it was Calum. But that wasn't the end of the story. A few days later, we admitted four more spays and since Calum was the only man around he anaesthetised them with nembutal instead of using our oxygen and ether apparatus and then did them himself. When I walked along to the operating room he was starting on the last one.

'I'm glad to see you, Jim,' he said. 'I've just done those three,' pointing at the sleeping cats. 'Did 'em in double quick time. Piece of cake. Anyway, I can show you what I mean now you're here.'

He inserted his forceps in the incision and pulled out, not the uterus, but the same string-like filament as before. He stared at it for a moment and then he tried again and then a third time but with the same result.

'I don't believe it!' he exploded. 'It's like black magic!'

I laughed and patted him on the shoulder. 'I'm sorry I can't wait, Calum. I just dashed along between jobs to see how you were getting on.'

'I was getting on fine till you came in,' he shouted as I went out.

When I think back, I realise this was one of the strange and unaccountable little episodes in my life, because on the third occasion, around a week later when I walked into the operating room I found my colleague bent over a sleeping cat.

He looked up and gave me an eager smile. 'Ah, here you are again, Jim. I've done a couple of spays like hot cakes and I'm just starting on this one. Now watch, and I'll show you how to do it.'

Quickly and confidently he reached inside with his forceps and instead of the expected uterus there appeared the same fine cord of baffling origin. He pushed it back and tried again, and again and again without success.

'Bugger it!' he yelled. 'What's going on? When it happened before I thought it was because I was too cocky, but now I know. It's you!' He stared at me, wild-eyed. 'You're a hoodoo! You put the evil eye on me every time!'

'Oh dear, I'm sorry, Calum,' I said, fighting the giggles. 'It's just unfortunate — but anyway, what *is* that thing you keep pulling out? Has it got a name?'

'It has now,' my colleague growled. 'It's called Herriot's duct.'

That passed into the language of the practice and, long after spaying had lost its novelty in the practice and become a regular, trouble-free routine, whenever that errant piece of tissue showed itself the cry went up.

'Hello, there goes Herriot's duct again!'

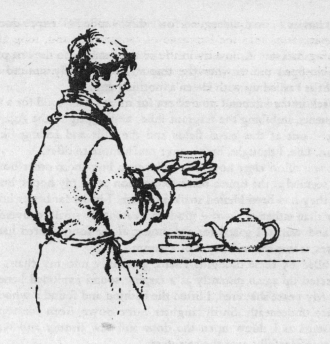

23

When I awoke on the first morning after our move to Rowan Garth, I found myself in the usual mental state of acute readiness, like a sprinter on his blocks, ready to hurl on my clothes and take off on my daily gallop round the icy acres of Skeldale House. I was so much in the groove that when my alarm went my legs started twitching, ready for the off. It took me a minute or two to realise that such things as the sessions of firelighting, wrestling with the anthracite stove and running to keep warm were all in the past.

Everything was to hand. Almost effortlessly, I donned a dressing gown and meandered down the few stairs to the little hall and then into the kitchen where a blissful warmth from the Aga cooker enveloped me. Dinah the beagle came wagging from her basket and as I patted her and exchanged the usual morning pleasantries I could discern an 'isn't this wonderful' expression in her eyes.

It was heaven. As in a trance, I slid the kettle onto the hot plate and dropped the tea into the teapot, and I hardly noticed the ascent as I sailed up with Helen's morning cup.

Back in the kitchen I poured tea for myself and stood for a few moments, imbibing the fragrant fluid, nestling up to the Aga as I looked out at the green fields and the hills and feeling like a sultan. Life, I thought, didn't have much more to offer.

It was all so clear now. My failures to buy those other houses had seemed at the time a black demolition of all my hopes, but in fact they had been blessed strokes of luck. I had a far better house now than either of them – modern, reasonably small, convenient ... and warm. I gazed for a moment at the long-desired hatch: oh yes, it was the realisation of a dream.

Lulled by these thoughts I sank gratefully into my chair, but rocketed up again instantly as a rasping sound exploded beneath me. My peace shattered, I lifted the cushion and found a whoopie device underneath. Shrill laughter came down from the top of the stairs as I threw open the door and saw Jimmy and Rosie hanging gleefully over the banisters.

'You young blighters!' I yelled as I stormed upwards. 'The very first morning! I'm coming to get you!' But they had locked themselves in their bedrooms by the time I arrived and I hadn't time to go further into the matter.

Sitting down for the second time I ruminated on the fact that I'd have to take extra care from now on. Playing jokes on dad was a hobby of my children – imitation ink blots, buns which squeaked when bitten, envelopes which emitted a terrifying buzz when opened – particularly in the mornings when my defences were down. Every time we visited my parents in Glasgow they made a bee-line for Tam Shepherd's joke shop in Queen Street to lay in further supplies and in this small house I was infinitely more accessible.

However it took only a few soothing draughts of tea before I slid back into my previous euphoria. I couldn't believe the warmth and comfort and the feeling that you could reach out and touch everything. Life was going to be so much easier for Helen.

The peace didn't last long. Within minutes of the children coming downstairs the kitchen was reverberating with deafening noise. Jimmy had rigged up an extension speaker on a shelf to play records from our beloved Murphy radiogram which was now stationed in the dining room next door and within minutes Elvis Presley was blasting his message into my ears.

I escaped for a few moments by taking up Helen's second cup. For a long time at Skeldale House it had been her only concession to my pleas to take things easier in the mornings and I was determined that this routine would continue in our new home. When I came downstairs I lifted the morning paper from the door, picked up my teacup and settled down again at the table.

Rosie, sitting next to me, was rocking back and forth in time with the music and she got so carried away that, on one of the ways down, she swivelled and the bottom of the chair leg crunched on to my slippered toe. She was a fat little girl at that time and very heavy, and I yelped in pain and my tea flew into the air and descended in a warm shower on my newspaper. As I leaped to my feet and hopped around in agony my son and daughter shrieked with laughter and Dinah set up a joyous barking to join in the fun.

Through my anguish I reflected that this was the second time within a few minutes that those two had had a good laugh at dad's expense. A memorable day for them.

Music was to be a regular pre-school routine every morning and at first it was torture because as a lifelong devotee of classical music, I found the pop scene bewildering. To me it was just a loud, unpleasant noise. But as the months passed at Rowan Garth and each day I was subjected to 'Blue Suede Shoes', 'Don't Be Cruel', 'Jailhouse Rock' and others, I developed something approaching affection for old Elvis, and now, forty years later, any of his songs coming over the radio can transport me back to those mornings in the kitchen at Rowan Garth with the children at their cornflakes, my dog at my side and the whole world young and carefree.

And yet ... there was at that time another pull on my emotions. Leaving Skeldale had been a far greater wrench than I had ever imagined. After the van had taken the last of our things away I roamed through the empty rooms which had echoed to my children's laughter. The big sitting room where I had read the bedtime stories and where, before all that, Siegfried, Tristan and I had sprawled in bachelor contentment, seemed to reproach me with its ageless charm and grace. The handsome fireplace with its glass cupboard above, and the old pewter tankard which used to hold our cash still resting there, the french window opening onto the long, high-walled garden with its lawns, fruit trees, asparagus and strawberry beds – these things were part of a great surging ocean of memories.

Upstairs, I stood in the large alcoved room where Helen and I had slept and to where we had brought our children as babies to sleep in the cot which once stood in that corner. I clumped over the bare boards to the dressing room which Jimmy and Rosie had shared, almost hearing their giggles and teasings which were the beginning of each new day.

I climbed another flight to the little rooms under the eaves where Helen and I had started our married life, where a bench against the wall and a gas ring once served as our only cooking arrangements; then I walked to the window and looked over the tumbled roofs of the little town to the green fells and swallowed a huge lump in my throat. Dear old Skeldale. I was so glad it was going to be kept on as the practice house and I would walk through its doors every day, but my family was leaving and I wondered if we could ever be as happy again as we had been here.

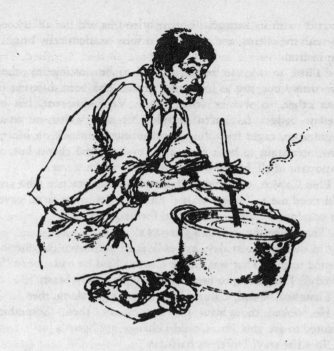

24

'Can I speak to the vet wi' t'badger?'

As I handed the phone to our new assistant, it struck me that this request was becoming common and it did me good to hear it. It meant that Calum was being accepted by the farmers. I didn't mind at all if some of them wanted him instead of me. What I dreaded hearing was 'Don't send that young bugger!' which I had heard about from some of my neighbouring vets when they employed new assistants.

We had been so lucky with John Crooks who had been an outstanding asset to our practice and it seemed to be asking too much of fate for a second top class man to come along. All the new graduates were better educated than I had been but there were other reasons why a few didn't make the grade. Some of them just couldn't face the long rough and tumble of general practice with its antisocial hours, others lacked the ability to get on with the clients, and one or two were academically bright but unpractical.

Calum, to my vast relief, seemed to be slotting into the job effortlessly but, just as John and Tristan had been different from each other, so was he from them. Very different. His ever-present badger fascinated people, his tall, walrus-moustached appearance, eager friendliness and unusual outlook on life made him interesting to both farm and small animal clients but, most important of all, he knew his stuff. He was a fine vet.

Phin Calvert, one of the characters in our practice who always addressed me as 'Happy Harry' on my visits to his farm, gave me his opinion of Calum in his usual forthright way.

'That feller,' he said, 'is a VITNERY!'

On this particular day, my colleague put down the phone and turned to me. 'That was Eddie Coates. Said he had a beast "a bit dowly". I'm getting to be an expert with dowly beasts.'

I laughed. 'Good, Calum. You'd better get along, then.'

He looked thoughtful for a moment, then, 'Something I wanted to ask you, Jim. Could I change my hours a bit?'

'In what way? Different half-day?'

'No, I'd like to start at six o'clock every morning and finish at two in the afternoon.'

I stared at him in amazement. 'What's the idea of that?'

'It would give me more opportunity to get about the country-side – find out more about the wild life and flora around here.'

'Well, I'm sorry, Calum. I know you're dead keen on that sort of thing, but those hours are just not practical. We can't do that – it wouldn't work.'

He shrugged philosophically. 'Okay,' and turned to go.

'Just a minute, Calum,' I said. 'While we're talking, I'd like to mention something else to you. You are a bit elusive.'

'Eh?'

'Yes. Difficult to find when we want you. As you know, quite a few of the small farms aren't on the phone and sometimes the only time I am able to get hold of an assistant is to catch him at mealtimes. But your eating habits are irregular and often you're in and out again without my knowing, and there might be something urgent waiting. So please, give me a ring whenever you do come in.'

Calum gave me a mock salute. 'Very good, sir, I will unfailingly report.'

We went out together to the dispensary and in the passage I was assailed by a dreadful stench. Sickly, horrible, it seemed to be coming from upstairs and I could see wisps of steam issuing from Calum's flat.

'Hell, Calum, that bloody awful stink! What's going on up there?'

He looked at me in mild surprise. 'Oh, I'm just boiling up some tripe for my animals.'

'Tripe! What sort of tripe?'

'Just ordinary cow's stomachs. Left overs at the butcher's. He says he'll let me have any tripe that's gone off a bit whenever I want it.'

I put my handkerchief over my face and shouted through the folds. 'Off-colour tripe! You're not kidding! For God's sake, get up there quickly and take that pan off. And cancel your order at the butcher's!'

I reeled into the back garden and took a few deep breaths and, as I leaned against the wall, a little thought swam in my mind. I was sure I was going to have a happy relationship with Calum, but nothing in the world was ever quite perfect.

Later that day, when I came in to lunch, it was confirmed that he had heeded my words of the morning. The phone rang and it was Calum's voice at the other end. 'Permission to eat, sir!'

'Granted, young man,' I replied, falling in gladly with his sally. I didn't know it then but throughout the time he stayed with the practice I would hear those words every day. He never ever came in at mealtimes without checking, and now when I look back over the years and think of him I seem to hear those words.

'Permission to eat, sir!'

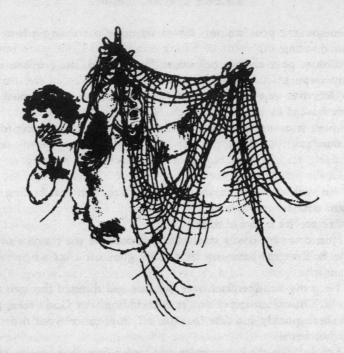

25

When we first set up house in Skeldale I often went to house sales to look for the many essential things we needed, but for some reason I repeatedly brought home useless objects. There was a long list of them – a fully-rigged sailing ship in a bottle, brass candlesticks, the little concertina of course and, on one memorable occasion, *The Geography of the World in Twenty-four Volumes.*

When we started in Rowan Garth, I was again eager to help. One big idea I had was to make a grass tennis court in the back garden, mainly for the children but also for Helen and myself since we were keen players – when we could find the time.

After mapping out the court, I realised that the big problem was to stop the balls from being knocked out of the garden and far away. Obviously a lot of high netting was required and I thought my problem was solved when a fisherman came to the door selling off yards of fishing nets. He had just gone out of business, he said, and he was selling off these superb nets at a giveaway price. I bought an enormous bundle of the things, tightly tied up with tarry rope, for £12 and proudly showed my purchase to Helen.

She was not impressed. 'Are you sure you haven't done something silly again, Jim? You know you are very easily taken in.'

I was indignant. 'Taken in? Impossible! You could see that this fisherman was as honest as the day. He was from Fraserburgh and was wearing a navy blue jersey. Cheerful, red, open face, I could smell the tar and salt off him. He said these were the last of the nets and he was selling them off extra cheap to get rid of them so that he can get back home.'

'Hmm. I don't like the sound of that, either,' Helen murmured. 'Did you look in his van to see if he had any more?'

'Well, no ... that was quite unnecessary. I assure you I've made a good buy this time. Come on, I'll prove it to you.'

We went out to the lawn and I began to untie the vast bundles of nets. As I opened them up, my spirits began to sink. They were a mass of enormous holes, some of them several feet in diameter. Helen began to giggle, and as I unrolled one holey net after another she staggered around, laughing helplessly.

'Oh dear,' she said, wiping away the tears, 'it's a good thing there's one practical person in this family. Thank heaven I never do silly things like this.'

Badly discomfited, I looked glumly at the useless things. 'Maybe I could patch up those holes with string,' I said.

'Oh stop it,' Helen said, beginning to fall about again. 'Don't start me off again. I feel weak.'

Those nets were a sore point and I kept away from the subject over the next few weeks, but I did, on several occasions, surreptitiously retire to the lawn when nobody was watching and have a go, unsuccessfully, at doing a bit of patching.

After this disaster I tried to win back a little credibility by thinking of some new ideas for the improvement of the garden. I noticed an advert in one of the Sunday papers for cloches to protect tender plants and it struck me that they would be an excellent thing in the harsh Yorkshire climate. The pictures showed the cloches standing in long trim rows, neat and functional, and they seemed extraordinarily cheap, too.

Without mentioning it to Helen I sent away for a substantial supply. I expected them to arrive in some enormous crate and was very surprised when the postman delivered a modest flat parcel. How could they possibly be the things I had seen in the picture?

The mystery was quickly solved because it turned out that what I had thought was rigid plastic was in fact ordinary floppy polythene sheeting. Not only that, but the rest of the outfit consisted of a mass of flimsy wires with ominous instructions to slide rod A into notch B and engage with flange C. I have never been any good with such things and spent maddening hours wrestling with the wires as Helen watched me curiously.

I was forced to confess my scheme to her and was irritated by the immediately sceptical reaction. She looked doubtfully at my tangled purchases and the corner of her mouth twitched as though she were fighting back a big grin. I fought on doggedly and at last had a row of the wires assembled and began to drape the polythene sheets over them.

The result was pathetic. Helen came out to have another peep just as I was surveying what looked like a long, low-slung line of washing with the polythene half attached to the wires and flapping disconsolately in the wind.

It was too much for my wife. She collapsed against the wall of the house and after a minute or two of unrestrained laughter had to go inside and sit down. I was left in the garden trying to muster a bit of dignity, but I couldn't bear to look at the cloches any more. I bundled them as quickly as I could into their original parcel and hid them away in the garage. It was another catastrophe and my stock plummeted even lower.

A week later I came in from my round and found Helen in an unusual mood. She was wide-eyed and excited, slightly breathless.

'Come in and look at this, Jim,' she said, leading me into the sitting room. The furniture had been pushed back to accommodate an extraordinary carpet, a huge, garish thing, thick and knobbly.

'What the devil's this?' I asked.

'Well,' she was more breathless than ever, 'a man came to the door this afternoon with this lovely carpet. It's a genuine Kasbah.'

'A what?'

'A Kasbah. It's a very rare oriental type of carpet.'

'Oriental?'

'Yes, this man's just come from India. He got it from a tribesman on the frontier.'

'A tribesman? The frontier?' My head was beginning to swim. 'What *are* you talking about?'

Helen drew herself up. 'It's surely quite simple. We have the opportunity to buy this beautiful carpet. It's something we need, and it's a bargain.'

'How much?'

'Twenty pounds'

'*What!*'

'It's very cheap,' said Helen, colouring. 'It's a genuine Kasbah. The man said it would cost hundreds of pounds, only he was lucky enough to meet this tribesman on the . . .'

'Don't start that again,' I said. 'I can't believe what I'm hearing. Where is this man?'

'He's coming back any minute now. I told him you'd want to see him.'

'I certainly do.' I bent down and felt the Kasbah. It seemed to be made of some spiky material and prickly strands came away and pierced my fingers painfully as I examined it. The violent colorations built up every few inches into mounds high enough for anybody to trip over. I had never seen anything remotely like it. Hot words were on my lips but I held my peace. I had a long record of this kind of boob and I wasn't on firm ground. I couldn't say it was a horrible carpet. Care had to be my watchword.

'Helen,' I said gently, 'are you really sure we want this? Look, it's so lumpy you can't close the door over it.' I demonstrated. 'And don't you think the colours are a bit bright?'

My wife began to look doubtful. 'Well . . . maybe I have been rather hasty . . . but I think that's the man at the door now.'

She led in the carpet specialist, a pleasant faced chap in his forties, radiating a powerful selling technique. Smiling warmly, he wrung my hand and presented a card to prove he was a seafaring man. Then, words pouring from him, teeth flashing, he extolled the Kasbah. His eyes never left mine and the effect was hypnotic. But when he started on about the tribesman on the frontier I managed to marshal my wits and stopped him.

'Many thanks, but we really don't want the carpet.'

He was astounded and indeed incredulous that we should throw away this heaven-sent opportunity, but I stuck grimly to my gentle refusals. He was fluent and persuasive, but as he lowered the price again and again, familiar ominous phrases began to creep in. 'Now, I'll tell you what I'll do for you,' and 'To be perfectly honest', 'I'll be very frank' until, finally, I managed to stop the torrent.

'I'll help you carry it out,' I said.

Clearly deeply disappointed in me, he inclined his head gravely. The thing was unbelievably heavy and we staggered out in a glum silence, shedding thousands of multi-coloured spicules on the way.

After he had gone I didn't say much about the incident and, in fact, I have kept pretty quiet about it ever since. With my record I cannot afford to be uppity. Helen is undoubtedly the sensible and practical member of our partnership and that carpet was her only aberration, but over the years whenever I landed in deeper than usual trouble it has been nice to have something up my sleeve. I have always been able as a last resort to bring up the subject of the genuine Kasbah.

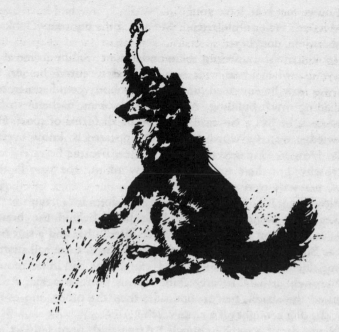

26

Bouncer was the only all-round canine games player I had ever met.

'Come on, lad,' cried his master, Arnold Braithwaite, 'let's see Lew Hoad's big serve.'

Eagerly, the dog, a handsome border collie, stood up on his hind legs, waved his right fore paw above his head and brought it down in an authentic sweep.

I laughed in delight. 'That's wonderful, Arnie. I didn't know he was a tennis player too.'

'Oh aye.' The big man bent and gazed at his pet with intense gratification, then bent over and fondled the shaggy head. 'There's nowt 'e can't do in that line. He's like his master – an expert at all sports. And I've been able to teach him that serve knowin' Lew Hoad like I do.'

'You've met him, have you?'

'Met 'im? He's an old friend. Me and 'im's big pals. Thinks a lot about me, does Lew.'

I looked at Arnie, feeling the wonderment welling in me as it always did when I was with him. He was a retired builder, or that was how he described himself, but nobody could remember him doing much building. A bulky, fit-looking bachelor in his late sixties, he had a fanatical devotion to all forms of sport. His knowledge was encyclopaedic and he appeared to know everybody. How he managed this was not clear because he rarely left Darrowby, but there seemed to be few among the world's top sportsmen who were not his friends.

'Now then, lad,' he said, addressing his dog, 'let's have a bit o' cricket.' We went out to the little lawn behind the house. 'You're fieldin' in the slips, right?' He lifted a bat and a soft ball and as Bouncer crouched in anticipation he struck the ball swiftly to one side of him. The dog leaped, caught the ball in his mouth and brought it back before taking up his position again. Arnie repeated the action, first to one side, then the other, and every time the dog brought off a clean catch.

'Never drops a catch,' chuckled Arnie with deep satisfaction. He held up the bat. 'That's the bat ah was tellin' you about. Len Hutton borrowed it a time or two for some of his big innings. I remember 'is very words. "A fine bit o' wood, Arnie, 'e said."'

I'd heard that one before. The legendary Len Hutton, later Sir Leonard, was at that time captain of England, holder of the record test match score, a household name throughout the world, and quite simply a god in cricket-mad Yorkshire.

'And these boots.' He held up a pair of well-blanco'd cricket boots. 'Them's the ones Len borrows, too. Borrows 'em a lot. Says they bring 'im luck.'

'Yes, I remember you saying so, Arnie.'

'Aye, ah've had some times in cricket.' His eyes took on a dreamy look and I knew he was going into one of his sporting reminiscences from the First World War. I had only dropped in as I was passing to clip Bouncer's nails, but I knew that would have to wait.

'Aye, it was when our battalion was playing the Gunners out

in France. Our bowlin' was getting knocked all over t'place and the score was mountin' fast. The colonel threw me the ball. "I'll have to call on you, Braithwaite," he said. "Things are looking bad." Well I did the hat-trick straight away.'

'You did?'

'Aye, three wickets, just like that. Then the colonel came over to me. "I'd better take you off, Braithwaite," he said. "That's kept the score down, but we don't want to push it too far the other way." Well, the same thing happened. Their batsmen started to clout our bowlers for sixes and fours, so the colonel came over to me again. "I'm sorry, Braithwaite," he said, "I'm going to have to call on you once more."'

Arnie paused and looked at me seriously. 'Well, I did it again.'

'You mean . . . another hat-trick?'

'That's right.'

'Extraordinary. Quite amazing.' I held up the nail clippers and clicked them a few times, but Arnie didn't seem to notice.

'Let's do your Tom Finney,' he cried, producing a football and rolling it along the grass. This was one of Bouncer's party tricks and I'd seen it before, but I still shared the big man's enjoyment as the dog dribbled the ball round the lawn, controlling it between his paws, weaving this way and that. 'Now score a goal!' shouted Arnie, and Bouncer made straight for two miniature posts at the edge of the lawn and knocked the ball between them with his nose.

We both laughed and clapped our hands and the big dog leaped up at us, wagging his tail furiously. It did me good to see Bouncer so sprightly because he was quite elderly; over nine years old.

'He loves that, doesn't he, Arnie?' I said.

'He does, there's nothin' he likes better than a bit of sport. He's never happier than when he's playin' one of his games.' He blew out his cheeks thoughtfully. 'It's a bit since I've seen Tom.'

Tom Finney was then at the peak of his glorious career. English international in three different positions and arguably the greatest English footballer of all time.

'You know him?' I said.

'Oh, I do, I do, we're great pals. Must get together with him soon. Hey, Bouncer,' he waved at his dog again, 'how about a bit o' golf. Let's see your Bobby Locke.'

I held up a hand. 'Some other time, Arnie. I must get this job done.'

'Okay, Jim, I don't want to keep you.' He smiled ruminatively. 'Just thinkin' about golf reminds me of the good times I've had with Bobby.'

'Another friend, eh?'

'Not half!'

As I snipped at Bouncer's nails I wondered if there were any of the world's famous sportsmen Arnie didn't know. At that time Locke was a giant in world golf, but just another chum for all that.

Like most dogs, Bouncer wasn't keen on having his nails done and as I grasped each paw he panted apprehensively, mouth wide, tongue lolling, but he was a good-natured animal and he resigned himself to his fate without any growling or snarling.

'These black claws are tricky,' I said. 'One can't see how far the quick comes down like one can on white claws and I'm having to go very carefully. You'd never forgive me if I got into the painful bit, would you, Bouncer?'

Despite his fear, the big dog lashed his tail briefly at the sound of his name, and as I patted his head at the end of the little operation, he leaped away and cantered around the lawn in relief.

'Come in and have a cup o' tea before ye go, Jim,' Arnie said.

I hesitated. I didn't have time for all this, but I knew he loved to talk and I always found he had interesting things to say. 'Well thanks, Arnie,' I said, 'but it'll have to be a quickie.'

It was a bachelor's kitchen, functional but comfortless, and when I saw Bouncer following his master around as he put on the kettle and fetched the cups I realised what a blessing his companionship must be. That kitchen would have been even more cold and bare without his shaggy presence, and Arnie chatted away to him as he pottered about. But there was no sign of poverty because Arnie always seemed to have enough money.

He sipped appreciatively at the steaming cup. 'There's nowt like a good cup o' tea, is there, Jim?'

'It's very refreshing, Arnie. But you've always loved your tea more than most, haven't you? You must have suffered during the war when you couldn't get it.'

He shook his head vigorously. 'Nay, not me. I 'ad no trouble. One or two Indian rajahs kept sendin' me supplies all the way through.'

'Rajahs, eh?'

'That's right. Durin' the first war ah was stationed in India for a bit and I got well in with a lot o' them rajahs. Nice fellers they were, too. And, by gum, they remembered me when t'second war broke out. I allus had plenty of tea.'

'Well, that's wonderful.' Arnie's army service had taken him to an amazing variety of countries. I'd heard about France, Belgium, Italy, Mesopotamia, Africa, Egypt and now India.

I finished my tea and left to continue my rounds. As I left, Arnie was starting a game of golf with his dog.

Apart from my professional duties I saw quite a bit of Arnie, as he was to be found every night in the same chair at the end of the bar at the Drovers. I was returning one evening from a calving during which I had lost a bit of sweat and dropped in for a thirst quencher. The big man was there in his usual place, Bouncer, as always, under his chair, and I sat down next to him.

'I've had a lovely day at Headingley,' he said. 'Saw some good cricket, too.'

'Lucky you. I wish I'd been there.' I had been listening to the Test Match on my car radio as I drove round the farms, and had been nourishing the thought that I might be able to go across to Leeds with Helen on the Saturday.

'Aye, it were right excitin', and you know, I was sittin' there on the front row when Denis Compton walked up to me. "Well Arnie, how nice to find you," he said. "I was hoping I'd see you. One of the lads said you would be here today and I've come to take you to lunch. I've been looking everywhere for you."'

'Oh, great,' I said, 'so you had lunch with the teams?'

'Oh aye, it was smashin'. There was Bill Edrich and Cyril Washbrook and all them great Australians. Keith Miller, Neil Harvey, Ray Lindwall and all the rest. They were right glad to see me again – I'd met them all before, of course.'

'Of course.'

Just then, Kenny Ditchburn, a beefy, red-faced young man, plumped himself down on the other side of my friend.

'Now then, Arnie,' he said, grinning, 'talkin' cricket, eh? Have you been lendin' Len Hutton your boots lately?'

Arnie turned an unsmiling face toward him and his eyes narrowed. 'Now then, Kenny,' he replied gruffly, then turned back to me.

His reminiscences had given him something of a reputation in the town and the younger element were at all times trying to take the mickey out of him, but he had become hyper-sensitive to the blunt approach and would clam up immediately. Throughout my many meetings with him, I had never ever initiated a conversation about his sporting experiences, never showed any particular interest in them, and it was then, when he was relaxed, with his guard down, that the fascinating tales came pouring out.

The poor man was a victim not only of teasing, but of a whole series of apocryphal anecdotes which were falsely attributed to him and bandied around among the locals. According to some, Arnie had described how, when serving in France in that first war, he had gained such a reputation as a football goalkeeper that finally a lot of famous dead shot players were lined up to take penalty kicks against him. For ages they booted that ball at him but they couldn't score. Arnie was impregnable. At last, in desperation, they loaded a football into a cannon and fired it at him. Apparently, Arnie's laconic ending to the tale was, 'Well, I saved it all right, but I broke a couple of ribs.'

It was also put about that he had told a story that, while on winter manoeuvres in Russia, the soldiers had organised a kicking contest. Arnie had won, and in fact he had sent the ball so high that it had snow on it when it descended. These and many other far-out yarns were put in Arnie's mouth by the local lads, but I personally had never heard them from him and so discounted them, as I did Arnie's reputed description of how, during a crisis in the Egyptian campaign, he had carried General Allenby across the Nile.

However, they all passed into local folk-lore, and I expect they will always be talked about. I remember one occasion at a charity concert in Darrowby's town hall when a comic violinist got up on the stage and declaimed, to loud laughter, 'I shall now play the second movement from a fantasy by Arnie Braithwaite.'

Never mind, I liked the old boy. I, too, was a sports buff and Arnie, when he wasn't reminiscing, talked with great knowledge of all aspects of the sporting scene. I always enjoyed his conversation. Also, he was an animal lover and devoted to his dog and that made another bond.

One sunny afternoon, a few weeks after the nail-clipping, I was walking my little beagle in the riverside fields when I saw Arnie with Bouncer. As usual, he was playing one of his games and the big dog was leaping around, chasing a ball under the great willows which overhung the water.

'He's lost a bit of weight, Arnie,' I said, looking at the hollows in Bouncer's flanks and his prominent ribs. 'Is he all right?'

'Oh aye, full of beans and eatin' like a horse. He's fit, that's all. In full training for the football season. Come on, lad, do your Stanley Matthews.'

Bouncer capered around with the ball, pushing it this way and that in a mazy dribble which did indeed make me think of the great man.

'Haven't seen Stan for a bit,' Arnie said ruminatively. 'He must be wondering where I'm hidin' myself.'

A month passed before I heard from the old man again. His voice on the telephone was strained. 'Wish you'd come and see my dog, Jim, he's right poorly.'

'What's he doing, Arnie?'

'Nowt, really. Got no life in 'im.'

The inseparable pair were in the garden when I called. I was shocked at Bouncer's appearance. He was emaciated, sitting motionless on the lawn, and he made no attempt to give me his usual greeting.

'My God, Arnie,' I said, 'why have you let him get to this state? He looks awful!'

'Well, I could see he was gettin' thinner, but he was eating so well, eatin' like a horse. I thought maybe he was just runnin' around too much. He's got suddenly worse over the last few days. I'm not one to neglect me dog, am I?'

'No, no, of course you're not. And he's still eating well, you say?'

'Aye, never better, that's what puzzles me.'

'And is he drinking a lot?'

'He is – allus at it.'

I began to examine Bouncer, but even before I started there wasn't much doubt in my mind. Loss of weight, voracious appetite, abnormal thirst, extreme lethargy. It could mean only one thing.

'Arnie,' I said, 'I think he has diabetes.'

'Oh 'ell, is that bad?'

'Yes, I'm afraid it is when it has got as far as this. It can be fatal.'

The big man stared at me, totally shocked. 'Oh, don't tell me that! Is he goin' to die?'

'I hope not. There's a lot we can do.'

'Can you start right away, Jim?' He ruffled his hair distractedly. 'I mustn't lose 'im.'

'I will, Arnie, but first I've got to make sure. I must eliminate one or two other things like kidney trouble. First thing tomorrow morning, I want you to get a urine sample from him. Stick a nice clean soup plate under him when he cocks his leg and put it in this bottle, and bring it straight round with Bouncer to the surgery.'

He nodded. 'Right . . . I will . . . but maybe he's not as bad as all that.' He picked up a football and rolled it up to the dog. 'Now, lad,' he cried eagerly, 'let's see you do your Tom Finney.'

Bouncer did not move. He touched the ball listlessly with his nose, then looked up at us with lack-lustre eyes. His master went over to him and stroked his head. 'Oh Bouncer, Bouncer,' he whispered.

Next morning I tested the sample. Positive for glucose.

'Now we know for sure, Arnie. It is diabetes, so this is what we do. I'm now giving him this injection of a small amount of insulin and you must come in every morning bringing Bouncer with a fresh sample which I will test. If still positive, I will slightly increase the dose of insulin until he is stabilised, that is when the urine is negative for glucose.'

'Aye, ah'll come in every day, for as long as it takes . . . that is, if he . . . if he stays alive.' The old man's face was a doleful mask.

I nodded. 'If he stays alive, Arnie.'

Sometimes in diabetes, the first shot of insulin brings a spectacular improvement, but it wasn't so with Bouncer. He was too far gone for that. For several mornings Arnie brought him round to the surgery and I looked in vain for even a hint of better things. The big dog was a woebegone, lifeless creature, so different from the all-round athlete of former days. Arnie, grim and resolute, was there on the dot of nine o'clock, and after ten days I commiserated with him.

'Arnie, it's tough on you having to do this day after day.'

He stuck out his chin, 'I'll come round here on me hands and knees till kingdom come if it'll save me dog.'

It was just around then that I sensed a difference in Bouncer. He was still as skinny as ever, still as apathetic, but there was the suggestion of a gleam in his eyes – they were losing something of their dead look. From then on my hopes grew as the big dog slowly began to show signs of his old vitality and after three weeks of the treatment the daily sample was negative and I had a happy, tail-wagging animal looking at me as though he was almost ready for a game.

'Arnie,' I said, 'he's stabilised at last. He's going to be all right. But it's over to you, now. You'll have to give your dog a shot of insulin every morning for the rest of his life.'

'Eh? Me inject him?' He didn't look very happy about that.

'Yes, you can do that, can't you? After his morning meal. It'll soon be part of your daily programme.'

He gave me a doubtful look, but didn't say anything and I supplied him with all he would require.

Once Bouncer had turned the corner his recovery proceeded at a galloping pace and Arnie after a few days brushed aside my doubts about his ability to carry out the injections. In fact it transpired that for a period he had been a sort of personal assistant to an army surgeon during the Balkans campaign and was very familiar with hypodermics.

My final happy memory of the diabetes episode was when I looked over the hedge into Arnie's garden and saw him wrestling with Bouncer on the grass.

'What *are* you up to, Arnie?' I cried.

'Doing a low tackle on Bouncer – teachin' him rugby,' came the reply.

As autumn stretched into winter, there was considerable excitement in Darrowby when it was announced that the important men's hockey match between the rival counties of Yorkshire and Lancashire was to be played on the local ground. They were two of the top teams and contained several international players. Everybody was looking forward to seeing these famous men in action and on the Saturday afternoon I got to the ground in what I had hoped would be good time. However, people were already standing several deep round the touchlines – I'd never seen such a crowd there – and I was wondering where I could find a vantage spot when I heard a voice calling.

'Hey, Jim, there's a spare seat over here.'

It was Arnie, comfortably settled in one of the seats in front of the club-house.

'Are you sure, Arnie?'

'Aye, ah've been keeping it for you. Sit down.'

Well, this was very nice. The game was just about to start and I had a perfect view. I felt something stirring against my trouser leg and saw that it was Bouncer's nose pushing at me. He was in his usual place under his master's seat and he seemed to be telling me that he was in top form again.

I tickled his ears while I watched the match. As expected, the standard of play was very high with the four internationals shining above the rest.

Arnie kept up a running commentary. 'That's Pip Chapman, Yorkshire captain and England centre forward – old pal of mine. And Greg Holroyd, captain of Lancashire and England winger – another good old mate, and those two other internationals, Tim Mowbray and Johnnie Hart, I know 'em all well, known 'em for years.'

At half time as the players gathered in the middle of the pitch, Arnie was in expansive mood. 'It's nice to see the winter games startin' again, but I keep thinkin' about that last cricket match of the season at the Scarborough cricket festival. I was just sittin' there enjoying the sunshine when Fred Trueman spotted me. "Arnie," he said, "I've been looking for you everywhere."'

This last remark attributed to another of cricket's immortals seemed to amuse a group of young men sitting behind us. After a few half-stifled giggles, one of them spoke up.

'Fred Trueman, Arnie? The *real* Fred Trueman? Looking for you everywhere?' Arnie, grim-faced, nodded slightly with the dignity born of long practice, and this evoked another outburst of sniggers with sotto voce repetitions of 'Looking for you everywhere,' a phrase which seemed to tickle them.

My friend ignored them, rigid in his seat, eyes gazing fixedly ahead, until another of the youths returned to the attack. 'I hear you've got some old pals out there on the field, too, Arnie? Those four top men – known 'em for years, eh?' Again Arnie nodded briefly and I felt a sharp twinge of apprehension. We were heading into deep water this time with the tangible evidence of his claims running around in front of us. Arnie was sitting on the end seat, right next to the aisle up which the teams would have to pass to get to the club-house; those men would be within touching distance of him. They couldn't fail to see him.

When the final whistle blew and the players began to make their way towards us, my throat tightened. Something awful was surely going to happen and I wished with all my heart that I was somewhere else.

Holroyd, the big, black-moustachioed Lancastrian, was the first to come clumping up the steps, face sweating, knees mud-spattered. He glanced at Arnie and brushed past him, then, as my stomach began to lurch, he stopped and took a step back. There was a pause as he looked down, then, 'It's Arnie Braithwaite!' he burst out. 'Hello! How are you old chap?' He began to pump my friend's hand and called out to his team mates. 'Hey, Pip, Johnnie, Tim, look who's here. It's our old chum!' There was a jam of players in the aisle as the four men gathered round Arnie, thumping his back, laughing and shouting. Bouncer jumped from under the seat and, as dogs like to do, began to add a joyful barking to the general merriment.

Pip Chapman gazed down at Arnie with warm affection. 'Do

you know, Arnie, we thought you might be here and we've been scanning the touchline all through the match. We've been looking for you everywhere.'

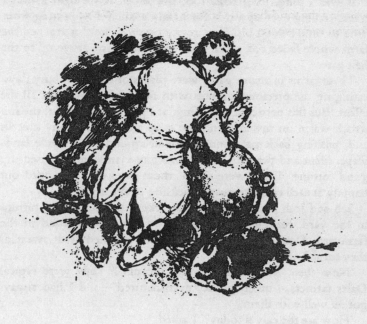

27

My clients' opinion of me varied widely, and although there were the odd one or two who thought I was brilliant, a large majority looked on me as a steady, reliable vet, while a few regarded me as of strictly limited ability. But I really think that only one family nourished the private conviction that I was not quite right in the head.

They were the Hardwicks, and it was a pity because they were some of my favourite people.

The situation was due to a few unfortunate little accidents and on this sharp and sunny January morning I had no inkling that I was going to sow the seeds of my image disintegration that very day. There had been just enough snow overnight to turn the world white and I could see the road to the Hardwick farm threading its way through a glittering frostiness under a sky of cloudless blue.

It was a long, long road too, not much more than a rough track, trailing ever upwards for nearly a mile, disappearing from time to time behind bluffs or rocky outcrops until it reached the farm whose faded red roofs were just visible as I drove up to the first gate.

These farms of many gates were places of dread on busy days, eating up the precious minutes with nothing to show for all the effort. But this particular morning, as I got out of the car, the sun struck warm on my face and the crisp air tingled in my nostrils and, pushing back gate one, I looked around at the wide landscape, silent and peaceful under its white mantle, and blessed my good fortune. There were six of these gates, and I hopped out happily at each one, the snow crackling under my feet.

Seb and Josh Hardwick were attacking a mountain of turnips in the yard, forking them up onto a cart which stood in the farmyard. Despite the cold, their faces gleamed with sweat as they turned smilingly to me.

'Now then, Mr Herriot, grand mornin'.' They were typical Dales farmers – quiet, polite, even-natured – and I had always got on well with them.

'How are the calves today?' I asked.

'Lot better,' Seb said. 'And thank 'eavens. We were a bit worried.'

I was relieved, too. Salmonella is a nasty thing – highly fatal to young animals and dangerous to humans – and when I had seen the calves a couple of days previously the whole picture had looked ominous.

I went into the fold yard with the brothers and over to the big pen at one end where my patients, twenty in all, were standing, and I felt a glow of satisfaction. Everything was different. Two days ago, there was an air of doom over that pen, with the little creatures, listless and dejected, hanging their heads as the diarrhoea trickled down their tails, but now they were brighter and livelier, looking at me with interest as I leaned over the rails.

Actually I was mentally patting myself on the back because I felt I had done rather well. I could easily have treated this as an ordinary case of scour, but the high temperatures and a tell-tale soft cough had alerted me. The rectal swabs I had taken had

confirmed my diagnosis. I had given them the usual combination
of chloromphenicol injections and furazolidone by the mouth
and it was clearly doing the job.

'Well, that's fine,' I said, climbing into the pen. 'So far, so
good. I'll repeat the injections and you must carry on with the
powders for another five days and I think all is going to be well.
And don't forget to wash your hands well after each time.'

Josh took off his cap and wiped his streaming face. 'That's
what we like to hear, Mr Herriot. It's a good job we got you in
right away or we'd have 'ad some dead 'uns lyin' about.'

After the injections, Seb waved me towards the house. 'We'll
all want a wash, and it's time for our ten o'clock, anyroad.'

Later, in the kitchen, as I sipped my tea and bit into a home-
made scone, the two attractive young wives, one dark, the other
a blazing redhead, chatted away to me. As I sat in the warmth of
the fire with a baby crawling round my feet and two toddlers
wrestling happily on the stone flags, I felt that life was pretty
good. I could have stayed there all day, but my other work was
pressing. The brothers, too, who had joined me for the tea, had
begun to fidget, no doubt thinking of all those turnips outside. It
was no good – I had to go.

In the yard, we made our farewells, the two men lifted their
forks and I put my hand on the car door, but nothing happened. I
tried to turn the handle but it wouldn't move. I went round, trying
the other doors, but the result was the same. I was locked out.

My little beagle, Dinah, was the culprit. While I was treating
the calves I had heard her barking at the farm dogs, which was
one of her hobbies, and in the process, as she had thrown herself
at each window, her paws must have pushed down the knobs
which locked the doors.

I called to the brothers. 'Look, I'm very sorry, but I can't get
into my car.'

'Oh aye, what's happened?' They came over and looked inside
and Dinah, tongue lolling, tail lashing delightedly, looked out at
them. Behind her, my keys hung in the ignition switch, just an
arm's length away but maddeningly inaccessible.

I explained the situation and Josh looked at me in surprise.
'You allus carry that little dog with you, don't you?'

'Oh, yes.'

'But you don't take your keys out when ye leave the car?'

'No . . . no . . . I'm afraid not.'

'Funny thing it's never 'appened before, then.'

'Well, yes, suppose it is, when you think about it. And it's a great pity it's happened away out here.'

'How's that?'

'Well, I'm afraid I'm going to have to ask you to give me a lift home to get my spare key.'

Seb's mouth fell open. 'Back to Darrowby?'

'Afraid so. Nothing else I can do.' I tried not to think of the ten miles.

The Hardwicks looked at each other in alarm, then at the vast heap of turnips and finally back at me. I knew what they were thinking. It wasn't only the turnips; there were always a thousand jobs to be done on a farm and I was about to wreck their chances of getting some of them done that morning.

But, nice fellows that they were, they didn't tell me what a daft bugger I was. Seb blew his cheeks out. 'Aye, well, we'd better get started then.' He turned to his brother. 'I'll 'ave to leave ye to it, Josh. When you've shifted them turnips you'd better get on with the muckin' out. We can move that lot o' sheep down to t'low garth this afternoon.'

Josh nodded and wordlessly seized his fork again while his brother got out the family car. Like a lot of the hill farmers' vehicles, it was very large and very old. We rattled down the track and as I opened each gate I was enveloped in a cloud of acrid fumes from the exhaust.

The road to Darrowby seemed very long, and longer still on the way back. I tried to pass the time with comments on sport, the weather and farming conditions but for the last half-hour the conversation languished. At the farm Seb opened the car door, gave me a hasty wave and trotted away to find his brother.

Dinah was in transports at my return, jumping all over me, licking at my face but, driving away, I had the strong feeling that I wasn't as popular with the humans I had left behind.

However, when I made my final check on the calves a week later, all seemed to be forgiven. I had no doubt been a damn nuisance, but the Hardwick brothers greeted me smilingly – although there was a bad moment when I got out of the car and both men shouted, 'Hey, get your keys out! Don't forget that!' as I was about to close the door.

Sheepishly, I complied, feeling foolish because ever since the previous incident I had made a point of doing just that.

I felt a lot better when I saw that the calves were completely recovered and after washing my hands and drinking the ritual cup of tea in the kitchen l felt that I could consign the whole silly episode to the past.

A few days afterward, Helen met me with a strange message on my return home. 'I've had a funny phone call from a Mrs Hardwick.'

'How do you mean, funny?'

'She says you've pinched her husband's spectacles.'

'What?'

'That's what she said.'

'How . . . how? I don't know what you're talking about.'

'Well, they've searched high and low for those spectacles and they're definitely not in the house and the only visitor they've had was you. She's convinced you've got them.'

'I've never heard anything so daft in my life. What the devil would *I* want with them?'

Helen spread her hands. 'I've no idea, but Mr Hardwick wants them badly. They're his reading glasses and he can't read *The Farmer and Stockbreeder*. He's quite upset. You'd better have a search.'

'This is crazy,' I said, but I went over to my working coat and began to go through the pockets. And there, among the little bottles and scissors and other veterinary odds and ends, was the spectacle case, lying next to the wallet in which I kept my thermometer and which it closely resembled.

I looked at it in disbelief. 'My God, it's here, right enough. I must have picked it up by mistake after I'd rinsed my thermometer in the kitchen.'

I rang the farm and apologised to Seb. 'Another silly thing I've done,' I said laughingly. He didn't disagree, but was still polite and declined my offer to bring the spectacles to him.

'No, it's awright, I'll come down for 'em now.' Clearly, *The Farmer and Stockbreeder* was waiting.

I was embarrassed at the thought of his long and needless journey on my account, and the feeling hadn't left me three days later when I looked in the appointments book and saw that I had another call to the Hardwicks' farm.

When I arrived I found the brothers in the cow byre, forking hay into the racks. They didn't give me the usual greeting. In fact, they seemed surprised to see me.

'I've come to see your lame cow,' I announced cheerfully.

They looked at each other expressionlessly, then back at me.

'We haven't no lame cow,' Josh said.

'But . . . there was a call from you this morning.'

Again the blank look between them.

'Well . . . there must be some mistake.' I tried a light laugh which wasn't reciprocated, and I couldn't help looking along the line of cows.

Seb raised a hand. 'Honest, Mr Herriot. There's none of 'em lame. You can examine them if you like.'

'No, no, no, of course not. I . . . somebody in the practice has got a message wrong. Do you mind if I use your phone?'

Seb led me into the kitchen and as I dialled the surgery it didn't make me feel any better when I saw him lift his spectacle case from the table and slip it unobtrusively into his pocket. When I got to Skeldale House, I found that I should have gone to the Borthwicks' farm, only half a mile away. But what was happening? Why did I have to keep making a fool of myself here?

I lifted the ballpoint by the side of the phone and wrote the name down so that I could not make any more mistakes, and turned to the two young wives. 'I'm terribly sorry, I'm always being such a nuisance to you.' I was about to leave when one of them held out her hand. 'Could we have our pen back, Mr Herriot?'

Hot-faced, I took it from my pocket and fled.

My embarrassment was acute when I was called back to the farm within a few days.

When I arrived, Seb was pointing gloomily at a young heifer lying on the cowhouse floor. 'She just can't get up,' he said, 'and that hind leg's stuck out, funny like.'

I bent over the animal and flicked her ear. 'Come on, lass, let's see you try.'

She replied by struggling briefly, then subsided on to the cobbles, and there was no doubt that her right hind leg was the cause of the trouble. It seemed to be useless.

I ran my hand up the shaggy limb and when I reached the pelvic region diagnosis was easy.

'She's got a dislocated hip, Seb,' I said. 'There's nothing broken, but the head of the femur is right out of its socket.'

'Are ye sure?' The farmer looked at me doubtfully.

'Absolutely positive. Here, feel this prominence. In fact, you can just about see it sticking up there.'

Seb didn't bother to take his hands out of his pockets. 'Well, ah don't know. I thought she'd maybe just strained 'erself. Maybe you could give me summat to rub on 'er – that might put her right.'

'No, I assure you. There's no doubt in my mind.'

'Awright, then, what do we do?'

'Well, we'll have to try to pull the joint back into place. It's not easy, but since it has only just happened I'd say there was a good chance of success.'

The farmer sniffed. 'Very well, then. On ye go.'

'I'm sorry,' I said, smiling, 'but it's quite a big job and I can't do it by myself. In fact, you and I can't do it. We'll need some help.'

'Help? I haven't got no 'elp. Josh is right over on the far field.'

'Well, I'm really sorry about that, but you'll have to get him back. And I hate to say it, but we'll also need one of your neighbours to lend a hand. And he'd better be a big strong chap, too.'

'Bloody 'ell!' Seb stared at me. 'What's all this for?'

'I know it seems a big fuss to you, but although she's only a young beast, she's big and strong and in order to get the joint back in place we have to overcome the muscular resistance. It needs a right good pull, I can tell you. I've done a lot of these jobs and I know.'

He nodded. 'Ah well, I'll go and see if Charlie Lawson can come over. You'll wait 'ere, then?'

'No, I'll have to go back to the surgery for the chloroform muzzle.'

'Chloroform! What the 'ell next?'

'I told you about the muscular resistance. We need to put her to sleep to overcome that.'

'Now, look 'ere, Mr Herriot.' The farmer lifted a portentous forefinger. 'Are ye sure we have to go through all this carry on? Don't ye think we could just rub summat on? A bit of embrocation, maybe?'

'I'm sorry, Seb, it's all necessary.'

He turned and strode out of the cowhouse, muttering, while I hurried across to my car.

On the journey to Darrowby and back, two thoughts were uppermost in my mind. This was one of the tricky jobs in veterinary practice but, when successful, it was spectacular. A hopelessly lame animal would rise and walk away, good as new. And I did feel I badly needed something to resuscitate my reputation on this farm.

When I returned with the muzzle, Josh and Charlie Lawson were waiting in the yard with Seb. 'Now, Mr Herriot,' 'Now then, Mr Herriot,' but they looked at me sceptically, and I could tell that the other brother had been voicing his doubts.

'It's good of you gentlemen to rally round,' I said cheerfully. 'I hope you're all feeling strong. It's a tough job, this.'

Charlie Lawson grinned and rubbed his hands. 'Aye, we'll do our best.'

'Okay, now.' I looked down at the heifer. 'We'd better move her nearer the door. You'll get a stronger pull that way. Then we'll get the chloroform muzzle on and rope the leg. You'll haul away while I put pressure on the joint. But first let's roll her over.'

As the farmers pushed against the animal's side, I tried to tuck the lame leg underneath her. As she rolled over there was a loud click, and after a rapid look around her she rose to her feet and walked out through the door.

The four of us watched her as she ambled across the yard and through a gate into the field. She was perfectly sound. Not the slightest trace of lameness.

'Well, I've never seen that happen before,' I gasped. 'The rolling movement and the pressure on the joint must have clicked it back. Would you believe it!'

The three farmers gave me a level stare. It was clear that they didn't believe it.

Retreating to my car, I heard Seb confiding to the other two. 'Might as well have rubbed summat on it.' And as I drove away past the heifer grazing contentedly on the green hillside, Siegfried's words at the beginning of our partnership came back to me. 'Our profession offers unparalleled opportunities for making a chump of yourself.'

How true that was. How true it would always be. But why, why, *why* did it have to happen this time at the Hardwicks'?

I couldn't believe it when I saw the Hardwick name on the book for another visit less than a week afterwards.

'Siegfried,' I said, 'I wish you'd go there. There's a jinx on me at that place.'

He looked at me in surprise. 'But it's one of your favourite spots. And they always ask for you personally.'

'Oh, I know, but I've got a feeling of doom at the moment.' I told him about my recent experiences.

'Nonsense, James!' He made a dismissive gesture. 'You're imagining things. These are tiny happenings.' He sat back in his chair and laughed. 'Amusing, I grant you, but of no importance. The Hardwicks are a grand family – they won't have given a thought to such details.'

'I'm not so sure. I know they're good people, but I'm convinced they think I've got a screw loose. A touch of kleptomania for a start.'

He laughed again. 'Oh, what rubbish! Off you go. It's only a sick pig. Nothing can go wrong this time.'

It was possibly my imagination, but I thought the brothers looked a little apprehensive as I got out of the car at the farm. The pig in question was a sow with a family of a dozen piglets squealing around her. She was lying in a dark corner of the fold yard, and the gloom was such that I could hardly see the animal, but I was used to this and had always done a lot of my work by touch and feel.

I climbed into the pen where the sow could only be seen as a dim bulk. I got out my thermometer and groped my way toward her rear end.

'Hasn't eaten today, you say?'

'Nay, not a thing,' replied Josh. 'And she hasn't moved from that spot. The little pigs look hungry, too – they don't seem to be gettin' much milk.'

'Yes . . . yes . . . yes . . . I see . . .' I was fumbling desperately to find the anus to insert my thermometer, but I just couldn't locate it. It was as black as pitch down there, but I had found many a pig's anus in the dark. I couldn't make it out. I could feel the tail and if I slid my hand down there, the thermometer would pop into the anus, but it didn't and when I found something lower down it was the vagina. The solution burst on me like a great light.

'This pig's got no backside!' I cried. For a moment it seemed like a triumphant scientific discovery to be shared with the world, but I realised suddenly that I was in the wrong place for such things.

The brothers were looking down at me in tight-lipped silence. Seb spoke with a touch of weariness in his voice. 'No what?'

I looked up at him from my crouched position. 'No backside, no anus. A very rare condition. Quite fascinating. Common enough in little pigs, but I've never seen it in an adult animal.'

'Oh aye,' said Josh, 'and if she 'asn't got no backside, where does all that muck come from? I 'ave to shovel a hell of a lot out of 'ere every morning.'

I replied eagerly, 'The faeces are coming through the vagina! That's what happens in this condition.'

'And she's been doin' that for all them years?'

'Yes, really she has. Look, bring me a torch and I'll show you.'

The brothers exchanged another look. 'It's awright, we believe you.' It was very obvious that they didn't.

I launched into further explanation, but I realised I was beginning to gabble and so desisted. In any case, when I rested my hand on the sow's belly I could feel her udder, inflamed and lumpy.

'Anyway, I don't need to take her temperature, she's got mastitis. Her udder's very hot and swollen. I'll give her a shot of antibiotic and I'm sure she'll be okay.' I was trying to be brisk and businesslike, but I wasn't impressing anybody.

Josh spoke again. 'So you don't 'ave to take the temperature?'

'That's right, there's no need.'

'Of course, there's no need,' he said, and they both nodded. 'Don't you worry, Mr Herriot. It doesn't matter.'

I felt my toes curling. They were trying to humour me. That was the worst part.

Mechanically, I gave the sow her antibiotic injection, hurried through my hand-washing and declined a cup of tea.

As I drove away, Seb and Josh, side by side on the cobbles of the yard, raised their hands gravely in farewell and I saw the young women watching from the kitchen window. I could read their thoughts.

Poor old Herriot. Not a bad chap, really. It was so sad to see him losing his mind like this.

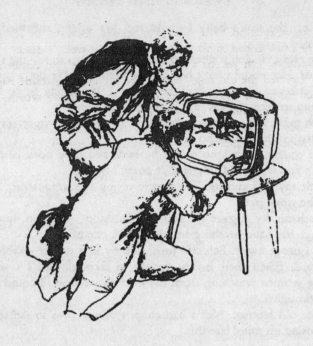

28

As I passed my stethoscope over the old dog's ribs, I wondered how much longer he could last.

'Don's heart isn't any better,' I said to old Mr Chandler, who sat hunched in the armchair by the kitchen fire.

I was doing my best to avoid being gloomy. The heart was definitely worse; in fact, I couldn't remember when I had listened to such a heart. It wasn't just the ordinary murmur of valvular incompetence, it was a swishing, squirting cacophony, filling me with amazement that the life-giving blood could possibly be driven round the organs of the old dog's body.

Don was fourteen, a shaggy collie cross, and with the heart weakness there was the inevitable chronic bronchitis adding its own bubblings and gurglings to the symphony within the chest.

'Aye, maybe so,' Mr Chandler leaned forward in his chair, 'but he's not so bad in other ways. Eats right well, 'e does.'

I nodded. 'Oh yes, he's happy enough, there's no doubt about that.' I patted the old dog's head as he lay on the fireside rug and the tail thumped vigorously as though to prove my words. 'He's not in any pain and still enjoying life.'

'If only it wasn't for that danged cough,' his master grunted. 'He's allus got it and it was worse than ever today. That's why I called ye out.'

'Ah well, he'll never get rid of that now, but I can help him when it gets really bad. I'll give him a shot now and leave some tablets for him.'

After the injection I counted out a supply of the faithful occytets.

'Thank ye, Mr Herriot.' The old man took the packet and placed it on the mantelpiece. 'What do you think his chances are?'

'It's very difficult to say, Mr Chandler.' I hesitated. 'I've seen dogs with bad hearts go on for years, but then – you never know. Anything could happen any time.'

'Aye . . . aye . . . I understand. I'll hope for the best. But it's a bit depressin' when you're an awd widower like me.' He scratched his head and smiled ruefully. 'I've 'ad a rotten night. The television's good company but even that's not workin'.' He pointed to the blank screen in the corner of the room. 'It started goin' funny at teatime. I've twiddled all the flippin' knobs, but it's no good. Do you know anythin' about these things?'

'Afraid not, Mr Chandler, I've only just bought a set myself.' Television was a new wonder in the early fifties and an impenetrable miracle to a non-mechanical mind like mine. However I went over and switched on the set. I began to play with the various dials and knobs, pushing in wires, flicking switches off and on.

I heard a sudden cry from the old man. 'Hey, it's back! The picture's back again!'

I stared unbelievingly at the screen. Sure enough, there was a posse thundering over the Texan plain. Somehow, I had done the trick.

'Eee, that's champion, Mr Herriot!' The old man's face was transfigured. 'That's really cheered me up.'

I felt an unaccustomed flush of triumph. 'Well, I'm glad I was able to help.' But I didn't feel so cheerful as I looked at the dog stretched out on the rug.

'You'll let me know if he gets any worse,' I said, and as I left the cottage I had a nasty feeling that I'd soon be hearing bad news from Mr Chandler. It would be the end of something, because I had become attached to old Don, one of my good-natured patients, a friendly tail-wagger I had treated for years.

I didn't have long to wait. It was seven o'clock in the evening, three days later, when the phone rang.

'It's Chandler 'ere, Mr Herriot.'

The voice was strained and anxious, and I steeled myself for what was coming next.

'I don't what to bother ye, Mr Herriot, but I wonder if ye'd slip out to my place?'

'Yes, of course, Mr Chandler, I'll come straightaway. I can hear how distressed you are.'

'Aye, it's a terrible thing but I know you can fix it.'

I remembered the sounds that had come through my stethoscope, and felt I had to be honest. 'Mr Chandler, fourteen years is a long time. The old valves do wear out, you know.'

'Fourteen? Damned thing is nobbut two!'

'*Two?*' Was the old man going soft? 'Don? Two?'

'Don? Ah didn't say Don. T'awd dog's fine since the tablets. It's that flippin' TV, gone off again. Do ye think ye could come and put it right for me?'

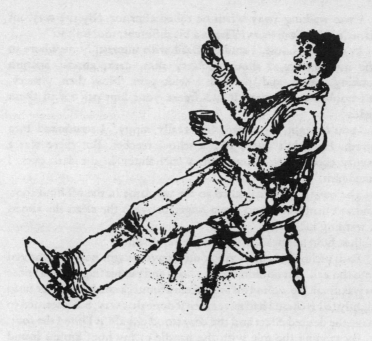

29

Farmer Whitehead rubbed his chin doubtfully.

'I don't really know what to make of this feller,' he said. 'He doesn't seem like a farm man, in fact he says he used to be a school teacher, but you can tell he knows something about stock keeping. Anyway, I'm givin' him a trial. It's a heck of a business finding men who'll work up here in this isolated spot, and I can't be too choosy. Let me know what you think about him.'

I nodded. 'Right, I will. Married man, is he?'

'Not half!' the farmer laughed. 'Seven kids, too.'

'Seven! That's quite a family.'

'Aye, it is. And I suppose it's one reason why I took him on. He seemed desperate for a place to live and we've got a good big cottage here. I felt a bit sorry for the chap.' He paused and looked thoughtfully across the yard. 'As I said, he's out of the ordinary.'

I was walking away when he called after me. 'By the way, his name's Basil Courtenay. That's a bit different, too, isn't it?'

In the cow house, I studied Basil with interest. Somewhere in the mid thirties, I thought. Very slim, dark, almost Spanish looking. He greeted me with a wide grin. 'Now then, vitnery, it's nobbut cold today. It 'ud freeze your lugs off out in them fields.'

'You're right,' I replied, 'it's really nippy.' I scrutinised him afresh. He didn't sound like a school teacher. But there was a jaunty cheerfulness about him, a friendliness in the dark eyes. I liked him.

The cow I had been called to see was lame in the off hind foot, and as I bent down and put a finger between the cleats she aimed a warning kick at me.

'Just hold her head, will you please,' I said.

Basil inclined his head graciously, gave a slight bow and moved into the stall. But he didn't grab a horn and put his fingers in the nose as was usual. He wound his arms round the neck and hugged the head tightly to his chest. I had never seen it done that way, but it seemed to have the desired effect and the cow stood quietly as I lifted the foot.

By tapping the sole with the handle of my hoof knife I found a tender area.

'There's a little abscess in there,' I said. 'I'll have to pare it out. It would be best to pull her leg up over that beam to do it. Can you fetch me a piece of rope, please?'

Again the little inclination of the head, the bow, and he went down the byre with long, graceful steps. When he returned he proffered the rope graciously, bending from the hips rather like a high-class tailor displaying his wares.

I tied the rope round the foot, threw the other end over the beam, and with Basil pulling cheerfully I began to pare the sole.

'I hear you've done a bit of teaching,' I said, as I scraped away at the hard tissue.

'Oh aye, I 'ave. Ah've done a good bit o' that in me time, ah can tell ye.'

'Really. What subjects did you teach?'

'Well now, a bit o' this and a bit o' that. There's nowt ah couldn't turn me 'and to, tha knows.'

'I see. And where did you teach? Which schools?'

'Oh, 'ere and there, 'ere and there. Ah got around a bit, like.'
Basil shook his head and smiled as though the words raised happy
memories.

As I worked on the foot he chattered away and, without being
at all specific, he suggested that he had also taught in universities.

'You actually lectured?'

'Oh aye, ah did, ah did.'

A feeling of unreality was beginning to envelop me, but I had
to ask.

'Which universities?'

'Well . . . 'ere and there, 'ere and there.'

The conversation was brought to a close by a trickle of pus
appearing under my knife, a happy outcome to my paring.

'There it goes.' I said. 'She'll be fine now. I'll give her a shot
and she ought to be sound in a day or two. But I'll want some
hot water to wash my hands.'

Basil made an expansive gesture. 'Ye can come into t'house
and 'ave a proper wash.'

I followed him to the cottage next to the farm buildings and
he threw open the door before ushering me ceremoniously
inside.

A table ran down one side of the big kitchen and the entire
family were at their Saturday dinner. Mrs Courtenay, very fat,
blonde and smiling, presided over an array of healthy-looking
children who were attacking the heaped plates with relish. In the
centre of the floor a sturdy infant was seated on a chamber pot
from whose interior a series of explosive poppings and splutter-
ings accompanied the child's expulsive efforts.

Basil waved a hand over the domestic scene. 'This is ma wife
and family, Mr 'erriot, and we're all right glad to meet ye.'

He did not exaggerate. There was an outburst of eager smiles
and nods from the children as their father looked on proudly. A
happy family indeed.

Basil led me to the kitchen sink which was filled to over-
flowing with the unwashed debris of several meals. In fact, it was
difficult to get my hands under the tap until Basil cleared a small
space for me, pushing greasy pans and dishes to one side, daintily

picking pieces of congealed bacon and sausage from around the soap dish.

As I washed, the toddler on the floor decided to vacate his seat on the chamber pot. Basil went over, lifted the vessel and surveyed the interior with satisfaction. Then he strode to the coke-burning cooker against the wall, lifted the lid and hurled the contents of the pot into the depths. And even this movement was performed with a graceful sweep of the arm.

Mrs Courtenay half rose from her seat. 'You'll 'ave a cup o' tea, Mr 'erriot?'

'No . . . er . . . no, thank you. I have a couple of visits waiting and I must get on. But thank you again, and it's been nice meeting you.'

I had to visit the farm several times over the next few months and Basil seemed to be coping reasonably well with his job. But I couldn't help noticing that he did things differently from all other stockmen I had known; his way of handling the animals was unusual, in fact, his whole approach had something strange about it. On one occasion, in order to get a halter on a loose heifer he hung upside down from a beam — it was as though he had a smattering of the farming business but not a lot of experience.

During my visits, Basil was always full of chat and his conversation was interspersed with shadowy references to his amazingly varied past. Little snippets emerged of his involvement in the acting world, in architecture and many other professions. It seemed, too, that at one time he had taught ballroom dancing. But all attempts to pin him down never got beyond the usual response of "ere and there.'

I also saw Basil a few times in Darrowby. He wasn't a big drinker but he liked to visit one of the local pubs on a Saturday evening, and when I first saw him there I was struck again by his distinctive behaviour. He was at a big table with a bunch of grinning farm men sitting behind tall pint glasses, but Basil wasn't drinking beer. He was lying back in his chair, legs outstretched, and he was holding a glass of red wine, cupped in his palm, the stem protruding beneath his fingers. I had seen people in films — foreign noblemen and the like — holding wine glasses in this way, but never anybody in a Yorkshire pub.

As always, he presented a picture of elegance and grace. Almost reclining in his seat, he was holding forth to his audience, waving a debonair hand to emphasise his points, sipping occasionally at his wine. And it was clear that the farm men were lapping it all up. The outbursts of laughter, the delighted nods, the expressions of amazement all testified to their enthralment in Basil's recital.

He soon became a celebrity among these men and I gathered that, although he was an object of mystery to them, the facet which had most intrigued them was his vague allusions to his university experiences. They christened him 'Professor Baz' and as such he was known throughout the agricultural community. The usual ''ere and there' was all anybody could elicit but, though various theories about him were bandied around, one thing was universal – everybody seemed to like him.

During the month of March I began to see quite a lot of Basil. It is the time of year when the health of livestock is at its lowest ebb. The animals have been confined to the buildings through the long winter and their resistance to disease has worn very thin. Calves especially are vulnerable at this time and the ones under Basil's care had been struck down by the dreaded scour – the highly fatal diarrhoea which has been one of the curses of calf rearing for generations, always lurking, always ready to strike. Any fault in feeding or environment brings trouble.

Fortunately, modern advances have put vastly improved weapons in the hands of the vets and at that time I was having good results with a granular mixture of antibiotics and sulphonamides, but I wasn't doing very well with these calves.

There were sixteen of them in a long row of pens and I looked at them with growing apprehension. They were miserable and depressed, many with whitish liquid faeces trickling down their tails, some prostrate in the straw.

'Basil,' I said, 'are you sure you're getting the right dose into them?'

'Oh aye, Mr 'erriot, just exactly wot you said.'

'And you're giving it to them last thing at night and first thing in the morning? That's important.'

'Definitely. You don't 'ave to worry about that.'

I dug my hands deeper into my pockets. 'Well, I don't understand it. They're not responding. And the next thing's going to be pneumonia. I don't like the look of them at all.'

I administered vitamin injections to back up the medication and left, but I had a nasty feeling that something very unpleasant was just round the corner.

It had been bitterly cold all day and the wind had that piercing quality which usually precedes snow. I wasn't surprised when, around eight o'clock that evening, the big white flakes began to drift down and within an hour the countryside was blanketed in white. The snow stopped then and I was grateful, because a heavy fall made it almost impossible to reach some of the high farms. A shovel was essential equipment.

When I had a call at 7 a.m. next morning to a calving at a remote smallholding at the top of the dale, I was relieved that no more snow had fallen during the night. I had finished the job by nine o'clock and as I drove home, warm with the satisfaction which the delivery of a live calf always gives me, I marvelled at the new world around me. It was always beautiful up there, but the snow had made a magical change, adding a white stillness and peace.

I was looking at the delicate roadside drifts which the wind had shaped so exquisitely in the night when I saw the gate to Mr Whitehead's farm. It was a good chance to check on those calves and I turned my car along the lane.

All was quiet when I reached the buildings and the first thing I noticed was that between Basil's cottage and the calf house stretched a long expanse of unbroken snow.

I knocked at the door and Basil answered, as cheerful and full of bounce as ever.

'Come in, Mr 'erriot! How ista this mornin'? Missus is upstairs makin' the beds. Ah'll shout 'er down and she'll get ye a cup o' tea.'

'No thanks,' I replied, 'I just dropped in to see those calves. How are they this morning?'

'Oh, about t'same, ah reckon.'

'And you've given them the granules?'

'Oh aye, I 'ave. Gave 'em before breakfast.'

I beckoned him to the kitchen window. 'Come over here, Basil.'

Together we looked out and he stood very still as he gazed at the carpet of virgin snow.

'You've never been out there at all, have you?' I said. 'And you weren't out last night, either. That snow stopped at nine o'clock and you were to dose them just before bedtime.'

He didn't say anything, but his head turned slowly towards me, and it was as though a mask had been stripped from his face. The jaunty smile had gone, leaving a terrible defencelessness. He looked at me with hunted eyes.

The transformation was so dramatic that my first anger dissolved. We stared at each other in silence for a few moments then I spoke slowly.

'Now look, Basil, I'm not going to tell your boss about this, but you've let me down badly. Will you promise me you'll do your job properly in future?'

He nodded dumbly.

'Right,' I said. 'Let's get over to the calves now.'

He sat down and began to pull on his wellingtons, then he looked up at me with a haggard expression.

'Ah tell ye, Mr 'erriot, ah don't mean no harm. Ah don't want to neglect them calves, but it's like me heart's not in the job. Ah'm not a proper farm man – never will be.'

I didn't say anything and he went on.

'Ah've spoken to t'boss about it and ah'll be leavin' soon.'

'Have you got another job to go to?'

'Aye ... aye ... ah've got summat in mind. But till ah go, you don't 'ave to worry. Ah'll look after them calves.'

He did, too. From that day the little creatures began to improve and, on my final visit, there was the warming sight of all sixteen of them, frisky and upright in their pens, poking their heads out into the passage as they looked for their food.

Shortly after this, Basil left the district, but the reputation of 'Professor Baz' lingered on, and his departure was bemoaned among the farming community. One cowman expressed the general sentiment to me.

'By gaw, he was a rum feller,' he said, 'but we 'ad some fun with 'im. You couldn't help liking 'im.'

I nodded. 'Yes, that's how I feel. I wonder where he's gone.'

The man laughed. 'Nobody knows, but I expect it'll be '"'ere and there".'

I thought I had seen the last of Basil, but I was wrong. One night, Helen and I drove into Brawton to celebrate her birthday. We had booked for dinner at one of the fine hotels in the town and the festive feeling was strong in us as we sat in the pillared splendour of the dining room, lapped around by the Victorian opulence which is one of Brawton's lasting charms.

It was a special treat for us and we enjoyed every bite of the meal, but as we sat over our coffee I noticed Helen staring intently across the vast room.

'That waiter, Jim, working right at the far end. You've had your back to him, but . . .'

I turned and looked. 'My God!' I said, 'it's Basil!'

I shifted my seat so that I could observe properly and there was no doubt. Basil it was. He was unbelievably elegant in white tie and tails and as he bent to serve an elderly couple it struck me forcibly that with his dark good looks, his courtly manner and his natural grace he was everything that a waiter should be.

I watched, spellbound. He was turning to the lady now, proffering vegetables with that inclination of the head I knew so well, smiling and bowing as she made her choice. He was talking, too, and I could imagine the same effortless flow which had entertained me so often in the cow house. The old couple were nodding and laughing, clearly captivated by him. I wondered what he was telling them. Was it about his colourful past? It looked very like it.

The coffee in my cup turned cold as I sat there. The more I watched him the more convinced I was that Basil had found his niche at last. The graceful way in which he glided among the tables, balancing plates along his arm as though he had been doing it all his life, his happy relaxed attitude, his obvious delight in dealing with his guests. This was really him. I found myself hoping, quite fervently, that there would be no further convolutions in the career of Professor Baz.

'Are you going to speak to him?' Helen asked.

I hesitated. 'No . . . no . . . better not.'

As we left the dining room, we passed within a few feet of the table where he was again attending the white-haired couple. They were all laughing, and the old gentleman raised a hand.

'By the way,' he asked, 'where was it that you were doing this?'

'Oh, 'ere and there,' Basil replied. "ere and there.'

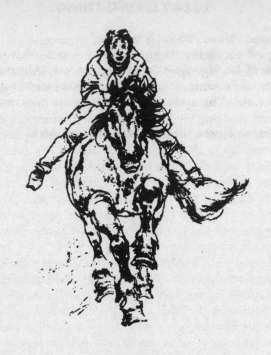

30

Calum gave me a friendly dig in the ribs. 'I wish you'd come with me to watch the deer one morning, Jim. I keep asking you, but I can never pin you down.'

We were sitting over a couple of pints in a cosy corner of the Drovers, and it was comparatively peaceful now that the regulars had become accustomed to the badger. At first, going for a beer with Calum almost caused a riot because he always brought Marilyn slung over his shoulder and the entire population of the bar would converge on us, but the situation had settled down to amused glances and cheerful greetings. The 'vet wi' t'badger' as the farmers called him was part of the local scenery now.

I took a pull at my glass. 'Oh, I will, Calum, I will. I promise you.'

'That's what you always say. Why not tomorrow?' He trained his dark-eyed stare on me and I felt trapped.

'Oh, I don't know. There's a lot doing tomorrow.'

'No, there isn't really. Doug Heseltine cancelled his tuberculin test, and it's left a big gap in the morning. It's an ideal chance.'

I didn't know what to say. Part of me wanted a glimpse of Calum's world of nature – he spent all his spare time roaming the countryside, studying the plants and flowers, observing the habits of the wild creatures – but I felt woefully ignorant by comparison. I had grown up in the big city of Glasgow and though I had fallen in love with the Yorkshire countryside I knew that a deep knowledge of flora and fauna was something best acquired in childhood. Siegfried had it, both my children had it and were always trying to educate me, but I knew I'd never be an expert. Certainly not like Calum. He was steeped in the things of the wild. It was his consuming passion.

'Tomorrow, eh?' As the level of my glass went down, my doubts began to evaporate. 'Well, maybe I could make it.'

'Great, great.' My colleague ordered two more pints. 'We'll go up to Steadforth Woods. I've built a hide there.'

'Steadforth Woods? Surely there aren't any deer in there.'

Calum gave me a secret smile. 'Oh yes, there are – lots of them.'

'Well, I'm amazed. I've passed those woods a thousand times. I've walked my dogs through them, but I've never seen a trace of a deer.'

'You'll see some tomorrow. Just you wait.'

'Okay. When do we start?'

He rubbed his hands. 'I'll pick you up at three o'clock.'

'*Three o'clock!* As early as that?'

'Oh yes, we've got to be up there before daybreak.'

As I finished my second pint the whole thing seemed pleasantly attractive. Up and away before the dawn to plumb the secrets of the woods. I couldn't understand my previous misgivings.

I felt different the next morning when the alarm blasted in my ear at 2.45 a.m. Years of being jerked from slumber in the small hours had bred in me a fierce love of my bed, and here I was deliberately quitting the warm nest to drive out into the cold darkness and sit in a wood – just for fun. I must be mad.

When I met Calum, it was clear he didn't share my feelings.

He was bubbling with enthusiasm and he laughed as he thumped me on the shoulder. 'You're going to love this, Jim. I've really been looking forward to doing this with you.'

I shivered as I got into his car. It was bitterly cold and the street was like a pitch black well. I huddled in the seat and Calum drove away, whistling.

He kept up a bright chatter on the way and it was easy to see that this was Calum in his natural element, roaming the countryside while the world was asleep, but after we had covered a few miles I knew something was wrong.

'Hey,' I said, 'this isn't the way to Steadforth Woods. We should have taken a left turn back there.'

He turned to me with a smile. 'We're going a different way. My hide is at the far end of the woods, a long way from the main road. We get to it from Fred Welburn's farm.'

'Fred Welburn's! My God, we'll have to walk about two miles!'

'Don't worry. I've arranged transport.'

'Transport . . . ? What *are* you talking about?'

Calum giggled. 'You'll see.'

We left the car near Fred Welburn's farm which was perched on high ground from which the field stretched away down a steep slope to a stream before rising again towards the edge of the distant woods. It was still dark and I knew this only from memory. In total bewilderment, I wondered about the transport.

Calum reached in to the back of the car and produced a bucket of corn.

I stared at him. 'What's that for?'

'It's for the horses.'

'Horses?'

'Yes. I'm going to tempt those two horses over to us so that we can ride them down into the woods.'

'What! You never said anything about that!' I burst out.

He smiled reassuringly. 'Oh, it's all right. It'll make everything much easier.' He rattled his bucket and my mouth fell open as two enormous Shires came trotting out of the gloom, their great hooves thudding on the grass.

'This is crazy!' I stared in disbelief at the animals. I was no equestrian, especially when it came to riding cart horses bare-backed.

'We can't ride those bloody great things! And what about Fred Welburn? What's he going to say?'

'All taken care of. I've got permission from Fred to use them whenever I want them. Come on, now, I'll give you a leg up.'

I was still protesting when he hoisted me on to the nearest animal and scrambled on to the other. He dug in his heels, gave a joyous whoop, and before I knew what was happening we were thundering down the grassy slope.

'Hang on,' cried Calum. 'There's a beck at the foot of the hill.'

He didn't have to tell me. I was hanging on as never before, gripping the mane tightly, eyes popping, absolutely certain that, within seconds, I would be cast from the great smooth back into the outer darkness. But somehow I kept my seat as our mounts leaped the stream like steeplechasers, then we were off again, galloping up the hill on the other side.

We were going at a terrifying pace, but it didn't seem to be fast enough for Calum who kept yelling encouragement at his steed. Dimly ahead, I saw him hurtling through a narrow gateway and I suffered a moment's panic at the certain thought that my fat animal would never get through that opening. I was partly right because the gatepost caught my knee such a fearful whack that I thought my leg had been torn off.

We made a hectic traverse of another long field, then my colleague pulled up and dismounted.

'My, that was great!' he breathed as I slithered groaning on to the grass. 'But you're lame! What's wrong?'

'Cracked my knee on the gate back there,' I grunted as I hobbled around, rubbing the painful joint.

'Oh, sorry about that, but it saved us a long walk. We're right up to the woods now.'

We climbed a fence and he led me for a long way among the dark trunks into the very heart of the wood, to his hide which he had built near a clearing. In the first pale light I could see that it was a well-hidden place, carefully constructed of branches of larch and spruce and tufts of grass.

'Sit here,' whispered my colleague. He was clearly in a state of high excitement, his eyes wide, a half smile on his face.

We hadn't long to wait. As the dawn light filtered through the branches, there was a rustling and a sound of movement among the trees, then, one by one, the deer began to appear in the clearing. Through all the years I had never seen a deer in these woods but here they were there in profusion; gentle does and majestic, antlered stags moving around, cropping the grass. It was a scene of indescribable peace and beauty, and with the feeling that I was a privileged observer I sat there enthralled, all my discomforts forgotten. There was a badger sett nearby and Calum pointed in delight as his favourite animals came out to play with their young.

Afterwards we walked through the scented silence of the woods, the pine needles soft under our feet, and he talked, not only about the deer, but about the other wild creatures of the forest and about the plants and flowers which flourished in those secret places. He seemed to know it all and I began to understand the depths of the interest which coloured his entire life. He held the key to a magic world.

As we reached the field the sun came out and, looking back, I could see long drifts of bluebells among the dark boles of the trees, and in the glades, where the first rays struck through the branches, primroses and anemones shone like scattered jewels.

By the time we had ridden back up the hill – slowly and gently at my request – and I had limped to the car, my knee had stiffened up and I groaned as I dragged my leg inside.

'Oh, bad luck about your knee.' Calum gave me a sympathetic smile, then his expression changed. 'But never mind, I've got a surprise for you.'

I could feel my eyes narrowing to slits as I looked at him. 'What kind of surprise?'

He grinned widely. 'I want you to come to dinner with me.'

'Dinner? Where?'

'In my flat. I know Helen's going to a meeting tonight and she was to leave you something to eat. Well, I've arranged it with her. I'm going to give you a meal. We're having roast duck.'

'Duck! Who's cooking it?'

'I am. It will be plucked and roasted by my own fair hand.'

My head began to swim a little. I knew he kept ducks at the bottom of the garden – an activity which Siegfried regarded with a jaundiced eye as being part of a 'menagerie' – but all this, coming from a man who had no interest in food and, in fact, seemed to eat only on rare occasions, was difficult to take in. But I was sure he was trying to be kind.

'Well, Calum . . . it's very good of you . . . what time do you want me?'

'Eight o'clock on the dot.'

At the appointed time I climbed the stairs to the flat and received an effusive welcome. Calum sat me down with a drink and as he went through to the kitchen I looked round the little sitting room. It was exactly as when he walked in that first day. Previous occupants had added or altered things according to their taste but Calum had not the slightest interest in carpets, curtains or furniture. The table was bare except for two sets of knives and forks and salt and pepper.

He was soon back again, banging down a plate for each of us, then a delicious aroma drifted in from the kitchen as he opened the oven door.

'Here we are, Jim!' he cried triumphantly as he carried in a roasting tin containing two ducks. He speared one bird with a fork and clumped it on my plate, then took the other for himself.

I was waiting for the vegetables and other trimmings, but Calum dropped into his chair and waved a fork at me. 'Wade in, Jim, I do hope you'll enjoy it.'

I looked down at my plate. Well, so this was dinner with Calum. A duck apiece with no adornment. He was eating busily and I started on my bird, but I was slowed down by the fact that my colleague had left quite a number of feathers on and I had to pick my way gingerly among the quills and crisped up plumage.

Nothing seemed to deter Calum, however, and he ate rapidly, then sat back with a sigh of deep contentment. I was surprised at his speed until it occurred to me that he probably hadn't bothered to have any food for the last twenty-four hours or so.

We didn't have dessert or coffee or anything like that and it wasn't long before he was ushering me out.

Around ten o'clock Helen came back from her meeting. 'Well, how was your day with Calum?' she asked as she took off her coat.

I rubbed my knee. Somehow it wasn't an easy question to answer. 'I enjoyed it. It was fun ... exciting ... quite fascinating ...' I was casting around for the word. 'It was different!'

She laughed. 'You've just about described Calum.'

'That's it,' I said, laughing too, 'it was a Calum day.'

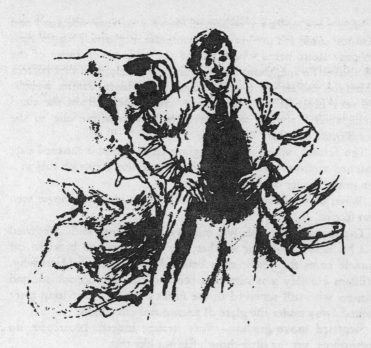

31

'That was old William Hawley,' Siegfried said as he put down
the phone. 'Sounded a bit agitated. One of his calves is laid out
unconscious, thinks it may be dying, and he hasn't many of
them, poor old lad. We'll have to get there quick.'

I looked up from the appointments book. 'But we've got to take
those tumours off Colonel Foulter's horse at ten this morning.'

'Yes, I know, but we can drop in at Hawley's place on the
way. It's in the same direction.'

It was a familiar situation as we drove off together. Siegfried
eagerly anticipating one of his equine operations; myself, his
anaesthetist, by his side and our enamel tray with all the freshly
sterilised instruments rattling behind us in the back. It was a fine
morning which was good, because the open fields were our
operating table.

After three miles we struck off down a narrow side road and soon we could see the Hawley farmhouse, not much bigger than the grey stone barns which dotted the wide green miles of the fell above. To me, those barns, squat and sturdy, and that pattern which the endless stone walls traced on the high pastures were at the very heart of the Dales scene. As I looked from the car I thought, as I always did, that there was nowhere else in the world quite like this.

The farmer, white hair straggling from under a tattered cap, watched anxiously as Siegfried bent over the prostrate calf in a pen in the corner of the cow house.

'What do ye make of it, Mr Farnon?' he asked. 'I've never seen owt like it.'

The appeal in his eyes was mingled with a deep faith. Siegfried was his hero, a wonder worker, the man who had brought off miracle cures for years, even before I had come to Darrowby. William Hawley was one of a breed of simple, unsophisticated farmers who still survived in the fifties but who have long since melted away under the glare of science and education.

Siegfried spoke gravely. 'Very strange indeed. No scour, no pneumonia, yet the little thing's flat out like this.'

Carefully and methodically he went over the little body with his stethoscope, auscultating heart, lungs and abdomen. He took the temperature, opened the mouth and peered at the tongue and throat, examined the eyes and ran his hand over the roan hairs of the coat. Then slowly he straightened up. His face was expressionless as he looked down at the motionless form.

Suddenly he turned to the old man. 'William,' he said, 'would you be so kind as to fetch me a piece of string.'

'Eh?'

'A piece of string, please.'

'String?'

'Yes, about this length.' Siegfried spread his arms wide. 'And quickly, please.'

'Right, right . . . I'll get ye some. Now where can I lay me hands on a bit that length?' Flustered, he turned to me. 'Can ye come and give me a hand, Mr Herriot?'

'Certainly.' I followed him as he hurried from the cow house and outside he clutched at my arm. It was clear he had only asked me to come with him to enlighten him.

'What does 'e want a piece of string for?' he asked in bewilderment.

I shrugged. 'I really have no idea, Mr Hawley.'

He nodded gleefully as though that was only what he expected. An ordinary vet couldn't possibly know what was in the mind of Mr Farnon, a man of legendary skill who was known to employ many strange things in the practice of his art – puffs of purple smoke to cure lame horses, making holes in jugular veins and drawing off buckets of blood to cure laminitis. Old William had heard all the stories and he was in no doubt that if anybody could restore his animal to health by means of a piece of string, it would be Mr Farnon.

But the maddening thing was that as we trotted round the buildings he couldn't find such a thing.

'Dang it,' he said. 'There's allus a coil of binder twine hangin' there, but it isn't there now! And I'm allus trippin' over bits o' string all over t'place, but not today. What'll he think of a farmer wi' no string?'

In a growing panic he rushed around and he was almost in tears when he saw a piece lying across a heap of sacks. 'How about this, Mr Herriot? Is it t'right length?'

'Just about right, I'd say.'

He grabbed it and ran as fast as his elderly limbs would carry him back to Siegfried.

'Here y'are, Mr Farnon,' he panted. 'Ah'm not too late, am I? He's still alive?'

'Oh yes, yes.' Siegfried took the string and held it dangling for a moment as he measured the length with his eye. Then, as we watched, wide-eyed, he quickly tied it round his waist.

'Thank you so much, William,' he murmured, 'that's much better. I couldn't work with that damned coat flapping open as I bent over. I lost a couple of buttons yesterday. Cow got her horn underneath them and tore them off – it's always happening to me.'

'But ... but ... the string ...' The old man's face was a picture of woe. 'Ye can't do anything for my calf, then?'

'Of course I can. Whatever makes you think I can't?'

'Well . . . do ye know what ails him?'

'Yes, I do. He's got CCN.'

'What's that?'

'Cerebrocortical necrosis. It's a brain disease.'

'It's a terrible big name. And his brain? It'll be a hopeless case?'

'Not a bit. I'm going to inject vitamin B into his vein. It usually works like a charm. Just hold his head for a moment. You see how it's bent over his back? That's called opisthotonos — typical of this condition.'

Siegfried quickly carried out the injection and got to his feet. 'One of us will be passing your door tomorrow, so we'll look in. I'd like to bet he'll be a lot better.'

It was I who called next day and indeed the calf was up and eating. William Hawley was pleased.

'Must have been wonderful stuff Mr Farnon gave 'im,' he said.

To him it was another miracle, but in his manner I sensed something of the deflation I had seen the day before when Siegfried tied up his coat. His favourite vet had done the trick again, but I knew that in his heart there was still the wistful regret that he hadn't done it with that piece of string.

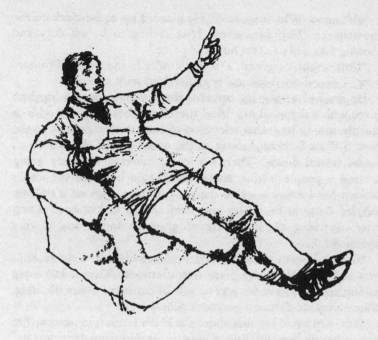

32

Siegfried, lounging by the fireside, was at his most expansive. 'Nice of you to drop in, James. Good to see you at any time – we don't get much chance to talk during the day, eh?'

I had called in at his home after an evening call nearby. He had pressed a drink on me and then flopped down in the armchair, exuding bonhomie. 'Any problems?'

'No, no. I've just been to a milk fever at John Lancaster's. The cow was up when I left.'

'Ah, splendid, splendid. He's a nice chap, is John.'

'Yes, a good bloke. He was really pleased when I slapped that beast on the rump and she staggered to her feet.'

'Excellent. The little triumphs of veterinary practice. I've had that sort of day, too – everything going well and, my word, isn't it grand to settle down by the fire on a cold night and relax with a quiet mind. What time is it?' He glanced up at the clock on the mantelpiece. 'Half past seven. Nice feeling to be off duty and looking forward to a few hours of peace.'

'That's right, Siegfried. I'm on. You're in the clear till tomorrow.' I sipped my drink and regarded him with affection.

He reached a long leg towards the fire and poked a log into place with a slippered toe. 'And there's another thing – it adds to the pleasure to have that television to look at.' He pointed to the new TV set flickering about at the other side of the hearth, its sound turned down. 'There's a lot of inverted snobbery going around – people talking about the goggle box and the idiot's lantern but I enjoy a lot of the programmes. I know it's a new fangled thing in the Dales but, I tell you, I've just been sitting here, watching an interesting programme and I find it very soothing.'

He sank lower in his chair and stretched his legs to the blaze. 'I was at Derek Mattock's place this afternoon. They'd had a pig killing and they gave me a great pile of cuttings – spare rib, liver, fillet – they are the most generous people.'

'Yes, you could say that about the Dales farmers in general. I'm always getting presents. Butter, eggs, vegetables from their gardens.'

Siegfried nodded. 'How true. I had a long talk with Derek and he mentioned something I'd better tell you about. You promised to do some de-hornings for him about a fortnight ago and he hasn't heard from you.' He gave me a quizzical look.

'Oh, damn, yes! I'll get on to him tomorrow. The beasts aren't taking any harm, anyway.'

He smiled again from down among the cushions. 'No, my boy – but you forgot, didn't you?'

'Yes, I suppose I did. But I'll put it right.'

'I'm sure you will, James.' He nodded gravely and was silent for a few moments. 'Strangely enough, there was something else in the same vein. Bob Hardy told me his tuberculin test was overdue. You said you'd do it last month.'

I shrugged. 'Oh, hell, that's right. But it's only a week or two overdue. Not serious. I'll see to it.'

Siegfried gave me the smile again and wagged a finger. 'But you forgot, didn't you?'

'Okay, okay, but as I say –'

'If you'll excuse me, James, for just a moment.' He held up a hand. 'You are inclined to forget things quite frequently. It is a tiny flaw in an otherwise excellent character. There is no more conscientious and capable veterinary surgeon than yourself and yet being forgetful can project quite a different image. People can think you're not concerned about their animals, that you don't care.'

'Wait a minute –'

'Let me finish, James. This is for your own good.' He put his fingertips together. 'Forgetfulness is a trait which can be easily cured if you know how to go about it. These unfortunate incidents can be prevented if you simply impress on your mind right at the beginning what it is you want to remember.'

'My God, this is really rich . . . what about . . . ?'

'One moment more, my dear chap. As I say, whenever you make an appointment, make a definite conscious effort to imprint that promise strongly on your mind. It's perfectly easy – I use this method regularly myself. You'll always remember that way.'

I was about to raise my strong objections to being lectured on forgetfulness by the most forgetful man in Yorkshire when the phone rang.

Siegfried extended a languid arm and picked up the receiver. 'Ah, how are you, Wilf, my old friend?' His eyes were half closed as he burrowed deeper in the cushions.

'I'm awright, Mr Farnon,' came the full-throated reply. It was Wilf Bramley, president of the local farmers' discussion group. He was one of the old school who considered it helped the voice to carry across the miles if they shouted and I could hear him clearly from where I sat. 'But I just 'ope you're awright, too.'

'I'm absolutely grand, Wilf,' Siegfried murmured, holding the receiver well away from his ear.

'Ah well, that's good. We just thowt something had happened to you.'

'Happened . . . ? Why is that?'

'Well, the hall's full – packed to t'doors and we were expectin' you half an hour ago. We worried you might have had an accident on your rounds.'

Siegfried snapped suddenly upright and his mouth fell open. 'Hall . . . ?'

'Aye, there must be two hundred of us 'ere. You gave us such a grand talk last year I knew there'd be a lot wantin' to hear you again and they're all waitin' patiently. We can't start without t'speaker, tha knows! Heh–heh–heh!'

Siegfried's expression was haggard. He seemed to have aged several years in those few moments. 'I really am frightfully sorry, Wilf, I . . .'

'Nay, nay, Mr Farnon, there's no need for you to apologise. A busy feller like you. You'll never know what's goin' to happen from one minute to the next. Rushed off your feet all the time. You can't help bein' a bit late now and again.' Wilf's voice swelled even more in volume. 'After all, we know you're not just sittin' there watchin' television! Heh–heh, heh–heh!'

Siegfried's eyes bulged. 'Yes, Wilf, yes, that's right . . . of course. Ha–ha–ha! What an idea. Ha–ha–ha!' The strangled laughter emerged with difficulty from the distraught face. 'I'm nearly ready – I'll be with you in a few minutes.'

My partner crashed the receiver down and catapulted from his chair. 'Got to go, James. See you in the morning.'

As he galloped towards the door, an unworthy impulse welled in me.

'Siegfried!' I called.

He stopped at the door and glared at me, wild–eyed.

I wagged a finger at him, feeling my features creasing into a leer. 'You forgot, didn't you?'

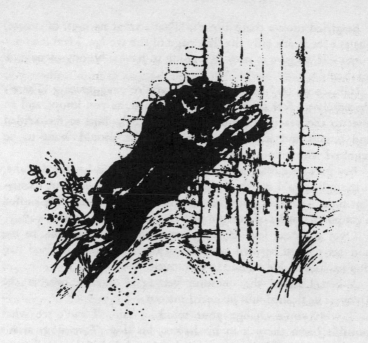

33

Siegfried caught my arm as I passed him coming out of the dispensary. He looked harassed.

'James,' he burst out, 'Calum wants another dog now! Has he mentioned it to you?'

'He did say something. Said he was going to speak to you about it. Apparently it's a dog he's had for some time. It's with his mother and he just wants to bring it to Darrowby. It's okay for him to do that, isn't it?'

My colleague stuck out his chin. 'I don't think it is. He started with a badger and a dog, now he's got two badgers and a dog, and on top of that he wants two badgers and two dogs up in that little flat. Anyway, I've told him it's not on.'

'Oh, I think you're being a bit hard, Siegfried. He's probably lonely, living on his own. He just wants his animals for company.'

Siegfried took a sharp breath. 'That's what he says, of course, but as I see it, it's only the thin edge of the wedge. I feel it in my bones – if we give in now he's going to have a bloody menagerie up there!'

'Oh, come on,' I said, laughing 'you're exaggerating. There's absolutely no fear of that. He's a good lad, as you know, and an asset to the practice. I think we should help him to feel settled and happy and it's only natural that he should want to be reunited with his other dog.'

My partner did some more rapid breathing as he stared at me. 'I thought you'd say that. You're too easily swayed. But I know I'm right – I'm not going to have it, and that's final.' He stuffed a couple of bottles of calcium into his pockets and strode away.

Over the next few days, Calum made several appeals to me and his request seemed perfectly reasonable, but Siegfried had dug his toes in. He refused to be moved.

When I raised the question yet again over a beer at the Drovers he flushed, but he heard me out.

'I wish you'd change your mind,' I said. 'I can't see what possible harm there is in his having his dog. Two dogs aren't much more trouble than one. And as I said, he's doing well and I think he should be encouraged. You've just got a thing about him – your worries are absolutely groundless.'

'Groundless, eh?' He choked a little in mid swallow, then put down his glass. 'I don't think so. I've got this feeling and it won't go away.' He paused and looked round the bar for a few moments. 'But you're beginning to wear me down and I'm tired tonight. I see you are both going to go on and on about this, so you can tell him to go ahead and do as he likes.'

I clapped him on the shoulder and laughed. 'Oh, thanks, Siegfried. I know it's the right thing. You'll never regret it.'

He gave me a weary smile. 'You may laugh, but I tell you, we'll be making a big mistake.' He waved a finger in my face. 'I'll regret it, all right. Mark my words!'

Next morning, Calum was delighted when I gave him the news and I felt a glow of satisfaction when, a few days later, I heard the sound of fresh barking from the top flat.

Siegfried was opening some letters in the office and I turned to him with a smile. 'Nice to hear that,' I said. 'Calum will be happy now.'

He gave me a cold look in return and just then our assistant walked into the office. By his side were two enormous Dobermann Pinschers.

'What the hell's this?' Siegfried enquired, rising to his feet.

'Oh, just my other dogs,' Calum replied with a light laugh. 'Meet Maggie and Anna.'

'*Dogs!*' Siegfried exploded. 'You said *dog* before!'

'Oh, I know. That was my intention. I was just going to bring Maggie, but poor Anna looked so pathetic, I hadn't the heart to leave her behind. They're such friends, and really, they're as gentle as old sheep.'

'They don't look so bloody gentle to me!' My partner's voice rose to a shout. 'You get round me to bring an extra dog here, then you walk in with these two killers!'

There was something in what he said. An air of quiet menace surrounded the Dobermanns, something unnerving in the way they stood motionless, tall and lean, looking thoughtfully from one strange man to the other. They gave me the impression that they could go into unpleasant action at any moment.

'This just isn't good enough!' Siegfried was working up into full cry, waving a hand in Calum's face, when the dogs, resenting the display of aggression, began to growl, softly but chillingly, their eyes fixed on my partner's face, their lips quivering, showing a lot of white teeth.

'Quiet!' rapped Calum. 'Sit!' Both dogs dropped immediately onto their haunches and looked up at him adoringly. Clearly, they, like all animals, were in his thrall.

'Well, there's a cow down at Jack Skinner's.' The young man consulted his list. 'I'd better get on.' He turned and left with the two big creatures trotting at his heels.

Siegfried looked at me wearily. 'Remember what I said? It's started.'

The following week I was coming down the garden path to the back of the house when I heard the sounds – a loud barking and snarling accompanied by a man's voice calling for help. There was a smaller yard immediately outside the operating room and the noise seemed to be coming from there. We didn't use this little yard very much – it held the surgery's dustbins, an outhouse and an ancient outside privy which had been there since the early days of the house.

There was a side door which led from the garden to the yard and I peered through. It was Siegfried's voice raised in frantic appeal that was coming from the old toilet whose door hung crazily on one hinge and to my horror I saw the two Dobermanns hurling themselves repeatedly at this flimsy bastion and baying for blood. My blood froze. My partner was in there and if that old door gave way something terrible was going to happen. There was nothing I could do. I am not afraid of dogs but I had a sure conviction that if I exposed myself to those two I wouldn't last very long.

I rushed from the garden and into the house. 'Calum! Calum!' I yelled.

He came running down the stairs and when he heard the uproar he galloped through with me to the back of the house. 'Maggie! Anna! You bad dogs! Come here at once!'

The noise was switched off immediately and the Dobermanns came slinking round Calum's feet, looking up at him furtively, their faces fixed in ingratiating grins. 'Get upstairs!' he shouted, and the dogs shot off into the house.

Wisely, Calum decided to follow them, leaving Siegfried to me. I dragged the broken door open to release one very cross veterinary surgeon. 'By God, James,' he said, wild-eyed, 'that was a near go! I was picking plums last night and I ate a few too many. Got caught short and had to make a dash for the nearest loo. I was just lowering myself on to the seat when those two man-eaters came roaring into the yard and I only just managed to jam the door with one foot against it. I'm bloody sure if I had moved that foot an inch they'd have had me! I've been stuck in there for ages!'

'Gosh. I'm sorry, Siegfried,' I said. I wasn't just sorry. I was riddled with guilt. This was my fault. I was the one who had persuaded my partner against his better judgment and he had been so right. The menagerie was on its way.

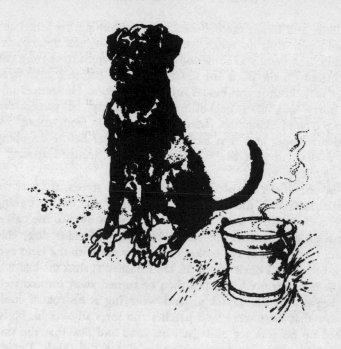

34

Eight o'clock on a Saturday evening and as I prepared to visit a sick calf the phone rang.

'This is Mr Birse, number 10 Ivy Street. I 'ave a dog bad, will you come?'

'What's the trouble, Mr Birse?'

'Doan't know. Won't eat. Will you come?' The voice was surly and impatient. It sounded as though the man had other, more pressing affairs to attend to.

'All right. I'll be along very soon.'

Bonk went the phone at the other end and I pondered, not for the first time, on the fact that vets weren't regarded as people. They had no interest in staying at home with their families on a Saturday night like others.

Number 10 was one of a long row of mean, brick-built

dwellings and I rang the bell and waited. Nothing happened and I tried again. Still no result, yet I could tell by the light in the window that there was somebody at home. I must have rung and hammered on the door for several minutes before a man aged about fifty, in shirt and braces, opened the door. He seemed in a big hurry and, after beckoning peremptorily, he turned and almost trotted along the passage and into the front room. He stabbed a finger at a dog basket in the corner before dropping into a chair to join the family who were grouped around a blaring television set.

Not one of the intent faces, staring at the screen, showed the slightest interest in me and when it was clear that I wasn't going to get a case history from any of them, I went over to the basket to inspect my patient. He was a big black labrador dog, chin resting on the rim of the basket looking at me with the kind eyes of his breed. As I knelt down his tail thrashed against the bedding and he licked at my hand, but then he turned away immediately and began a frantic scratching and worrying at his coat. I could see now that there were bald patches and sores all over his body. I lifted up his fore leg and then his hind and saw that the skin inflammation was most intense under elbow and thigh. Typical sarcoptic mange, but in this case neglected until the sheer misery of the irritation had put the poor animal off his food.

I was pretty sure of my diagnosis but decided to take the routine skin scraping. Nobody took any notice as I went out to the car for scalpel and slide, leaving the door ajar. Back inside, I scraped a little of the inflamed tissue onto the glass slide and slipped it into an envelope as the dog gazed at me patiently and the television boomed.

When I had finished I went into the kitchen and washed my hands at a sink filled with dirty dishes to which congealed vegetables and Yorkshire pudding adhered. Back in the living room I looked round the unheeding group. Father, mother, and a son and daughter in their twenties all puffing cigarettes, all gaping wide-eyed at the bawling screen. I had to communicate somehow and I chose father.

'Your dog has mange,' I shouted into his ear. For an instant his eyes flickered toward me, then, as the screen belched out a screech of brakes and a volley of shots, they resumed their hypnotic stare.

I held out two packets of my activated sulphur mange wash. More modern treatments for external parasites were coming on to the market, but I had always had great results with my beloved Number Three Wash as we called it and I remained faithful to it.

'Follow the directions on the packet,' I bellowed. 'Give him a really thorough bath tomorrow and be sure to get into every nook and cranny of his body. Repeat with the other pack in a week and then I'll have another look at him.'

Mr Birse nodded, glassy-eyed. It didn't seem as though I could do anything more, so I put the packets on the sideboard and let myself out.

In the dark street I leaned on my car for a moment. Strange things happened in veterinary practice, but this was really very strange. All that time in there without a word spoken and why, after they had let that nice dog get into such a state which must have taken several weeks, had they decided to call assistance on a Saturday night? Ah well, part of the rich tapestry. I got into the car and drove away.

The sick calf was at Mr Farrow's farm, two miles outside Darrowby. I walked into the fold yard where the farmer was forking straw to bed up a group of young heifers. When he saw me he put down his fork and opened his arms wide in delight. 'Well, Mr Herriot, well, well, well.'

He spoke the words slowly, almost reverently and a delighted smile transfigured his face. 'I'm sorry to bother ye on a Saturday night, but it is lovely to see you again. It's been a long time!' His tall son went by with a sack of meal on his shoulder and he, too, grinned and waved.

I was about to turn into the calf house when Mr Farrow held up a hand. 'Nay, nay, you'll 'ave to come and see t'missus first.' He hurried with me to the farm kitchen.

'Edith, Edith!' he called out eagerly. 'Here's Mr Herriot come to see us again!'

Mrs Farrow was a shy lady, but she got up from her chair and gave me a gentle smile. 'Well, Mr Herriot, it's a bit since you were here. You're a sight for sore eyes. I'll put t'kettle on and you'll come in for a cup o' tea when you're done, won't you?'

'Yes, thank you very much, I will.' I went out into the yard, feeling the cold air on my face but warmed inside by the welcome. The Farrows were always like that but it was particularly sweet after my visit to the Birse household.

The difference in their concern for their animal, too, was marked. The calf was suffering from a congestion of the lungs which could easily have progressed into pneumonia and after I had injected it, the farmer and his son, without my telling them, began to thread binder twine through the corners of a thick sack and by the time I was ready to leave, the little creature's chest was warmly wrapped.

'That's good to see,' I said. 'With all these new sulpha drugs and antibiotics it's easy to forget the nursing of animals, but it's still so important.'

Back in the surgery I put my skin scraping under the microscope and the nasty little *Sarcoptes scabei* looked up at me; the unpleasant, bristly-legged mite which was burrowing pitilessly into the skin of that nice dog and making his life a torment. However, it was better than the other horror, the cigar-shaped Demodex which sounded the death knell of so many dogs.

Demodectic mange was often incurable, but my trusty Number Three Wash would clear up this present case, bad as it was. And yet, over the weekend, the thought kept recurring; would those Birses have done the job properly? Would they have done it at all? Somehow, the solicitude of the Farrows with their calf seemed to make the situation almost unbearable.

By Monday morning I could stand it no longer and I rang the doorbell at 10, Ivy Street. 'Good morning, Mrs Birse,' I said breezily. 'I was just passing and thought I'd have another look at your dog.'

'Aye, well . . .' The woman seemed a little nonplussed, but as she hesitated I slipped past her and into the front room.

The big dog was still in his basket and my two white packets were on the sideboard where I had put them.

'We've been a bit busy,' she muttered. 'We'll get 'im done tonight.'

I looked at the dog. I have always thought that there is a special beauty in the lustrous coat of a black labrador but this was a desecration. The ravaged skin looked even worse in the daylight and the hind legs moved convulsively in response to the constant itching.

'What's his name?' I asked.

'Jet.'

I bent down and stroked the dog's head. 'Poor old Jet,' I said. 'You are in a state.' And as the tail thumped and the tongue reached for my hand I made up my mind.

'Give me a bucket of warm water, will you please, Mrs Birse. I'll give him his first treatment. It'll only take a minute or two.'

'Come on, lad,' I said, and Jet trotted obediently after me into the back garden where a few tired-looking Brussels sprouts stood among a jungle of weeds. I tipped the packet into the water and stirred the mixture rapidly, feeling an irrational compulsion to get at those mange mites. I felt a bit awkward, too, because I had never done this on a client's premises before but I decided I didn't care and slapped the thick liquid on to Jet's coat with a kind of savage joy.

As I rubbed the stuff into the dog's skin, working it deeply into the clefts of thigh and elbow, he looked up at me happily, his tail waving. Dogs in my experience hate being bathed, but it seemed as though the big animal was only too pleased to have any sort of attention. He was enjoying the whole thing.

As I worked I became aware of a head watching me over the garden hedge. I looked up and an elderly man nodded cheerfully.

'Mornin'. You'll be t'vitnery.'

'That's right.'

He blew out his cheeks. 'By gaw, you must be a busy feller goin' round washin' all them dogs all the time.'

I smiled at his idea of a veterinary surgeon's life. 'Oh, yes, it's quite a job.'

I was aware of his intent gaze as I completed my shampoo and began a brisk towelling, happy in the knowledge that I had delivered the first blow against those malignant little beasties in the skin.

'Grand dog, that,' said the old man.

'He is indeed.'

The man lowered his voice to a conspiratorial whisper. 'Them folks don't bother with 'im, tha knows. He's in a 'ell of a state.'

I didn't say anything, but the sight of Jet standing bedraggled and half bald like a canine scarecrow bore out his words.

'Can ye cure 'im?'

'I think so, but it's going to take time and regular bathing with this stuff of mine. Every week until he's right.'

'Next week for a start, eh?'

'That's right. I'm going to ask Mrs Birse to do it next Monday.'

'You'll be lucky,' the old man grunted and his head moved away from the hedge.

In the kitchen I passed on my instructions to Mrs Birse and she sniffed. 'Ah see you've been talkin' to awd Howell. He's a nosy awd bugger. Allus watchin' ower that hedge.'

Nosy or not, I thought, he was a lot more concerned about her dog than she was. And as I took my leave with a last look back at Jet wagging his tail cheerfully despite his plight, I knew that I'd be back at No 10 next Monday.

And, feeling daft but determined, I was duly there on the day, ringing that bell. Mrs Birse displayed her usual lack of enthusiasm and beckoned me unsmilingly into the house. She led me into the back garden and jerked her head in the direction of the hedge.

'Them next door's doin' 'im.' She turned and went back into the house.

I looked over the hedge. In the middle of a tidy little garden Jet was standing by a steaming bucket while Mr Howell and his wife busily rubbed the mange wash into his coat.

The old man looked up at me and grinned. 'Now then, vitnery, we're doin' your job. Them Birses would never bath 'im every week like you said so I asked if we could have a go. We like this dog.'

'Well . . . that's fine. You're doing a good job, too.'

Jet looked up at me and although his face was thickly smeared with my concoction his eyes danced with pleasure and his tail lashed. This, he was telling me, is great. As the two old people worked, they were talking to him all the time. 'Now then, a bit more on 'ere, Jet, lad.' 'Let's have hold of that other leg, old feller.' The friendly murmurings went on, and the big dog was lapping up the unaccustomed affection.

I watched until they were finished and as they towelled my patient I spoke again. 'That's absolutely terrific. You've done him properly, you haven't missed an inch.'

The old lady smiled. 'Aye, well, we heard what you said at t'start. We want to get 'im better.'

'Good ... good ... you're going the right way about it.' I looked at Jet, still as bare and scruffy as ever. 'You understand that it's going to be a long time before his coat gets back to normal, if it ever does, but the main question is – is he scratching less?'

'Oh aye,' replied Mr Howell. 'He still does a bit, but nothing like before. He's much less itchy now, and he's eatin' well again.'

'Fine, fine. So far, so good, but there's a lot of work still to do. Are you prepared to do this for several weeks? After all, he isn't your dog.'

'Oh, we'll do 'im all right,' said the old lady eagerly. 'We'll stick to 'im – you needn't worry about that.'

I looked at the two Howells in wonder. 'You're real dog lovers, aren't you. And yet you haven't got a dog of your own?'

There was a silence. 'Oh, we did 'ave,' said the old man. 'Had 'im for twelve years, but you never saw him, Mr Herriot, because he never ailed a thing.' He paused and swallowed. 'But he was knocked down and killed just a month ago.'

I gazed for a few moments at the stricken faces. 'I'm so sorry, I know what it's like. It's awful. But ... you didn't think of getting another dog? It's the only thing to do, you know.'

Mrs Howell shrugged. 'We understand that and we thought about it, but we're both in our seventies and if we got a pup now and anythin' happened to us he'd be left and we'd never know if he was properly looked after.'

I nodded and looked at the old couple with renewed respect. It was the attitude of caring people.

'Anyway,' I said, 'you've got a good friend in Jet for the time being. I can see that he appreciates all you're doing for him. I'll leave you a few more packets of the wash and I know he'll be in good hands.'

My confidence was such that I didn't bother to call at the house and it was three weeks before I saw Jet again. The Howells were shopping in the market place and Jet was by their side. He was cheerful, but his skin was still wrinkled and hairless with many half-healed sores.

'You've got him out, then,' I said.

'Aye, we have.' The old lady clutched my arm. 'He's ours now.'

'Yours?'

'Yes. Mrs Birse said 'e was still bare and scabby and she didn't think he'd ever get better and she didn't want a big vet bill with all them visits and packets of stuff. She said her husband and her wanted Jet put down.'

'Oh dear . . . what then?'

'Well, I said we'd tek 'im and we'd pay the bill.'

'You did?'

'Aye. She wasn't sure at first but I said it would be a whackin' big bill and you'd charge double for comin' out that Saturday night.'

I looked at her for a moment and detected the suggestion of a twinkle in her eye.

'We don't do that. Maybe we should, but we don't. But . . . maybe you wanted to persuade her, eh?'

'Well . . .' It was indisputably a twinkle.

I smiled. 'Anyway, Jet has moved next door and I'm sure it's a good thing for everybody. Even the Birses — they didn't seem to have any interest in him.'

'Aye, that's right, and he's lovely. They never took 'im out for a walk — just let him wander about by himself. I don't know why some people have dogs at all.'

'And how about what you were saying to me before. About your fears about being too old?'

She squared her shoulders. 'Oh well, we talked that over, and we thought that after all, Jet isn't a pup — he's six now, so . . . the three of us will just potter on together.'

'That's great. Grow old along with me! The best is yet to be.'

They both laughed, and Mr Howell held up a finger. 'Yes, that's just it. That poem's got it right. It's so grand havin' Jet — it was awful being without a dog after we lost our Nobby. We've always had one and now we're happy.'

They did indeed look happy as did Jet, laughing up at me and lashing his tail.

It was many weeks before I saw them again. I was walking along one of the many bridle tracks which wound among the fields around Darrowby. The sun was blazing from a cloudless sky and even from a distance it was easy to see the rich black gloss of Jet's coat. When I came abreast of them I bent and stroked the big dog's head.

'Well, what a handsome dog you are!' I said, running my hand over the flawless sheen of the neck and ribs. I turned to the old couple. 'There's not a bare patch anywhere – I can nearly see my face in his coat. You've done wonderfully well with him.'

The Howells smiled modestly and Jet, perfectly aware that we were talking about him, wagged his entire rear end and capered around in panting delight.

'Oh, it's been worth it,' said the old lady. 'We're having a great time with 'im – we can't believe our luck having such a dog.'

I watched them as they went their way along the green path and under the overhanging branches of an oak tree. Jet was chasing a stick and I could hear the cheerful voices of the Howells as they shouted their encouragement to him.

I thought again of Browning's lines, and as I watched the trio until a patch of woodland hid them from view I felt a strong conviction that the best was yet to be for those three.

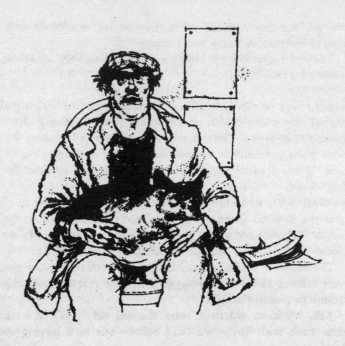

35

'Right, Mr Busby,' I said, feeling a rising tension in response to the urgency of the voice at the other side of the phone, 'I'll be out very soon.'

'Well, see that you are! Ah don't like the look of this cow at all. She's sunken-eyed and gruntin' and she won't look at 'er hay. She could die. Don't be long!'

As I listened to the aggressive harangue I could almost see the red-haired man shouting, bulging-eyed, into the receiver. He had told me all the symptoms several times over to make sure they penetrated my thick skull. Mr Busby wasn't a bad chap, but he had a temper to go with his hair and always seemed to operate on the edge of panic. I knew I'd better hurry.

I looked at my list, then at my watch. It was 9 a.m. and there weren't any really urgent calls. I could do Mr Busby first and keep him happy.

I grabbed my bag and trotted to the front door. Young Mrs Gardiner was standing on the step with her terrier under her arm. She looked upset.

'Oh, Mr Herriot, I was just going to ring your bell. Something has happened to William. He went out this morning and jumped over the garden gate and now he can't use one of his front legs.'

I managed a strained smile. 'All right, bring him in.'

We went through to the consulting room and I lifted the little dog on to the table. It took only a quick feel to tell me that there was a fracture of radius and ulna.

'He's broken his leg, I'm afraid.'

'Oh dear,' the lady wailed, 'how awful!'

I tried to be cheerful, 'Oh, don't worry. It's a clean break and it's a lot easier on a fore leg. We'll soon put him right.'

William, trembling and anxious with his leg dangling, looked up at me with a mute appeal. He was hoping somebody would do something for him, and soon.

'Has he had any breakfast?' I asked as I fished the plaster of Paris bandages out of the cupboard.

'No, nothing yet today.'

'Good. I can go ahead with the anaesthetic.' As I filled the syringe, the old feeling came back that this was the sort of thing which gave vets ulcers. Mr Busby would have to wait and I could picture him stamping round his farmyard and cursing me.

A few ccs of nembutal sent William into a peaceful sleep and I began to soak the bandages in tepid water. Mrs Gardiner held the shaggy leg straight while I carefully applied the bandages. Normally, this was a job I enjoyed, seeing the plaster hardening until it formed a firm supporting sheath and knowing that the little animal would wake up to find his pain gone and his leg usable, but at this moment I was conscious mainly of the passage of time.

I tapped the plaster. It had set like a rock.

'Right,' I said, lifting the sleeping dog from the table, 'he'll have to keep that on for at least a month, then you must bring him back. If you're worried before that, give me a ring, but I'm sure he'll be fine.'

I deposited William on the back seat of the lady's car and looked at my watch – 9.45 a.m. I picked up my gear again and set off for the second time.

It took me half an hour's hard driving along the narrow, drystone-walled roads to reach the Busby farm and as I approached I could see the farmer standing, hands on hips, legs splayed on the cobbled yard, a menacing picture against the squat buildings and the bracken-clad fells behind. When I got out of the car the farmer looked exactly as I had imagined him. His eyes were glaring and the ginger fringe thrusting from under his cap seemed to bristle with rage.

'Where the bloody hell have you been?' he yelled. 'You said you were coming straight out.'

'Yes, I know, but I had to attend to a dog just as I was leaving.'

I thought Mr Busby would explode. 'A dog! A bloody dog! Ma good cow's a lot more important than any bloody dog!'

'Well, yes, but I had to treat him. He had a broken leg.'

'I don't give a bugger what he had. This cow's my livelihood. If she dies it's a serious loss for me. The other thing's just a flippin' pet, a lapdog.'

'Not a lapdog, Mr Busby, a tough little terrier and he was in pain. The lady owner is very fond of him.'

'Fond, fond! What does that matter. It's not touching her pocket, is it? It isn't costing her anything?'

I was going to say something about her heart being touched and about the importance of pets in the lives of people, but Mr Busby's feet had begun to twitch and then to move up and down on the cobbles. I had never seen a man actually dancing with rage and I didn't want to start now. I made for the cow house.

I was vastly relieved to find that the cow only had a mild stasis of the rumen and it turned out that she had been in the fold yard earlier in the morning and had stolen a few extra turnips. But as I examined and injected her, the farmer kept up a grumbling monologue as he held the tail.

'Ah've got to live on a little spot like this and you don't think one cow is important. Where do you think I'm gettin' the money to buy another? Ah'll tell ye, it's a job makin' ends meet

on a little hill farm, but you don't seem to 'ave any idea. Dogs
... bloody dogs ... flippin' pets ... this is my livin' ... you
don't care ...'

I was fundamentally a cow doctor and I made the greatest part
of my own personal living from hill farmers whom I regarded as
the salt of the earth, but I held my peace.

When I called again the following day, I found the cow
completely recovered, but Mr Busby was still sulky. He hadn't
forgiven me.

It was a few weeks later that Helen stopped me as I was
leaving to start the morning round.

'Oh, Jim. I've just taken a call. There's a dog coming in. It's
crying out in pain. I didn't get the name – the man put the
phone down quickly.'

I rubbed my chin. In those days we were almost totally a large
animal practice and had no set surgery hours, certainly not in the
morning.

'Whoever it is will have to wait,' I said. 'Rod Thwaite has a
bullock bleeding badly – knocked a horn off. I'll have to go there
first.'

Trying to be in two places at once was a constant problem in
our job. I did my best not to think about the dog and sped into
the hills at top speed.

It was a typical broken horn with a pretty ornamental fountain
of blood climbing several feet into the air and onto anything
near. Mr Thwaite and I were soon liberally spattered as we tried
to hold the beast still while I packed the stump with sulphona-
mide, applied a thick pad of cotton wool and bandaged it in a
figure of eight to the other horn. It all took quite a time as did
the cleaning-up process afterward, and more than an hour had
gone by before I declined Mrs Thwaite's offer of a cup of tea and
headed back towards Darrowby.

At Skeldale House I hurried down the passage and pushed
open the waiting room door. I halted there in surprise. It was Mr
Busby. He was sitting in the far corner with a little corgi on his
knee and his face bore exactly the same expression as when I paid
the first visit to his cow.

'Where the bloody 'ell have you been?' he barked. The words

were the same too. 'I've been sittin' here for a bloody hour! And I made an appointment!'

'I'm very sorry, Mr Busby. I had a bleeding bullock. I just had to go.'

'A flippin' bullock! And how about ma poor dog, waitin' here in agony! That doesn't matter, does it?'

'Of course it does, but you know as well as I do that that beast could have bled to death. It would have been a big loss to the farmer.'

'A big loss? Aye, a big loss o' money, you mean. But what if me good dog dies? He's worth more than any money. You couldn't put a price on him!'

'Oh, I do understand, Mr Busby. He looks a grand little chap to me.' I hesitated. 'I didn't know you had a pet beside your farm dogs.'

'Of course, I 'ave. This is Dandy. Missus and me think the world of 'im. If anything happens to 'im, it 'ud break our hearts! And you neglect 'im for a flippin' bullock!'

'Oh, come on, now, it's not a case of neglecting him. You must appreciate that I couldn't leave that beast to go on bleeding – it's the farmer's livelihood.'

'There ye go again! Money! It's all you can think about!'

I bent down to lift the little dog and almost as soon as I touched him he screamed out.

Mr Busby's eyes popped further. 'Listen to that! I told you he was in a desperate state, didn't I?'

I carried the corgi along the passage, feeling his muscles as tense and rigid as a board. Already I was sure I knew what was wrong with him. On the table I gently squeezed his neck and the dog yelped again, with Mr Busby moaning in response.

The temperature was normal, in fact everything was normal except the rigidity and the pain.

'Is he goin' to die?' The farmer stared into my face.

'No, no, he's got rheumatism. It's a terribly painful thing in a dog, but it does respond well to treatment. I'm sure he'll soon be well again.'

'I hope you're right,' the farmer grunted. 'I just wish you'd seen 'im sooner instead of leaving 'im to suffer while you run off to a bullock. It's all right you harpin' on about money, but love and companionship mean a lot more than that, you know.'

I filled my syringe. 'I quite agree, Mr Busby. Just hold his head, will you.'

'There's more things in life than money, young man. You'll find that out as you grow older.'

'I'm sure you're right. Now give him one of these tablets night and morning and if he's not a lot better by tomorrow, bring him back.'

'I will and I 'ope you'll be here if I do.' Mr Busby's rage had subsided and was replaced by a lofty sanctimoniousness. 'I would ha' thought that a chap like you would know what it means to have a pet. Material things ain't everything.'

He tucked the corgi under his arm and made for the door. With his hand on the knob he turned. 'And I'll tell tha' summat else.'

I sighed. The lecture wasn't over yet.

He waved a finger. 'Man shall not live by bread alone.'

As he walked along the passage, Dandy turned his head and looked back at me. He seemed better already. Mercifully, rheumatism, though terrifying in its onset, is just as dramatically curable.

Yes, Dandy would soon be himself again, but I knew his master would remember only my mercenary outlook and my heartlessness.

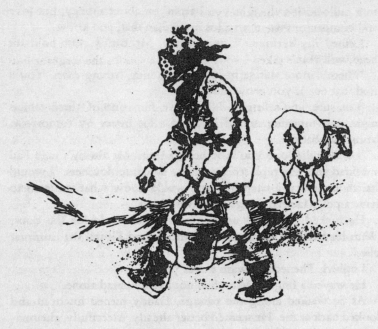

36

It was late when the Darrowby police sergeant's voice came on the telephone.

'I think we have a criminal character here, Mr Herriot. Found him skulking down Docker's Alley in the dark, wearing a face mask. Asked him what he was doing there at ten o'clock at night and he said he was on the way to the fish and chip shop. That sounded a bit thin to me – we've had a lot of petty break-ins and thieving lately – so we've brought him in to the station.'

'I see. But where do I come in?'

'Well, he insists he's innocent and says you can vouch for him. Says his name's Bernard Wain and he has a little farm out on the moors near Hollerton.'

All became suddenly clear and I laughed. 'And the face mask is a red-and-white spotted handkerchief?'

'Yeah! How the heck did you know?'

'Because that's the Cisco Kid you have there.'

'What!'

It would have taken a long time to explain to the sergeant but it all fitted in.

Bernard was in his forties and he shared a smallholding with his redoubtable elder sister. It would be wrong to say that he ran the place because he simply did as he was told, Miss Wain's opinion of him being summed up in her favourite word, 'useless'.

For some years now I had become accustomed to her constant refrain on my visits. 'Aye, well, you'll 'ave to manage as best you can, Mr Herriot. Bernard won't be much good to you. He's useless.'

I recounted to the sergeant the events surrounding my visit to the Wains earlier that evening. It had been a ewe lambing. Miss Wain rang from the village kiosk. 'She's been on all afternoon. Bernard's had 'is hand in and he says there's summat far wrong but I don't suppose you'll 'ave much trouble. It doesn't take much to flummox Bernard. He's useless.'

There were three gates on the rough track to the farm and as I drove into the yard, Bernard was standing there in the headlights' beam. Small, dark, perpetually smiling as I had always known him.

He rubbed his hands and, ever anxious to please, bowed slightly as I got out of the car. 'Now then, Mr Herriot.' But he didn't make any sort of move until his sister came strutting from the house, her bandy legs carrying her dumpy little frame rapidly over the cobbles.

She was at least ten years older than her brother, and her jaw jutted as she looked at him. 'Come on, don't just stand there. Take this bucket and show Mr Herriot where t'ewe is. Eee, I don't know.' She turned to me. 'We've got 'er in the stable, but I think he's forgotten!'

As I stripped off in the makeshift pen and soaped my arms I looked at the ewe. She stood knee deep in straw, straining occasionally, but she didn't look unduly distressed. In fact, when Bernard made a clumsy grab at the wool of her neck she skipped away from him.

'Oh, can't you even hold the thing for Mr Herriot?' his sister wailed. 'Go on, get your arms round her neck properly and haul her in the corner. Eee, you're that slow! Aye, that's it, you've got 'er at last. Marvellous! And where's that towel I gave you to bring? You've forgotten that, too!'

As I slipped my hand into the ewe's vagina, Miss Wain folded her arms and blew out her cheeks. 'Ah don't reckon you'll have any problems, Mr Herriot. Bernard can't manage, cos 'e's got no idea about lambin' a ewe. In fact, 'e's got no idea about anything. He's useless.'

Bernard, standing at the animal's head, nodded and his smile widened as though he had received a compliment. He wasn't really feeble-minded, he was just a supremely ineffectual, vague man, a gentle soul, totally unfitted for the rough farming life.

Kneeling on the straw, I reached forward into the ewe and Miss Wain spoke again. 'Ah bet everything's all right in there.'

She was right. Everything was fine. Sometimes this first exploration revealed a single, over-sized lamb, maybe dead, with no room for the hand to move and everything dry and clinging; little wonder that the farmer was unsuccessful, however long he had tried doing the job himself. But on this occasion, there was all the room in the world, with at least two tiny lambs lying clean and clear and moist in the large uterus, beautifully lubricated by the placental fluid. The only thing that was stopping them from popping out was that two little heads and a bunch of legs were trying to enter the cervix at the same time. It was simply a case of repelling a head and relating the legs to the relevant lamb and I'd have them out, wriggling in the straw in one minute flat. In fact, I had corrected the legs with one finger while I was thinking about it, then I realised that if I did a lightning job Bernard was going to be in big trouble.

He could, of course, have done the whole thing easily but anything so earthy as guddling round inside a ewe was anathema to him. I could just imagine his single, shuddering exploration before he capitulated.

I looked up and detected a trace of anxiety in the smiling face. There was no doubt about it; I was going to have to hold these lambs in for a little while.

I gasped and grunted as I rotated my arm and the first lamb moved his tongue against my hand.

'My word, Miss Wain, this is a right mix up. Could be triplets in here and all tangled up together. It's a tricky business, I can tell you. Now let's see . . . which lamb does that leg belong to? . . . no . . . no . . . gosh, it isn't easy.' I gritted my teeth and groaned again as I fought my imaginary battle. 'This is a real vet's job, I can tell you.'

As I spoke, Miss Wain's eyes narrowed. Maybe I was overdoing it. Anyway, Bernard was in the clear now. I hooked a finger round the tiny legs which were first in the queue and drew out lamb number one. I deposited him in the straw and he raised his head and shook it vigorously; always a good sign, but possibly he was puzzled at the delay.

'Now then, what else have we got?' I said worriedly as I reached back into the ewe. The job was as good as over now, but I was still making a meal of it for Bernard's sake and I did a bit more panting and grunting before producing a second and then a third lamb. They made a pretty sight as they lay wriggling and snuffling in the straw. The first one was already making efforts to rise on wobbly legs. It would soon be on its way to the milk bar.

I smiled up at Miss Wain. 'There you are, then. Three grand lambs. I'll put in a couple of pessaries and that's that. It was a complicated business, though, with the legs all jumbled up together. It's a good job you called me or you might have lost these three.'

Arms still folded, her head sunk on her chest, she regarded me unsmilingly. I had the impression that part of her was sorry she had been deprived of another opportunity of castigating her brother. However, she had another line of attack.

'Tell ye what,' she said suddenly, 'there's a cow been hanging her cleansin' for five days. You might as well take it away while you're here.'

This was the kind of routine job which you didn't usually do at nine o'clock at night, but I didn't demur. It would save another visit.

'Okay,' I said. 'Will you bring me some fresh water, please?'

It was then that I noticed the alarm flickering in Bernard's eyes. I remembered that he couldn't stand smells, and in the odoriferous trade of country vetting, removal of the bovine afterbirth is the smelliest. And he would have to hold the tail while I did it.

When he came back with the steaming bucket, he set it down and whipped out a large red-and-white spotted handkerchief from his pocket. Carefully he tied it round his face, knotting it tightly at the back of his neck, then he took up his place by the side of the cow.

As I put my arm into the animal and looked at Bernard's big eyes smiling above the mask, I thought again how fitting was our nickname for him. It was Tristan who had first christened him the Cisco Kid because of his uncanny resemblance to the famous bandit. In all the unpleasant procedures which assailed Bernard's nostrils – stinking calvings, autopsies, releasing the gas from tympanitic cows – the handkerchief came out and, in fact, in every image I had of him he was wearing that mask.

It seemed to give him a feeling of security, because he was able to make cheerful, if muffled, replies to my attempts at conversation, although occasionally he closed his eyes in a pained manner as though some alien whiff had got through to him.

Fortunately this was an easy cleansing and it wasn't long before Bernard was waving me good-bye as I drove away. In the darkness of the yard he still had the handkerchief round his face – the Cisco Kid to the life.

I felt I had managed to put the police sergeant in the picture.

However, he still wasn't quite convinced.

'But he still wouldn't be wearing that mask when he came into Darrowby.'

'Bernard would.'

'You mean he just forgot to take it off?'

'Absolutely.'

'Well, he's a rum sort of feller.'

I could understand his wonderment, but to me Bernard's actions were quite in character. He'd had a traumatic evening with the lambing and the cleansing and it was totally understandable that he would jump on his bike and pedal into the town to seek solace in a parcel of fish and chips. I knew for a fact that they were his greatest pleasure. A little matter like removing the handkerchief would easily slip his mind.

'Aye well,' the sergeant said, 'I suppose I can take your word about him.'

'Sergeant,' I said, 'that man you have there is the most harmless character in North Yorkshire.'

There was a pause. 'Okay, then, we'd better get the handcuffs off him.'

'What! You haven't . . .'

'No, no, heh–heh–heh! Just having a bit o' fun with you, Mr Herriot. You did it to me with your flippin' Cisco Kid, so I'm giving it back to you.'

'All right, fair enough.' I laughed in return. 'Is Bernard very upset?'

'Upset? Not him. Not a care in the world. His only worry is that the fish and chip shop might be closed.'

'Oh dear. And is it?'

'No, I'll be able to reassure him about that. They're stayin' open till eleven o'clock tonight.'

'Good, good, so it's a happy ending for Bernard.'

'Guess so.' The sergeant laughed again as he put down the receiver.

But it could have been so different. If the little farm had been on the phone, Miss Wain would have received that call. My mind reeled at the thought of her reaction when she learned that Bernard couldn't even go out for fish and chips without landing in the hands of the police.

I could imagine her exasperated cry. 'Useless! Quite useless!'

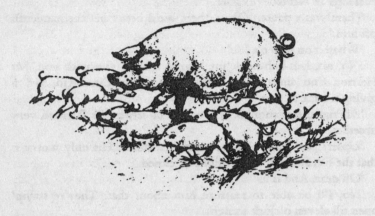

37

There are few sights more depressing than a litter of dying piglets.

'Looks pretty hopeless, Mr Bush,' I said as I leaned over the wall of the pen. 'And what a pity, it's a grand litter. Twelve of them, aren't there?'

The farmer grunted. 'Aye, it allus happens like that.' He wasn't a barrel of laughs at any time but now his long, hollow-cheeked face was set in gloom.

I looked down at the little pink creatures huddled in a heap, liquid yellow faeces trickling down their tails. Neonatal scour, the acute diarrhoea which afflicts new-born piglets and was nearly always fatal unless treated quickly.

'When did they start with this?' I asked.

'Pretty near just after they were born. That were three days ago.'

'Well, I wish I'd seen them a bit sooner. I might have been able to do something for them.'

Mr Bush shrugged. 'I thought it was nowt – maybe t'milk was too rich for 'em.'

I opened the door and went into the pen. As I examined the little pigs, their mother grunted as if in invitation. She was stretched on her side, exposing the long double row of teats, but her family weren't interested. As I lifted and laid the limp little bodies I felt sure they would never suckle again.

However, I just couldn't do nothing. 'We'll give it a go,' I said. 'You never know, we might manage to save one or two.'

The farmer didn't say anything as I went out to the car. I couldn't remember ever having seen him smile and his hunched shoulders and sombre features added to the general atmosphere of doom.

For my part I was disappointed I hadn't been called earlier because I had a new product with me which might have helped. It was a Neomycin mixture contained in a plastic bottle which enabled the antibiotic to be squirted into the mouth. I'd had some good results with it in calves but hadn't had the chance to try it on pigs, but as I handled the unresisting little creatures, giving each one a shot onto its tongue and laying it, apparently lifeless, back on the floor, I felt I was wasting my time.

I supplemented the treatment with a small injection of a sulpha drug, and having satisfied my conscience with the feeling that I had done everything, I prepared to leave.

I handed the Neomycin bottle to the farmer. 'Here, if there's any alive tomorrow, give them a squirt. Let me know if you manage to save any – it isn't worth my paying another visit.'

Mr Bush nodded wordlessly and walked away.

After three days I had heard nothing and presumed that my unhappy prognostications had been correct, but it was on my mind that I ought to have given the farmer some advice for the future. There were some preventive *E.coli* vaccines which could be given to the sow before farrowing and he had a couple of other sows which ought to be protected.

Since I happened to be passing right by Bush's farm on my way home from another visit, I turned in at the gate. As I got out of the car the farmer was sweeping up in a corner of the yard. He didn't look up and my spirits sank. At the same time I felt a little annoyed; it wasn't my fault he had lost his litter. He didn't have to ignore me – I had done my best.

Since he still didn't pay any attention to me, I walked into the piggery and looked into the pen.

At first I thought I was looking in the wrong place, but no, I recognised the sow – she had a small nick out of one ear. What my mind could hardly grasp was the sight of a pink jumble of little creatures fighting to get hold of the best teat. It was difficult to count them in the scramble but finally they settled down to a rapt sucking, each contented with his lot. And there were twelve of them.

I looked out of the doorway. 'Hey, Mr Bush, they're all alive! Every one of them!'

The farmer walked slowly across the yard, trailing his brush and together we looked down into the pen.

I still couldn't believe it. 'Well, that's marvellous. A miracle. I thought they'd all die – and there they are!'

There was no joy in Mr Bush's face. 'Aye,' he muttered, 'but they've lost a bit o'ground.'

With Mr Bush's unimpressed line still groaning in my ear, I drove out to Lord Gresham's farm.

It was only when I was in the RAF with the SP's bawling, 'Hey, you, c'mere!' that I realised that the quiet respect I usually received as a veterinary surgeon on the Yorkshire farms was something I had taken for granted and yet it was very special in my life. It was nothing to do with success or failure in my work – things sometimes went wrong and occasionally I was ticked off by my clients – but behind it all there was the feeling that I was a professional man doing my best for the animals and I was esteemed accordingly.

But I never got any more respect from Lord Gresham's men than I did from Mr Bush. Danny, Bert, Hughie and Joe regarded me with a total detachment which I always found disquieting. It wasn't that they disliked me or were rude in any way, it was the fact that no matter what I did they were totally unimpressed, not, seemingly, even interested.

This was strange because, as every vet knows, there are some places where everything goes right and others where everything goes wrong and Lord Gresham's place was one of the former. I always felt that my good fairy was watching over me there, because every single case had gone like a breeze and in fact I had pulled off a long succession of cures that warmed my heart.

Today, after climbing out of my car and walking into the fold yard, I believed I would do it again. I looked at the cow standing alone and disconsolate in the deep straw. She was a pathetic sight with, it seemed, half her insides hanging out of her. Prolapsed uterus. It was a scene to wipe the smile from any veterinary surgeon's face – a promise of hard labour with the animal's life at stake. But with the passage of years it had lost a lot of its dread and, although I was naturally apprehensive, I had the feeling that with my new knowledge and equipment I could restore this poor cow to normal. But at the same time I knew I would get no credit for it, no respect. Not on this farm anyway.

By bringing up a tractor and, using the recently invented Bagshaw hoist clamped on the cow's pelvis, I raised the cow's back end so that I was working downhill. I administered a spinal anaesthetic and replaced the uterus with none of the labour of past years.

The cow walked away, good as new, and while I felt delighted at the magical return to normal, the men were completely unmoved and strolled off without a word. It was always like this here.

Shortly after this, I attended some sheep going round in circles with listeriosis. An injection of penicillin and they were right within a couple of days – quite a spectacular cure. Same reaction from the men. No interest. Not a scrap of respect.

A week later, I was called to a cow with a twisted uterus. She was unable to calve and was lying straining, distressed, on the point of exhaustion. Without my help she would have had to be slaughtered, but by rolling her over several times I righted the twist and produced a beautiful live calf. As I looked wonderingly and with deep satisfaction at the result of my work, the men offered no comment but went phlegmatically about the business of clearing up after the operation. For the umpteenth time I wondered what I had to do to get through to them.

I was putting on my jacket when an envelope fell out of my pocket. It was from Liverpool, from the football pools firm and, just for the sake of breaking the silence, I said, 'Ah, my winnings for this week.'

The effect was electric and the previous apathy was replaced by acute interest. They studied the enclosed postal order, which was only for two pounds, with total absorption. 'By gaw, look at that!' 'We can't do any good with them things!' 'Fust time I've ever seen a winner!' The remarks flew thick and fast. Then Danny, the foreman, said, 'De ye often win?'

Carried away by the excitement and the unprecedented interest, I replied casually, 'Oh yes, regularly,' which was an exaggeration because I very rarely won but the remark was received with open-mouthed fascination. For the first time ever I was the centre of concentrated attention.

After a few moments, Danny cleared his throat. 'Mr Herriot, the lads and me do the three draws every week – we each put on a shillin' – and we've never 'ad a touch yet. Will you fill up our coupon for us?'

With a wistful feeling that my sudden popularity would be soon exploded I took the coupon and, using the cow's back as a desk, I did as they asked.

It was a winner and, during that week, Danny appeared at my surgery. 'We've got thirty bob apiece, Mr Herriot. It's never happened before and t'lads are over the moon. Will ye do t'same again?'

'Certainly,' I replied airily and put my crosses in the little squares. It won again, and this time all four of the men turned up at the surgery, smiling and triumphant. 'Another thirty bob each, Mr Herriot! It's champion! We're goin' to put a bit more on this week.'

I felt that things were getting out of hand. 'Look, chaps, I'd really rather not do this again. I don't want to lose you a lot of money and you will if you start putting on bigger stakes. Anyway, I'm no expert at this – I was only kidding when I gave you the idea that I won every week.'

A hush fell upon the room and four pairs of eyes narrowed to slits. They didn't believe a word.

Helplessly I looked from one to the other but they stood there as though carved from stone, waiting for me to make my move.

'I tell you what,' I said at length, 'I'll do your coupon this week, but it will be for the last time. All right?'

There were nods all round. 'Aye, that'll do us fine,' Danny said.

'Just this week and never n'more.'

Once more I entered the crosses in the squares and as I handed over the coupon I made my final appeal. 'And you'll never ask me to do this again?'

Danny raised a hand. 'Nay, never n'more, Mr Herriot. That's a promise.'

For the third successive week, their coupon was a winner. Even as I write, I feel I can hardly ask anybody to believe it, but it is a true story. And a growing sensation of the eerie workings of fate was strengthened when I myself had my biggest ever win – seventy-seven pounds four shillings and elevenpence – on the treble chance. The sum is engraven on my memory until the end of time.

That evening I showed the postal order tremblingly to my partner. 'Look at this, Siegfried. All this money! And if I had had just one more draw I'd have won the first prize – sixteen thousand pounds!'

Siegfried whistled as he studied the postal order. 'James, this calls for a celebration. Let's get over to the Drovers.'

In the bar, Siegfried bustled to the counter. 'Two large whiskies, Betty,' he cried. 'Mr Herriot's just won sixteen thousand pounds on the pools!'

'No, no . . .' I protested, trying to restrain my ebullient colleague. 'It wasn't as much as that . . .'

But it was too late. The barmaid's eyes popped, the other occupants nearly choked on their beer and the damage was done. The news swept through Darrowby like a prairie fire. Sixteen thousand pounds was a vast fortune in those days and wherever I went over the next few weeks I was greeted with secret smiles and knowing winks. It happened nearly forty years ago, but to this day there are many people in our little town who are convinced that Herriot became rich on the pools.

The next time I had to visit Lord Gresham's farm was to carry out the tuberculin test on the cattle. I didn't have to do anything clever to the beasts – just clip a couple of inches of hair from the necks and inject into the skin, but there was a different atmosphere altogether from the previous occasions when I was pulling off miracle cures, saving animals' lives with my veterinary skill. The four men seemed to hang on my every word, treating my requests with the greatest deference. 'Yes, Mr Herriot.' 'Right you are, Mr Herriot.' And, whereas before they had always acted as though I weren't there, they now watched my smallest move with the greatest concentration. It became clear to me that I was forever enshrined in their minds as the one man to whom the mysteries of the football pools were an open book, to be manipulated as the fancy took me, and as I looked round the four men I could read something in their eyes which I had never seen before.

It was respect – deep, abiding respect.

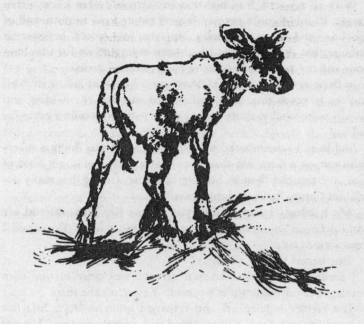

38

I was in a familiar position. Lying flat on my face on a hard
cobbled floor with my arm up to the shoulder inside a straining
heifer. I had been doing this for over an hour and was beginning
to despair. There was a huge live calf in there and the only thing
stopping the delivery was that there was a leg back – normally a
simple malpresentation and easily corrected. That was the cause
of my frustration – I couldn't believe that such a thing could beat
me, but the trouble was that this was a very small heifer and
there was no room to work. Time and again, I had managed to
reach the calf's foot but I could only get a couple of fingers
round it and as soon as I tried to pull, it slipped away from me.
And on top of this, the heifer was giving me hell with her
expulsive efforts, trapping my hand painfully between the calf's
head and the pelvic bones.

With all my soul, I wished that my arm had been a few inches longer. If only I could get my fingers beyond the smooth wall of the hoof and grasp the hairy leg, the job would be over in minutes, but this was what I had been trying to do for that long hour and my arm was becoming paralysed and useless.

In these situations I would often get a big farm lad to strip off and try to reach inaccessible places for me, but Mr Kilding and his son were stocky, short-armed chaps – they wouldn't get as far as I had.

Suddenly I remembered something. Calum was doing a tuberculin test on a farm less than a mile away. If I could get hold of him my troubles would be over because among his many attributes Calum had very long arms.

'Mr Kilding,' I said, 'could you phone the Ellertons and ask Mr Buchanan to come round and give me a hand. I'm afraid I need a bit of help.'

'Buchanan? Vet wi' t'badger?'

I smiled. Calum was known as such not only in our own practice but for many miles beyond. 'Yes, that's the man.'

The farmer hurried off and returned quickly. 'Aye, he's just finished the test. Says 'e'll be round in a minute or two.' He was a nice man, and wasn't complaining at my long, unproductive rolling about on his byre floor, but he couldn't hide his anxiety. 'I 'ope you'll be able to do summat, Mr Herriot, I've been really lookin' forward to getting this calf.'

A few minutes later Calum strode into the byre. He looked down at the prostrate animal and grinned. 'Having a little trouble, Jim?' His manner, as always, was breezy.

I explained the situation and he quickly whipped off his shirt. We lay down together on those cobbles which had been getting steadily harder. I inserted my left arm until I could feel the calf's muzzle against the palm of my hand and Calum pushed in his right arm alongside mine.

'Right,' I said, 'I'll push the head back while you try to get hold of that foot.'

'Okay,' he replied. 'Fire away.'

I pushed and just as the head moved away, making the vital room we needed, the heifer gave a mighty strain and pushed it back at me. Calum yelped as his fingers were trapped. 'Ouch, that hurt! You'll have to do a bit better than that.'

I gritted my teeth and tried again, bracing my arm desperately against the heifer's expulsive efforts.

'I'm nearly there,' grunted Calum. 'Nearly ... nearly ... push, you're not pushing!'

'I *am* pushing, dammit!' I gasped, 'but she's stronger than I am, and I've been doing this for an hour, you know. My arm's like spaghetti.'

We tried again, several times, groaning and panting, then Calum let his head slump onto his shoulder. 'I know. Let's have a rest for a few seconds.'

I was all for that and I relaxed, feeling the calf's rough tongue licking at my palm. He was still alive, anyway.

As we lay there, practically cheek to cheek, arms still inside the heifer, my colleague put on a bright smile. 'Well, now, what shall we talk about while we're resting?'

I didn't feel like light conversation, but I tried to fall in with his sally. 'Oh, I don't know. Have you any interesting news?'

'Well, yes. As a matter of fact I have. I'm going to get married.'

'*What!*'

'I said I'm going to get married.'

'You're joking!'

'No. I assure you, I am.'

'When?'

'Next week.'

'Well ... well ... Anybody I know?'

'No, no. Girl who works in the surgery department at the London College. I met her there while I was taking the course.'

I lay there, thunderstruck. I found it difficult to take in. I had never imagined that a chap like Calum would ever entertain dreams of domestic bliss. I was still trying to sort out my thoughts when he brought me back to reality. 'Come on, let's have another go.'

And it seemed as though the shock to my system had brought a surge of adrenalin with it, because this time I gave a great, pop-eyed heave and was able to hold the head back until I heard Calum's triumphant cry. 'I've got it!'

And, having got it, he wasn't going to let go. Eyes closed, teeth bared, he pulled until the elusive foot appeared at the vulva. His sweating face broke into a delighted grin. 'That's a lovely sight!'

It was indeed. We had two legs and a head now, although nearly everything was still inside. I slapped the heifer's rump. 'Come on, old girl. This is when we need you. You can push as much as you like now.'

As if in reply, the heifer gave us enthusiastic help as we pulled on the legs and soon the muzzle appeared, nostrils twitching, the big, wide brow and the eyes – which, I imagined, held a glimmer of disapproval at the delay – then, the rest of the head and body till we had a fine calf wriggling on the straw.

I felt good – I always did – but on this occasion something else was crowding in my mind. Calum's bombshell about his impending nuptials.

I could hardly wait to see what kind of girl Calum would bring back. He was such an unusual chap with ideas so far different from the ordinary man that the new woman could be anything – ugly, eccentric, fat, skinny – my mind played restlessly with the possibilities.

I was put out of my pain quite soon. I opened the sitting room door one afternoon and my young colleague was there with a girl at his side. 'This is Deirdre,' he said.

She was quite tall, and the first words which came to me were 'kind' and 'motherly'. But I would like to banish any thought that being kind and motherly meant that she wasn't attractive. Dierdre was very attractive indeed and now, nearly forty years later, when I think of her wonderful family of six young Buchanans I feel I deserve full marks for intuition.

As we shook hands, her smile was wide and warm, her voice gentle, and it struck me that Calum had done it again – with all his funny ways he seemed to get the fundamental things right, and now, when it came to choosing a wife he had found the kind of girl any young man would be glad to see first thing every morning.

Any notion we might have harboured of celebrating an exciting wedding was soon quashed, and in a way which I realised was typical of them. They slipped away quietly to Keeler church and the ceremony was carried out there without fuss.

I have never in my travels through Britain seen anything quite like Keeler. It is an ancient church of great beauty built by the Normans around 1100, standing quite alone among surrounding fields. There is a farm nearby but the nearest village is two miles away. It is on the borders of our practice area, but it can be clearly seen from the main road and whenever I drive past I always slow down to look yet again at that lovely building, solitary among the fields with the hills rising behind. To me, it is a romantic, thrilling sight.

Throughout the centuries, services have been conducted regularly there with a small congregation drawn from the surrounding farms and nearby villages, so that the church has been preserved in all its glory. Its beauty is a stark beauty of massive stone with nothing like the traceried battlements and buttresses of Darrowby's splendid church which is famed to such an extent that it is often referred to as a little cathedral. Helen and I were married there and have never ceased to be enthralled by its sheer magnificence.

However, Calum and Deirdre went to Keeler in its wild and lonely setting and I could understand its appeal which would reach out to them. There was a brief honeymoon and that was all.

Whenever I pass the old church standing in its solitary dignity looking over the empty fields and the long line of hills as it has done for nine centuries, I think again how fitting it was that those young Buchanans should pledge their future life within its walls.

I had the good feeling that Deirdre would add the woman's touch to Calum's flat – introduce a little more comfort in the way of her own individual furniture and decorations – but it was not to be. Deirdre didn't care any more about that side of life than Calum – her interests were all outside. Like his, in the creatures, the plants and flowers of North Yorkshire.

The flat stayed spartan – no chintz covers on the furniture or anything like that – but she seemed perfectly happy as she padded round up there, very often in slacks and bare feet, her mind completely in tune with her new husband's.

When they had time off together they spent it in rambling and observation in the woods and hills, and if Calum's work prevented him from doing something important in his world of exploration, Deirdre would happily stand in for him. I saw an example of this one balmy summer evening around dusk when I had to send the young man to a call.

'Calum,' I said, 'there's a colic at Steve Holdsworth's – will you get there as soon as you can?'

'Certainly,' he replied. 'Just give me a few minutes to put Deirdre up a tree and then I'll be on my way.'

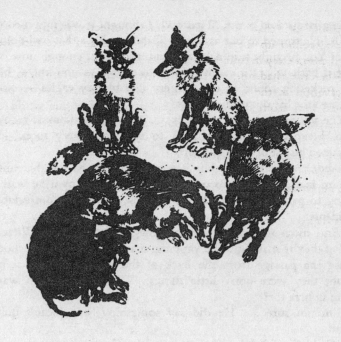

39

It was around the time when Calum's third badger arrived that an uncanny sense of the inevitable began to settle on me.

The new badger was called Bill and Calum didn't say much about his unheralded advent. He did mention it in an off-hand way to me, but prudently failed to take Siegfried into his confidence. I think he realised that there wasn't much point in upsetting my partner further – it seemed only reasonable to assume that Siegfried was getting a little punch-drunk with the assorted creatures milling around and wouldn't even notice.

I was discussing the day's work with my colleagues in the doorway of the dispensary when Siegfried ducked down. 'What the hell was that?' he exclaimed as a large feathery body whizzed past, just missing our heads.

'Oh, it's Calum's owl,' I said.

Siegfried stared at me. 'That owl? I thought it was supposed to be ill.' He turned to our assistant. 'Calum, what's that owl doing here? You brought it in days ago and it looks fit enough now, so take it back where it came from. I like birds as you know, but not rocketing round in our surgery like bloody eagles – could frighten the life out of the clients.'

The young man nodded. 'Yes . . . yes . . . she's almost recovered. I expect to take her back to the wood very soon.' He pocketed his list of visits and left.

I didn't say anything, but it seemed certain to me that once Calum had got his hands on an owl of his very own he wasn't going to part with it in a hurry. I foresaw some uncomfortable incidents.

'And listen to those fox cubs!' Siegfried went on. 'What a racket they're making!' The yapping, snarling and barking echoed along the passage from the back of the house. There was no doubt they were noisy little things. 'What does Calum want them in here for?'

'I'm not sure . . . He did say something, but I can't quite recall . . .'

'Well,' Siegfried grunted, 'I just hope he'll remove them as soon as the problem is over.'

Later that day, Siegfried and I were setting a dog's fractured radius when Calum walked into the operating room. Marilyn, as usual, was on his shoulder, but today she had company; seated comfortably in the crook of the young man's arms was a little monkey.

Siegfried looked up from his work. He stopped winding the plaster of Paris bandage and his mouth fell open. 'Oh, my God, no! This is too much! Not a bloody monkey now! It's like living in a bloody zoo.'

'Yes,' replied Calum with a pleased smile. 'His name is Mortimer.'

'Never mind his name!' Siegfried growled. 'What the hell is he doing here?'

'Oh, don't worry, this isn't a pet – in a way, he's a patient.'

Siegfried's eyes narrowed. 'What do you mean – in what way? Is he ill?'

'Well, not exactly ... Diana Thurston has asked me to look after him while she's away on holiday.'

'And you said yes, of course! No hesitation! That's just what we need here – bloody monkeys roaming the place on top of everything else!'

Calum looked at him gravely. 'Well, you know, I was in a difficult position. Colonel Thurston is a very nice man and one of our biggest clients – large farm, hunting horses and umpteen dogs. I couldn't very well refuse.'

My partner recommenced his winding. The plaster was setting and I could see he wanted time to think. 'Well, I see your point,' he said after a few moments. 'It wouldn't have looked so good.' He glanced up at Calum. 'But it's definitely just while Diana's on holiday?'

'Oh, absolutely, I promise you.' The young man nodded vigorously. 'She's devoted to the little chap and she'll pick him up as soon as she returns.'

'Oh, well, I suppose it'll be all right.' Siegfried shot a hunted look at the monkey which, open-mouthed, teeth-bared and chattering, was apparently laughing at him.

We lifted the sleeping dog from the table and carried him to one of the recovery kennels. My partner seemed indisposed to speak and I didn't break the silence. I had no desire to discuss Calum's latest acquisition because I happened to know that Diana Thurston wasn't just going to Scarborough for a fortnight – she was off to Australia for six months.

I was called out that evening and went to the surgery for extra drugs. As I walked along the passage I could hear a babel of animal sounds from the end of the house and, on opening the door to the back room, I found Calum among his friends. The three badgers were nosing around the food bowls, the owl flapped lazily onto a high shelf. Storm, vast and amiable, waved his tail in welcome, while the Dobermanns regarded me contemplatively. Mortimer the monkey, clearly already under Calum's spell, leaped from a table into the young man's arms and grinned at me. In a corner, the fox cubs kept up their strange yapping and growling and I noticed two cages containing a couple of rabbits and a hare – apparently new arrivals.

Looking round the room I realised that Siegfried had been right from the very beginning. The menagerie was now firmly installed. And as I opened the door to leave I wondered just how big it was going to grow.

I had stepped into the passage when Calum turned from the table where he was stirring some nameless comestible in a large bowl.

'Before you go, Jim, I've got some very exciting news!' he cried.

'Oh, what's that?'

He pointed to one of the Dobermanns. 'Anna's having pups next month!'

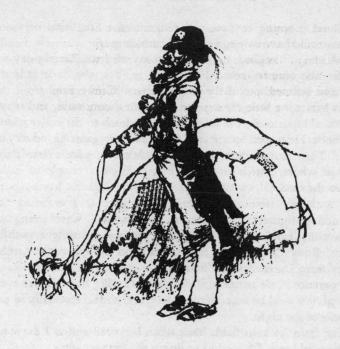

40

As I got out of my car to open the gate to the farm, I looked
with interest at the odd-looking structure on the grass verge; it
was standing in the shelter of the dry-stone wall, overlooking the
valley. It seemed as though sheets of tarpaulin had been stretched
over metal hoops to make some kind of shelter. It was like a big
black igloo, but for what?

As I wondered, the sacking at the front parted and a tall,
white-bearded man emerged. He straightened up, looked around
him, dusted down his ancient frock coat and donned the kind of
high-crowned bowler hat which was popular in Victorian times.
He seemed oblivious of my presence as he stood, breathing
deeply, gazing at the heathery fellside which ran away from the
roadside to the beck far below. Then after a few moments he
turned to me and raised his hat gravely.

'Good morning to you,' he murmured in the kind of voice which could have belonged to an archbishop.

'Morning,' I replied, fighting with my surprise. 'Lovely day.'

His fine features relaxed in a smile. 'Yes, yes, it is indeed.' Then he bent and pulled the sacking apart. 'Come, Emily.'

As I stared, a little cat tripped out with dainty steps, and as she stretched luxuriously the man attached a leash to the collar round her neck. He turned to me and raised his hat again. 'Good day to you.' Then man and cat set off at a leisurely pace towards the village whose church tower was just visible a couple of miles down the road.

I took my time over opening the gate as I watched the dwindling figures. I felt almost as though I were seeing an apparition. I was out of my usual territory because a faithful client, Eddy Carless, had taken this farm almost twenty miles away from Darrowby and had paid us the compliment of asking our practice if we would still do his work. We had said yes even though it would be inconvenient to travel so far, especially in the middle of the night.

The farm lay two fields back from the road and as I drew up in the yard I saw Eddy coming down the granary steps.

'Eddy,' I said, 'I've just seen something very strange.'

He laughed. 'You don't have to tell me. You've seen Eugene.'

'Eugene?'

'That's right. Eugene Ireson. He lives there.'

'What?'

'It's true — that's 'is house. He built it himself two years ago and took up residence. This used to be me dad's farm, as you know, and he used to tell me about 'im. He came from nowhere and settled in that funny place with 'is cat and he's never moved since.'

'I wouldn't have thought he would be allowed to set up house on the grass verge.'

'No, neither would I, but nobody seems to have bothered 'im. And I'll tell you another funny thing. He's an educated man and the brother of Cornelius Ireson.'

'Cornelius Ireson, the industrialist?'

'The very same. The multi-millionaire. Lives in that estate you pass about five miles along the Brawton road. You'll have seen the big lodge at the gates.'

'Yes . . . I know it . . . but how . . . ?'

'Nobody knows the whole story, but it seems Cornelius inherited everything and his brother got nowt. They say that Eugene has travelled the world, living rough in wild countries and havin' all kinds of adventures, but wherever he's been he's come back to North Yorkshire.'

'But why does he live in that strange erection?'

'It's a mystery. I do know he has nowt to do with 'is brother and vice versa and anyway 'e seems happy and content down there. Me dad was very fond of 'im and the old chap used to come up to the farm for the odd meal and a bath. Still does, but he's very independent. Doesn't sponge on anybody. Goes down to the village regularly for his food and 'is pension.'

'And always with his cat?'

'Aye.' Eddy laughed again. 'Allus with his cat.'

We went into the buildings to start the tuberculin test, but as I clipped and measured and injected over and over again, I couldn't rid my mind of the memory of that odd twosome.

When I drew up at the farm gate three days later to read the tuberculin test Mr Ireson was sitting on a wicker chair in the sunshine, reading, with his cat on his lap.

When I got out of the car, he raised his hat as before. 'Good afternoon. A very pleasant day.'

'Yes, it certainly is.' As I spoke, Emily hopped down and stalked over the grass to greet me, and as I tickled her under the chin she arched and purred round my legs.

'What a lovely little thing!' I said.

The old man's manner moved from courtesy to something more. 'You like cats?'

'Yes, I do. I've always liked them.' As I continued my stroking, then gave her tail a playful tug, the pretty tabby face looked up at me and the purring rose in a crescendo.

'Well, Emily seems to have taken to you remarkably. I've never seen her so demonstrative.'

I laughed. 'She knows how I feel. Cats always know – they are very wise animals.'

Mr Ireson beamed his agreement. 'I saw you the other day, didn't I? You have some business with Mr Carless?'

'Yes, I'm his vet.'

'Aah . . . I see. So you are a veterinary surgeon and you approve of my Emily.'

'I couldn't do anything else. She's beautiful.'

The old man seemed to swell with gratification. 'How very kind of you.' He hesitated. 'I wonder, Mr . . . er . . .'

'Herriot.'

'Ah yes, I wonder, Mr Herriot, if, when you have concluded your business with Mr Carless, you would care to join me in a cup of tea.'

'I'd love to. I'll be finished in less than an hour.'

'Splendid, splendid. I look forward to seeing you then.'

Eddy had a clear test. No reactors, not even a doubtful. I entered the particulars in my testing book and hurried back down the farm road.

Mr Ireson was waiting by the gate. 'It is a little chilly now,' he said, 'I think we'd better go inside.' He led me over to the igloo, drew back the sacks and ushered me through with old world grace.

'Do sit down,' he murmured, waving me to what looked like a one-time automobile seat in tattered leather while he sank down on the wicker chair I had seen outside.

As he arranged two mugs, then took the kettle from a primus stove and began to pour, I took in the contents of the interior. There was a camp bed, a bulging rucksack, a row of books, a Tilly lamp, a low cupboard and a basket in which Emily was ensconced.

'Milk and sugar, Mr Herriot?' The old man inclined his head gracefully. 'Ah, no sugar. I have some buns here, do have one. There is an excellent little bakery down in the village and I am a regular customer.'

As I bit into the bun and sipped the tea, I stole a look at the row of books. Every one was poetry. Blake, Swinburne, Longfellow, Whitman, all worn and frayed with reading.

'You like poetry?' I said.

He smiled. 'Ah, yes. I do read other things – the van comes up here from the public library every week – but I always come back to my old friends, particularly this one.' He held up the dog-eared volume he had been reading earlier. *The Poems of Robert W. Service.*

'You like that one, eh?'

'Yes. I think Service is my favourite. Not classical stuff perhaps, but his verses strike something very deep in me.' He gazed at the book, then his eyes looked beyond me into somewhere only he knew. I wondered then if Alaska and the wild Yukon territory might have been the scene of his wanderings and for a moment I hoped he might be going to tell me something about his past, but it seemed he didn't want to talk about that. He wanted to talk about his cat.

'It is the most extraordinary thing, Mr Herriot. I have lived on my own all my life but I have never felt lonely, but I know now that I would be desperately lonely without Emily. Does that sound foolish to you?'

'Not at all. Possibly it's because you haven't had a pet before. Have you?'

'No, I haven't. Never seemed to have stayed still long enough. I am fond of animals and there have been times when I felt I would like to own a dog, but never a cat. I have heard so often that cats do not dispense affection, that they are self-sufficient and never become really fond of anybody. Do you agree with that?'

'Of course not. It's absolute nonsense. Cats have a character of their own, but I've treated hundreds of friendly, affectionate cats who are faithful friends to their owners.'

'I'm so glad to hear you say that, because I flatter myself that this little creature is really attached to me.' He looked down at Emily who had jumped onto his lap and gently patted her head.

'That's easy to see,' I said and the old man smiled his pleasure.

'You know, Mr Herriot,' he went on, 'when I first settled here,' he waved his hand round his dwelling as though it were the drawing room in a multi-acred mansion, 'I had no reason to think that I wouldn't continue to live the solitary life that I was accustomed to, but one day this little animal walked in from nowhere as though she had been invited and my whole existence has changed.'

I laughed. 'She adopted you. Cats do that. And it was a lucky day for you.'

'Yes . . . yes . . . how very true. You seem to understand these things so well, Mr Herriot. Now, do let me top up your cup.'

It was the first of many visits to Mr Ireson in his strange dwelling. I never went to the Carless farm without looking in through the sacks and if Eugene was in residence we had a cup of tea and a chat. We talked about many things – books, the political situation, natural history of which he had a deep knowledge, but the conversation always got round to cats. He wanted to know everything about their care and feeding, habits and diseases. While I was agog to hear about his world travels which he referred to only in the vaguest terms, he would listen with the wide-eyed interest of a child to my veterinary experiences.

It was during one of these sessions that I raised the question of Emily in particular.

'I notice she is either in here or on the lead with you, but does she ever go wandering outside by herself?'

'Well, yes . . . now that you mention it. Just lately she has done so. She only goes up to the farm – I make sure she does not stray along the road where she may be knocked down.'

'I didn't mean that, Mr Ireson. What I was thinking about was that there are several male cats up there at the farm. She could easily become pregnant.'

He sat bolt upright in his chair. 'Good heavens, yes! I never thought of that – how foolish of me. I'd better try to keep her inside.'

'Very difficult,' I said. 'It would be much better to have her spayed.'

'Eh?'

'To let me do a hysterectomy. Remove the uterus and ovaries. Then she'd be safe – you couldn't do with a lot of kittens in here, could you?'

'No . . . no . . . of course not. But an operation . . .' He stared at me with frightened eyes. 'There would be an element of danger . . . ?'

'No, no,' I said as briskly as I could. 'It's quite a simple procedure. We do lots of them.'

His normal urbanity fell away from him. From the beginning he had struck me as a man who had seen so many things in life that nothing would disturb his serenity, but now he seemed to shrink within himself. He slowly stroked the little cat, seated, as usual, on his lap. Then he reached down to the black leather volume of *The Works of Shakespeare* with its faded gold lettering which he had been reading when I arrived. He placed a marker in the book and closed it before putting it carefully on the shelf.

'I really don't know what to say, Mr Herriot.'

I gave him an encouraging smile. 'There's nothing to worry about. I strongly advise it. If I could just describe the operation, I'm sure it would put your mind at rest. It's really keyhole surgery – we make only a tiny incision and bring the ovaries and uterus through and ligate the stump . . .'

I dried up hurriedly because the old man closed his eyes and swayed so far to one side that I thought he would fall off the wicker chair. It wasn't the first time that one of my explanatory surgical vignettes had had an undesirable effect and I altered my tactics.

I laughed loudly and patted him on the knee. 'So, you see, it's nothing – nothing at all.'

He opened his eyes and drew a long, quavering breath, 'Yes . . . yes . . . I'm sure you're right. But you must give me a little time to think. This has come on me so suddenly.'

'All right. I'm sure Eddy Carless will give me a ring for you. But don't be too long.'

I wasn't surprised when I didn't hear from the old man. The whole idea obviously terrified him and it was over a month before I saw him again.

I pushed my head through the sacks. He was sitting in his usual chair, peeling potatoes and he looked at me with serious eyes.

'Ah, Mr Herriot. Come and sit down. I've been going to get in touch with you – I'm so glad you've called.' He threw back his head with an air of resolution. 'I have decided to take your advice about Emily. You may carry out the operation when you think fit.' But his voice trembled as he spoke.

'Oh, that's splendid!' I said cheerfully. 'In fact, I've got a cat basket in the car so I can take her straight away.'

I tried not to look at his stricken face as the cat jumped on to my knee. 'Well, Emily, you're coming with me.' Then as I looked at the little animal, I hesitated. Was it my imagination or was there a significant bulge in her abdomen?

'Just a moment,' I murmured as I palpated the little body, then I looked up at the old man.

'I'm sorry, Mr Ireson, but it's a bit late. She's pregnant.'

His mouth opened, but no words came, then he swallowed and spoke in a hoarse whisper. 'But . . . but what are we going to do?'

'Nothing, nothing, don't worry. She'll have the kittens, that's all and I'll find homes for them. Everything will be fine.' I was putting on my breeziest act, but it didn't seem to help.

'But Mr Herriot, I don't know anything about these things. I'm now terribly worried. She could die giving birth – she's so tiny!'

'No, no, not at all. Cats very rarely have any trouble that way. I tell you what, when she starts having the kittens – probably around a month from now – get Eddy to give me a ring. I'll slip out here and see that all is well. How's that?'

'Oh, you are kind. I feel so silly about this. The trouble is . . . she means so much to me.'

'I know, and stop worrying. Everything will be absolutely okay.'

We had a cup of tea together and by the time I left he had calmed down.

The next time I saw him was under unimagined circumstances.

It was about two weeks later and I was attending the annual dinner of the local Agricultural Society. It was a formal affair and the company consisted of an assortment of farmers, big landowners, and Ministry of Agriculture officials. I wouldn't have been there but for my elevation to the Milk Sub-Committee.

I was having a pre-prandial drink with one of my clients when I almost choked in mid swallow. 'Good heavens! Mr Ireson!' I exclaimed, pointing to the tall, white-bearded figure, immaculate in white tie and tails standing among a group at the far end of the room. The usually untidy bush of silver hair was sleeked back and shining over his ears and, glass in hand and with a commanding air, he was rapping out his words to the group who were nodding deferentially.

'I can't believe it!' I burst out again.

'Oh, it's him, all right,' my friend grunted. 'Miserable bugger!'

'What!'

'Aye, he's a right old sod! He'd skin 'is own grandmother.'

'Well, that's funny. I haven't known him long, but I like him. I like him very much.'

The farmer raised his eyebrows. 'I reckon you're about the only one as does,' he muttered sourly. 'He's the hardest bugger I've ever known.'

I shook my head in bewilderment. 'I can't understand this. And those clothes – where the heck did he get them? I've only seen him in his roadside hut and he seems to have no more than the bare essentials.'

'Hey, wait a minute!' The farmer laughed and punched me in the chest. 'Now I get it. You're talkin' about his brother, old Eugene. That's Cornelius over there!'

'My God, how amazing! The likeness is incredible. Are they twins?'

'Nay, there's two years between them but, as you say, you can hardly tell 'em apart.'

As though he knew we were discussing him, the tall man turned towards us. The face was almost Eugene's, but where there was gentleness, there was aggression, where there was softness and serenity there was a fierce arrogance. I had only a chilling glimpse before he turned away and began to harangue his companions again. It was an uncanny experience and I continued to stare at the group until my friend broke in on my thoughts.

'Aye, a lot of people have made that mistake, but they're only alike in appearance. You couldn't find two people more different in character. Eugene's a grand old lad, but as for that bugger – I've never seen 'im smile.'

'Do you know Eugene?'

'As well as most people, I reckon. I'm nearly as old as him and my farm's on the Ireson estate. Cornelius was left everything when the father died, but I don't think Eugene would've been interested in running the textile empire and the estate. He was a dreamer and a wanderer – kind and friendly, but somehow unworldly. Money or social position meant nothing to him. Went to Oxford, you know, but soon after that he took off and nobody knew if he was alive or dead for years.'

'And now he's back in that little place by the roadside.'

'Aye, it's a rum 'un, isn't it?'

It was a rum 'un indeed – one of the strangest stories I'd ever heard, and it was never far from my mind over the following weeks. I kept wondering how the old man and his cat were getting on in that igloo, and if the kittens had arrived yet? But they couldn't have – I was sure he would have let me know.

I did hear from him at last one stormy evening.

'Mr Herriot, I am telephoning from the farm. Emily has not yet produced those kittens, but she is . . . very large and has lain trembling all day and won't eat anything. I hate to trouble you on this horrible night but I know nothing about these things and she does look . . . most unhappy.'

I didn't like the sound of that, but I tried to sound casual. 'I think I'll just pop out and have a look at her, Mr Ireson.'

'Really – are you sure?'

'Absolutely. No bother. I'll see you soon.'

It was a strange, almost unreal scene as I stumbled through the darkness and parted the sacks forty minutes later. The wind and rain buffeted the tarpaulin walls and by the flickering light of the tilly lamp I saw Eugene in his chair, stroking Emily who lay in the basket by his side.

The little cat had swollen enormously – so much as to be almost unrecognisable and as I kneeled and passed my hand over her distended abdomen I could feel the skin stretched tight. She was absolutely bursting full of kittens, but seemed lifeless and exhausted. She was straining, too, and licking at her vulva.

I looked up at the old man. 'Have you some hot water, Mr Ireson?'

'Yes, yes, the kettle has just boiled.'

I soaped my little finger. It would only just go into the tiny vagina. Inside I found the cervix wide open and a mass beyond, only just palpable. Heaven only knew how many kittens were jammed in there, but one thing was certain. There was no way they could ever come out. There was no room for manoeuvre. There was nothing I could do. Emily turned her face to me and gave a faint miaow of distress and it came to me piercingly that this cat could die.

'Mr Ireson,' I said, 'I'll have to take her away immediately.'

'Take her away?' He said in a bewildered whisper.

'Yes. She needs a Caesarean operation. The kittens can't come out in the normal way.'

Upright in his chair, he nodded, shocked and only half comprehending. I grabbed the basket, Emily and all, and rushed out into the darkness. Then, as I thought of the old man looking blankly after me, I realised that my bedside manner had slipped badly. I pushed my head back through the sacks.

'Don't worry, Mr Ireson,' I said, 'everything's going to be fine.'

Don't worry! Brave words. As I parked Emily on the back seat and drove away, I knew I was damn worried, and I cursed the mocking fate which had decreed that after all of my airy remarks about cats effortlessly giving birth I might be headed for a tragedy. How long had Emily been lying like that? Ruptured uterus? Septicaemia? The grim possibilities raced through my mind. And why did it have to happen to that solitary old man of all people?

I stopped at the village kiosk and rang Siegfried.

'I've just left old Eugene Ireson. Will you come in and give me a hand? Cat Caesar and it's urgent. Sorry to bother you on your night off.'

'Perfectly all right, James, I'm not doing a thing. See you soon, eh?'

When I got to the surgery Siegfried had the steriliser bubbling and everything laid out. 'This is your party, James,' he murmured. 'I'll do the anaesthetic.' I had shaved the site of the operation and poised my scalpel over the grossly swollen abdomen when he whistled softly. 'My God,' he said, 'it's like opening an abscess!'

That was exactly what it was like. I felt that if I made an incision the mass of kittens would explode out in my face and, indeed, as I proceeded with the lightest touch through skin and muscle, the laden uterus bulged out alarmingly.

'Hell!' I breathed. 'How many are in here?'

'A fairish number!' said my partner. 'And she's such a tiny cat.'

Gingerly, I opened the peritoneum which, to my relief looked clean and healthy, then, as I went on, I waited for the jumble of little heads and feet to appear. But with increasing wonderment I watched my incision travel along a massive, coal black back and when I finally hooked my finger round the neck, drew forth a kitten and laid it on the table, I found that the uterus was otherwise empty.

'There's only one!' I gasped. 'Would you believe it?'

Siegfried laughed. 'Yes, but what a whopper! And alive, too. He lifted the kitten and took a closer look. 'A whacking great tom – he's nearly as big as his mother!'

As I stitched up and gave the sleeping Emily a shot of penicillin, I felt the tensions flow away from me in happy waves. The little cat was in good shape. My fears had been groundless. It would be best to leave the kitten with her for a few weeks, then I'd be able to find a home for him.

'Thanks a lot for coming in, Siegfried,' I said. 'It looked like a very dodgy situation at first.'

I could hardly wait to get back to the old man who, I knew, would still be in a state of shock at my taking away his beloved cat. In fact, when I passed through the sacking doorway, it looked as though he hadn't moved an inch since I last saw him. He wasn't reading, wasn't doing anything except staring ahead from his chair.

When I put the basket down by his side, he turned slowly and looked down wonderingly at Emily who was coming round from the anaesthetic and beginning to raise her head, and at the black newcomer who was already finding his private array of teats interesting.

'She's going to be fine, Mr Ireson,' I said, and the old man nodded slowly.

'How wonderful. How simply wonderful,' he murmured.

When I went to take out the stitches ten days later, I found a carnival atmosphere in the igloo. Old Eugene was beside himself with delight, while Emily, stretched in the back with her enormous offspring sucking busily, looked up at me with an expression of pride which bordered on the smug.

'I think we ought to have a celebratory cup of tea and one of my favourite buns,' the old man said.

As the kettle boiled, he drew a finger along the kitten's body. 'He's a handsome fellow, isn't he?'

'He certainly is. He'll grow up into a beautiful cat.'

Eugene smiled. 'Yes. I'm sure he will, and it will be so nice to have him with Emily.'

I paused as he handed me a bun. 'But just a minute, Mr Ireson. You really can't do with two cats here.'

'Why not?'

'Well, you take Emily into the village on a lead most days. You'd have difficulty on the road with two cats, and anyway you don't have room in here, do you?'

He didn't say anything, so I pressed on. 'A lady was asking me the other day if I could find her a black kitten. Many people ask us to find a specific pet for them, often to replace an older animal which has just died, and we always seem to have trouble obliging them, but this time I am delighted that I was able to say I knew the very one.'

He nodded slowly, and then after a moment's cogitation, said, 'I'm sure you're right, Mr Herriot. I hadn't really thought about it enough.'

'Anyway,' I said, 'she's a very nice lady and a real cat lover. He'll have a very good home. He'll live like a little sultan with her.'

He laughed. 'Good ... good ... and maybe I'll hear about him now and then?'

'Absolutely. I'll keep you posted regularly.' I could see I had got over the hurdle nicely and I thought I'd change the subject. 'By the way, I meant to tell you, I saw your brother for the first time not so long ago.'

'Cornelius?' He looked at me expressionlessly. We had never mentioned the subject of his brother before. 'And what did you think of him?'

'Well . . . he didn't look very happy.'

'He wouldn't. He is not a happy man.'

'That's the impression I got. And yet he's got so much.'

The old man smiled gently. 'Yes, but there are so many things he hasn't got.'

I took a sip at my tea. 'That's right. For instance, he hasn't got Emily!'

'Very true! In fact I was about to say that but I thought you might think me silly.' He threw back his head and laughed. A merry, boyish laugh. 'Yes, I have Emily, the all-important thing! I'm so glad we agree about that. Come now, do have another bun.'

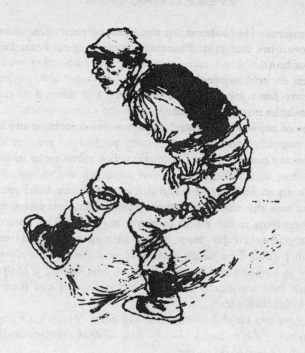

41

'Ooh! Aaah! Ooooh! Ya bugger, 'erriot! What the hell 'ave ye done?' Nat Briggs staggered round the calf pen clutching his left buttock, and glaring at me in fury.

'Sorry, Nat,' I said, holding up the syringe loaded with Strain 19 abortion vaccine. 'I'm afraid you fell right on to my needle.'

'Fell on? You stuck the bloody thing right up me arse, that's what you mean!' He was a big man with a habitually glowering expression, but at the moment he looked positively murderous. He had been holding the calf's head as I was about to make the injection and the animal had swung round at the wrong moment.

I tried a placatory smile. 'No really, Nat. It was just a little prick.'

'Don't give me that!' The big man arched his back, kneaded his buttock and groaned. 'Ah felt it go right in!'

283

His rage was not allayed by the peals of merriment from his comrades, Ray and Phil. The three were long-time workers on Sir Eustace Lamburn's farm and we knew each other well, but Nat was the odd man out. The other two were always cheerful and ready for a joke but Nat was surly and seemed to carry a permanent chip on his shoulder.

A lot of my work consisted of preventive injections and in the many wrestling matches with beasts packed in pens or down passages my needles did occasionally score a bull's-eye in human rather than animal flesh. The most common victim was myself because my patients rarely stood still and with one hand pinching the skin and the other poising the syringe an inch away, it was the easiest thing in the world to pierce my hand. The vet coming to grief either in this way or by getting toes stood on was invariably good for a laugh and there was always an outburst of hilarity as I yelped and hopped around, but having it happen to the dour Nat was nearly as good, especially as I had found my target in his backside.

'Aye, ye can laugh,' snarled the big man, 'but what's goin' to happen now? Ah've had a bloody dose of that abortion stuff, and what's that goin' to do to me?'

'You're not in calf are ye, Nat, lad?' giggled Phil. 'They say that vaccine's only dangerous to pregnant cows, but ah can't see you slippin' your calf.' There was another eruption of mirth from the two.

Briggs stuck out his jaw. 'It's awright you talkin' but that's mucky stuff. It could do summat inside me.'

'Look, Nat,' I said, 'you haven't had a dose of anything.' I held up the syringe showing the full 5 cc dose within. 'You've just had a prick from the needle. You might be a bit sore and I do apologise, but it can't do you any harm.'

'That's what you say, 'erriot, but we'll see. Any road, I'm keepin' clear of you. Somebody else can hold the rest of the buggers.'

Ray clapped him on the shoulder. 'Never mind, Nat. You've just got married, so you'll be well looked after. Your new missus'll get you a cushion whenever you want to sit down.'

There was no doubt that the little accident made the day for

Phil and Ray, but for a long time afterwards I had to suffer complaints from their cantankerous colleague every time I visited the Lamburn farm. It transpired that the buttock had swelled up and remained painful for a long time, causing immense inconvenience, but I was sure the rigmarole was exaggerated and I paid little attention until one day a vastly more serious charge was laid at my door.

Nat Briggs pushed his irascible face close to mine. 'Ah'm goin' to tell tha summat, 'erriot. You've stopped me ever havin' a family.'

'What!'

'Aye, ah'm not jokin'. Missus and me have been trying for a long time but there's no sign of anything happenin'. The doctor doesn't know why, but ah do! It's your bloody injection!'

'Oh, come on, Nat, that's ridiculous. How could that little accident possibly have such an effect?'

'How could it? Ah'll tell you! That bloody stuff you injected into me was to do with abortion and breedin' and all that sort o' thing. It stands to reason that you've stopped me and the missus ever havin' kids!'

I couldn't believe what I was hearing. I pleaded and expostulated, but the man was in deadly earnest. I had ruined his life and he'd never forgive me.

His mates didn't help.

'Don't listen to 'im, Mr Herriot,' cried Ray. 'He can't do it properly – he's only makin' excuses.' More laughter and coarse comments followed.

Despite the jocularity, I found the thing upsetting because it wasn't only on the farm that I had trouble. I never knew when I was going to run into the man. I received dirty looks from Briggs in Darrowby market place, and in the evenings when I was sipping a soothing beer in some country inn it shattered my peace when I found his disapproving gaze trained on me.

Over many months my visits to the Lamburn farm were uncomfortable. The leg-pulling had stopped, but I sensed the hostility from Briggs at all times. He rarely mentioned the matter, but the thing was accepted between us. I was responsible for his permanent sterility and that was that.

★

A long time after the abortion incident I was back on the farm treating a batch of beasts with pneumonia. It was the usual rodeo with about twenty strong young cattle packed in a penned-off corner of the fold yard. I was poising my syringe charged with antibiotic as the men squeezed their way among the crush. Briggs was hanging on to a particularly wild stirk, his back towards me and I'll never know if he was thrown back or if one of the other men nudged my arm because, next moment, he let out an anguished yell.

'Ya rotten bugger, 'erriot, you've done it again!' He staggered about, clutching his behind and staring wide-eyed at me.

I couldn't believe it. Surely history couldn't repeat itself so exactly. But there was no doubt about it, the scene was the same. Briggs bellowing and clutching his buttock, the other two men falling around laughing, myself transfixed in horror.

Still grasping his backside, Briggs turned on me, his fifteen stones hanging over me menacingly. 'What's *this* stuff goin' to do to me, eh?' he barked. 'You've done me enough damage, ya bugger, with that fust lot, but what am I goin' to suffer now?' He glowered at me.

'Nat, I'm truly sorry, but I can only tell you again that it can't possibly do you any harm. There's only antibiotic in the syringe – like penicillin only stronger.'

'Ah don't care a bugger what it is – it's meant to go into the bloody beast, not me. Ah'm bloody fed up with you, 'erriot, doin' the same thing to me again.'

'It's not the same, Nat,' cried Phil. 'You got it in the right cheek this time. Mr Herriot's just levellin' you up – I've allus said he was a tidy worker and it's only natural 'e would want to square the job up.' He and Ray abandoned themselves to helpless mirth.

After that incident, I was grateful that Sir Eustace's livestock had a long spell of good health and I was able to pass the few visits which came up on to Siegfried. It was nearly a year later before the three men and I were together again. As we carried on with our work, I was relieved to find that Briggs was not particularly unfriendly. Whereas the last time I thought he had been going to hit me, now he caught and held the struggling animals without comment.

During a moment's respite, as I refilled my syringe, Ray piped up. 'We've got a bit o' news for you, Mr Herriot.'

'Oh yes?'

'Aye, red 'ot news. Nat's become a dad!'

'Hey, that's great! Congratulations, Nat! What is it – boy or a girl?'

Fatherhood seemed to have mellowed the big man because a sheepish smile spread over his face. 'Twins,' he said proudly. 'Boy and a girl!'

'Well – terrific. You can't do better than that!'

Phil broke in. 'We've been tellin' him, Mr Herriot. He blamed you for stoppin' the job with that first injection you gave 'im. Well, the second jab must have been the antidote!'

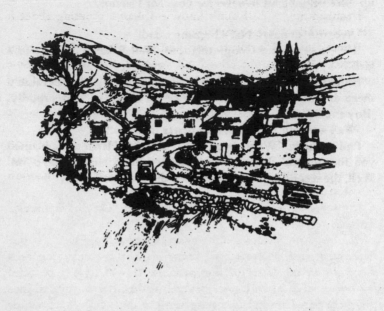

42

'Something for you to think about, James,' Siegfried said one day as he closed the appointments book and rose from the desk.

He was unusually serious and I looked at him in surprise. 'What's that?'

'Well, I know you've had many happy years at Rowan Garth but you've always had an ambition to live right out in the country in a village.'

'That's right – some time in the future, anyway.'

'Well, there's a grand little place – High Field House – coming up for sale in Hannerly and I think it's something special. I'm sure it will soon be snapped up – maybe you'd care to have a look.'

It gave me a jolt. I had certainly nourished this idea for a long time, but as one who hated change of any kind I had never got further than regarding it as a distant dream. Now I was suddenly brought right up against it.

I rubbed my chin. 'I don't know – I wasn't thinking about it yet for a while. Maybe some day . . .'

'James, it takes a lot to stir you into action.' My partner wagged a finger at me. 'But I tell you this, that day will come some time and when it does you will start to thrash around and you'll never find anything better than this place I'm talking about. There isn't a prettier village than Hannerly and the house is ideal for you.'

I felt trapped at the suggestion. Siegfried knew me so well. But as the hours passed and my mind went through its usual gradual adjustment I finally came round sufficiently to mention the proposition to Helen.

My wife was much less diffident than me. 'Let's have a look,' she said.

We did have a look, right away, spurred by Helen's better developed sense of urgency. I knew Hannerly well, sitting as it did right in the heart of our practice. It was tiny; a peaceful backwater of a dozen houses, several of them farms, tucked into the sheltering fellside and strung along a quiet little road which led nowhere in particular. It was beautiful, but not with the chocolate box prettiness of the tourist villages. No shop, no pub, no street lights. To me, it was a secret corner of Yorkshire, a little tableau in stone of that stern and lovely county.

The doctor who was leaving showed us round. The house was modest but charming, resting on the face of its own field, a steeply sloping pasture where sheep grazed. An extensive lawn stretched down to a swiftly running beck which widened into a pond where a score of mallard duck floated serenely and great willows bent their branches towards the water.

Afterwards, in the May sunshine, Helen and I climbed with our dog Dinah behind the house, up the grassy bank, past trees heavy with blossom, then over a stile to a lofty green plateau which seemed to overlook the whole world.

We flopped on to the grass and from our eyrie we looked down past the sheep unhurriedly cropping the grass to the house lying below us. Behind us was a great crescent of tree-covered hillside with the rim of the high moorland peeping above the trees. This majestic sweep curved away to a headland where a tall cliff dominated the scene – a huge friendly slab of rock gleaming in the sunshine. Away in the other direction, over the roofs of the hamlet, there was a heart-lifting glimpse of the great wide plain of York and the distant hills beyond.

After a cold spring, the whole countryside had softened and the air had a gentle warmth, rich with the scents of May blossom and the medley of wild flowers which speckled the grass. In a little wood to our right a scented lake of bluebells flooded the shady reaches of the trees.

As we sat there, three squirrels hopped one after another from a tall sycamore and, pursued optimistically by fat Dinah, flitted, quick and light as air, over the greensward and disappeared behind a rise, leaving her effortlessly behind.

Helen voiced my thoughts. 'Living here would be heaven.'

We almost ran down the hill to the house and closed the deal with the doctor. There were none of the traumas of our previous house-buying efforts; a shake of the hand and it was over.

Helen's words were prophetic. It was a sad moment when we had to leave the happy memories of Rowan Garth behind, but once we were installed in High Field we realised that living in Hannerly was heaven indeed. At times I could hardly believe our luck. To be able to sit outside our front door, drinking tea in the sunshine and watching the mallard splashing and diving on our pond; with the hillside before us aflame with gorse and, away above, that changeless cliff face smiling down. And to live always in a quiet world where the silence at night was almost palpable.

Picking my torchlit way with Dinah on our nocturnal strolls I could hear nothing except the faintest whisper of the beck murmuring its eternal way under the stone bridge. Sometimes on these nightly walks, a badger would scuttle across my path, and under the stars I might see a fox carrying out a stealthy exploration of our lawn.

One morning on an early call just after dawn, I surprised two roe deer in the open and watched enthralled as they galloped at incredible speed across the fields and, clearing the fences like steeplechasers, plunged into the woods.

EVERY LIVING THING

Here in Hannerly, just a few miles from Darrowby, there was the ever present thrill for Helen and me that we were living on the edge of the wild.

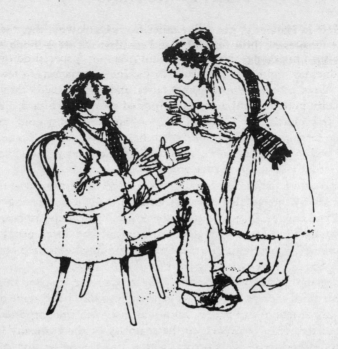

43

'By God, ah's sweatin'!' Albert Budd gasped as he collapsed his
sixteen stones onto a chair next to me and wiped his face with a
bright red-spotted kerchief. Then he gave me an anguished look,
'And ah know ah'm goin' to start fartin' in a minute.'

'What!' I stared at him in alarm. We had just finished a set of
quadrilles at Calum's newly formed Highland dancing club in
the village hall, and I was puffing, too, as I rested down next to
the young farmer. 'Really? Are you sure?'

'Aye, nothin' surer. When Calum roped me in for this dancin',
I didn't know there'd be all this jumpin' and jogglin', and I've
just had a bloody good feed with three Yorkshire puddin's. This
is murder!'

I didn't know what to say but I tried to be reassuring. 'Just sit
quietly for a bit – I expect you'll be all right.'

Albert shook his head. 'No chance! I can feel it comin' on..
He's a bugger is Calum. He came in and grabbed me as soon as
I'd finished me dinner. Me mother allus gives me a special do on
a Wednesday night after I get back from Houlton market – a few
good slices o' beef, sprouts and taties and, like I said, three
Yorkshire puddin's and a smashin' spotted dick and custard. I'd
had a few pints at the Golden Lion, too, and I was just goin' to
put me feet up for half an hour when he walked into the house.
Said I had to come with him, but I thought the dancin' would be
like Victor Sylvester on the television.'

The stab of pity I felt for the poor chap's predicament was
sharpened by the fact that everybody else in the hall was having a
wonderful time. Calum's persuasive energies had obviously been
successful and there was a good turnout of the local people
forming up for an eightsome reel as the gramophone poured out
Jimmy Shand's foot-twitching beat.

Helen and I had gladly fallen in with the dancing idea and this
was our third visit. With my Glasgow upbringing, I had done it
all before at school and parties, but I was rusty and had forgotten
some of the steps. However, to the majority of the company –
farmers, school-teachers, doctors, and a good cross-section of
local people – the whole business was strange and new. But they
were definitely fun to learn, and at times the loud laughter
almost drowned the music.

I could understand that Albert didn't find it funny at all. He
was about twenty-five and lived with a doting mother who
looked after him far too well. He was one of the many young
farmers who had formed a friendship with the ebullient new vet
and were eager to join him in his activities, but this Scottish
dancing was definitely not his scene.

I had often noted that there weren't many fat chaps among the
farmers but Albert was a striking exception. Six feet three,
beacon-faced and with an enormous belly which he somehow
managed to carry round his milking, hay-making and other
farming chores. His appetite was legendary in the district and he
was a constant menace to those carvery restaurants where you
could pay a set amount and eat as much as you liked.

He looked acutely uncomfortable at this moment, resting his

hands on his vast stomach and gazing at me with intensely worried eyes.

I could sympathise with him. I had seen his streaming face bouncing aimlessly above the crowd in the quadrilles and there was no doubt he must be suffering.

'Ah tell ye this, Jim,' he went on, 'if I have to do any more jumpin' around I've had it. I'm goin' to start fartin', and when ah do ah can't stop!'

'Oh dear, I'm sorry, Albert. It's a bit awkward for you with all these ladies around.'

I hadn't meant to be cruel but he stared at me in horror. 'Oh 'ell!' he groaned, then, 'By God, I'm startin'! I'm gettin' out – I'm off 'ome!'

He was about to heave himself off his chair when the curate's young wife came over.

'Really, Mr Budd,' she said, with mock disapproval, 'we can't have you sitting against the wall when we need a man for this reel.'

Albert gave her a ghastly smile. 'Nay . . . nay . . . thank ye. I was just . . .'

'Oh, come now, you mustn't be shy. Most of us are still learning.' She put out her hand and Albert gave me a last despairing glance before he was led onto the floor.

His eyes registered acute anxiety as he was stationed between the curate's wife and a pretty young teacher from Darrowby Infants' School, but there was no escape. The gramophone sounded the opening chord, they bowed, then they were off, skipping round hand in hand one way and then the other. I watched in morbid fascination as he halted and faced his partner. On my God, they were starting the pas de bas! That was fatal! For a few moments I watched the tortured face bob–bob–bobbing up and down, the great belly quivering like a blancmange as the music reverberated round the hall then I just couldn't look any longer.

I tore my eyes away and as I searched for some distraction among the dancing throng, it struck me that all this jollity was another example of something new which Calum had brought to Darrowby. These people were just a few of the many on whom he had laid his hand. I looked at him now, the tall, black-moustached figure, magnificent as any highland chieftain in his kilt, leaping high, kicking out his feet, toes pointed in the classical manner while Deirdre, tartan-sashed and graceful, glided expertly among the stumbling rookies.

The thought recurred that Calum had an irresistible attraction for a large number of people and he had brought fresh, meaningful angles into their lives, yet there seemed always to be a faint spice of danger for those who followed closely in his beguiling wake – whether it be myself on that bare-backed cart horse, Siegfried with the Dobermanns and now the hapless Albert jogglin' in agony out on that floor.

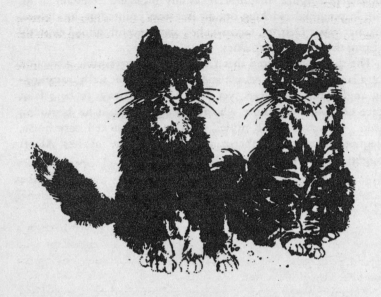

44

'Look at that, Jim! Surely that's a stray cat. I've never seen it before.' Helen was at the kitchen sink, washing dishes, and she pointed through the window.

Our new house in Hannerly had been built into a sloping field. There was a low retaining wall, chest high, just outside the window and, behind, the grassy bank led from the wall top up to some bushes and an open log shed perched about twenty yards away. A lean little cat was peering warily from the bushes. Two tiny kittens crouched by her side.

'I think you're right,' I said. 'That's a stray with her family and she's looking for food.'

Helen put out a bowl of meat scraps and some milk on the flat top of the wall and retired to the kitchen. The mother cat did not move for a few minutes, then she advanced with the utmost caution, took up some of the food in her mouth and carried it back to her kittens.

Several times she crept down the bank, but when the kittens tried to follow her, she gave them a quick 'get back' tap with her paw.

We watched, fascinated, as the scraggy, half-starved creature made sure that her family had eaten before she herself took anything from the bowl. Then, when the food was finished, we quietly opened the back door. But as soon as they saw us, cat and kittens flitted away into the field.

'I wonder where they came from,' Helen said.

I shrugged. 'Heaven knows. There's a lot of open country round here. They could have come from miles away. And that mother cat doesn't look like an ordinary stray. There's a real wild look about her.'

Helen nodded. 'Yes, she looks as though she's never been in a house, never had anything to do with people. I've heard of wild cats like that who live outside. Maybe she only came looking for food because of her kittens.'

'I think you're right,' I said as we returned to the kitchen. 'Anyway, the poor little things have had a good feed. I don't suppose we'll see them again.'

But I was wrong. Two days later, the trio reappeared. In the same place, peeping from the bushes, looking hungrily towards the kitchen window. Helen fed them again, the mother cat still fiercely forbidding her kittens to leave the bushes, and once more they darted away when we tried to approach them. When they came again next morning, Helen turned to me and smiled.

'I think we've been adopted,' she said.

She was right. The three of them took up residence in the log shed and after a few days the mother allowed the kittens to come down to the food bowls, shepherding them carefully all the way. They were still quite tiny, only a few weeks old. One was black and white, the other tortoiseshell.

Helen fed them for a fortnight, but they remained unapproachable creatures. Then one morning, as I was about to go on my rounds, she called me into the kitchen.

She pointed through the window. 'What do you make of that?'

I looked and saw the two kittens in their usual position under the bushes, but there was no mother cat.

'That's strange,' I said. 'She's never let them out of her sight before.'

The kittens had their feed and I tried to follow them as they ran away, but I lost them in the long grass, and although I searched all over the field there was no sign of them or their mother.

We never saw the mother cat again and Helen was quite upset.

'What on earth can have happened to her?' she murmured a few days later as the kittens ate their morning meal.

'Could be anything,' I replied. 'I'm afraid the mortality rate for wandering cats is very high. She could have been run over by a car or had some other accident. I'm afraid we'll never know.'

Helen looked again at the little creatures crouched side by side, their heads in the bowl. 'Do you think she's just abandoned them?'

'Well, it's possible. She was a maternal and caring little thing and I have a feeling she looked around till she could find a good home for them. She didn't leave till she saw that they could fend for themselves and maybe she's returned to her outside life now. She was a real wild one.'

It remained a mystery, but one thing was sure: the kittens were installed for good. Another thing was sure: they would never be domesticated. Try as we might, we were never able to touch them, and all our attempts to wheedle them into the house were unavailing.

One wet morning, Helen and I looked out of the kitchen window at the two of them sitting on the wall, waiting for their breakfast, their fur sodden, their eyes nearly closed against the driving rain.

'Poor little things,' Helen said, 'I can't bear to see them out there, wet and cold, we *must* get them inside.'

'How? We've tried often enough.'

'Oh, I know, but let's have another go. Maybe they'll be glad to come in out of the rain.'

We mashed up a dish of fresh fish, an irresistible delicacy to

cats. I let them have a sniff and they were eager and hungry, then
I placed the dish just inside the back door before retreating out of
sight. But as we watched through the window the two of them
sat motionless in the downpour, their eyes fixed on the fish,
but determined not to go through the door. That, clearly, was
unthinkable.

'All right, you win,' I said and put the food on the wall where
it was immediately devoured.

I was staring at them with a feeling of defeat when Herbert
Platt, one of the local dustmen, came round the corner. At the
sight of him the kittens scurried away and Herbert laughed.

'Ah see you've taken on them cats. That's some nice stuff
they're gettin' to eat.'

'Yes, but they won't come inside to get it.'

He laughed again. 'Aye, and they never will. Ah've know'n
that family o' cats for years, and all their ancestors. I saw that
mother cat when she first came, and before that she lived at awd
Mrs Caley's over the hill and ah remember that 'un's mother
before her, down at Billy Tate's farm. Ah can go back donkey's
years with them cats.'

'Gosh, is that so?'

'Aye, it is, and I've never seen one o' that strain that would go
inside a house. They're wild, real wild.'

'Ah well, thanks, Herbert, that explains a lot.'

He smiled and hoisted a bin. 'Ah'll get off, then, and they can
finish their breakfast.'

'Well, that's it, Helen,' I said. 'Now we know. They're always
going to be outside, but at least we can try to improve their
accommodation.'

The thing we called the log shed, where I had laid some straw
for them to sleep, wasn't a shed at all. It had a roof, but was open
all down one side, with widely spaced slats on the other three
sides. It allowed a constant through-wind which made it a fine
place for drying out the logs but horribly draughty as a dwelling.

I went up the grassy slope and put up a sheet of plywood as a
wind-break. Then I built up a mound of logs into a protective
zariba around the straw bed and stood back, puffing slightly.

'Right,' I said. 'They'll be quite cosy in there now.'

Helen nodded in agreement, but she had gone one better. Behind my wind-break, she put down an open-sided box with cushions inside. 'There now, they needn't sleep on the straw any more. They'll be warm and comfortable in this nice box.'

I rubbed my hands. 'Great. We won't have to worry about them in bad weather. They'll really enjoy coming in here.'

From that moment the kittens boycotted the shed. They still came for their meals every day, but we never saw them anywhere near their old dwelling.

'They're just not used to it,' Helen said.

'Hmm.' I looked again at the cushioned box tucked in the centre of the encircling logs. 'Either that, or they don't like it.'

We stuck it out for a few days, then, as we wondered where on earth the kittens could be sleeping, our resolve began to crack. I went up the slope and dismantled the wall of logs. Immediately the two little creatures returned. They sniffed and nosed round the box and went away again.

'I'm afraid they're not keen on your box either,' I grunted as we watched from our vantage point.

Helen looked stricken. 'Silly little things. It's perfect for them.'

But after another two days during which the shed lay deserted, she went out and I saw her coming sadly down the bank, box in one hand, cushions under her arm.

The kittens were back within hours, looking round the place, vastly relieved. They didn't seem to object to the wind-break and settled happily in the straw. Our attempts to produce a feline Hilton had been a total failure.

It dawned on me that they couldn't bear to be enclosed, to have their escape routes cut off. Lying there on the open bed of straw, they could see all around them and were able to flit away between the slats at the slightest sign of danger.

'Okay, my friends,' I said, 'that's the way you want it, but I'm going to find out something more about you.'

Helen gave them some food and once they were concentrating on the food, I crept up on them and threw a fisherman's landing net over them and after a struggle I was able to divine that the tortoiseshell was a female and the black and white a male.

'Good,' said Helen, 'I'll call them Olly and Ginny.'

'Why Olly?'

'Don't really know. He looks like an Olly. I like the name.'

'Oh, and how about Ginny?'

'Short for Ginger.'

'She's not really ginger, she's tortoiseshell.'

'Well, she's a bit ginger.'

I left it at that.

Over the next few months they grew rapidly and my veterinary mind soon reached a firm decision. I had to neuter them. And it was then that I was confronted for the first time with a problem which was to worry me for years – how to minister to the veterinary needs of animals which I was unable even to touch.

The first time, when they were half grown, it wasn't so bad. Again I slunk up on them with my net when they were feeding and managed to bundle them into a cat cage from which they looked at me with terrified and, I imagined, accusing eyes.

In the surgery, as Siegfried and I lifted them one by one from the cage and administered the intravenous anaesthetic, I was struck by the fact that although they were terror-stricken at being in an enclosed space for the first time in their lives and by being grasped and restrained by humans, they were singularly easy to handle. Many of our domesticated feline patients were fighting furies until we had lulled them to sleep, and cats, with claws as well as teeth for weapons, can inflict a fair amount of damage. However, Olly and Ginny, although they struggled frantically, made no attempt to bite, never unsheathed their claws.

Siegfried put it briefly. 'These little things are scared stiff, but they're absolutely docile. I wonder how many wild cats are like this.'

I felt a little strange as I carried out the operations, looking down at the small sleeping forms. These were my cats yet it was the first time I was able to touch them as I wished, examine them closely, appreciate the beauty of their fur and colourings.

When they had come out of the anaesthetic, I took them home and when I released the two of them from the cage, they scampered up to their home in the log shed. As was usual following such minor operations, they showed no after effects, but they clearly had unpleasant memories of me. During the next few weeks they came close to Helen as she fed them but fled immediately at the sight of me. All my attempts to catch Ginny to remove the single little stitch in her spay incision were fruitless. That stitch remained for ever and I realised that Herriot had been cast firmly as the villain of the piece, the character who would grab you and bundle you into a wire cage if you gave him half a chance.

It soon became clear that things were going to stay that way because, as the months passed and Helen plied them with all manner of titbits and they grew into truly handsome, sleek cats, they would come arching along the wall top when she appeared at the back door, but I had only to poke my head from the door to send them streaking away out of sight. I was the chap to be avoided at all times and this rankled with me because I have always been fond of cats and I had become particularly attached to these two. The day finally arrived when Helen was able to stroke them gently as they ate and my chagrin deepened at the sight.

Usually they slept in the log shed but occasionally they disappeared to somewhere unknown and stayed away for a few days and we used to wonder if they had abandoned us or if something had happened to them. When they reappeared, Helen would shout to me in great relief, 'They're back, Jim, they're back!' They had become part of our lives.

Summer lengthened into autumn and when the bitter Yorkshire winter set in we marvelled at their hardiness. We used to feel terrible, looking at them from our warm kitchen as they sat out in the frost and snow, but no matter how harsh the weather, nothing would induce either of them to set foot inside the house. Warmth and comfort had no appeal for them.

When the weather was fine we had a lot of fun just watching them. We could see right up into the log shed from our kitchen, and it was fascinating to observe their happy relationship. They were such friends. Totally inseparable, they spent hours licking each other and rolling about together in gentle play and they never pushed each other out of the way when they were given their food. At nights we could see the two furry little forms curled close together in the straw.

Then there was a time when we thought everything had changed for ever. The cats did one of their disappearing acts and as day followed day we became more anxious. Each morning, Helen started her day with the cry of, 'Olly, Ginny' which always brought the two of them trotting down from their dwelling, but now they did not appear, and when a week passed and then two we had almost run out of hope.

When we came back from our half day in Brawton, Helen ran to the kitchen and looked out. The cats knew our habits and they would always be sitting waiting for her but the empty wall stretched away and the log shed was deserted. 'Do you think they've gone for good, Jim?' she said.

I shrugged. 'It's beginning to look like it. You remember what old Herbert said about that family of cats. Maybe they're nomads at heart – gone off to pastures new.'

Helen's face was doleful. 'I can't believe it. They seemed so happy here. Oh I hope nothing terrible has happened to them.' Sadly she began to put her shopping away and she was silent all evening. My attempts to cheer her up were half-hearted because I was wrapped in a blanket of misery myself.

Strangely, it was the very next morning when I heard Helen's usual cry, but this time it wasn't a happy one.

She ran into the sitting room. 'They're back, Jim,' she said breathlessly, 'but I think they're dying!'

'What? What do you mean?'

'Oh, they look awful! They're desperately ill – I'm sure they're dying.'

I hurried through to the kitchen with her and looked through the window. The cats were sitting there side by side on the wall a few feet away. A watery discharge ran from their eyes which were almost closed, more fluid poured from their nostrils and saliva drooled from their mouths. Their bodies shook from a continuous sneezing and coughing.

They were thin and scraggy, unrecognisable as the sleek creatures we knew so well and their appearance was made more pitiful by their situation in the teeth of a piercing east wind which tore at their fur and made their attempts to open their eyes even more painful.

Helen opened the back door. 'Olly, Ginny, what's happened to you?' she cried softly.

A remarkable thing then happened. At the sound of her voice, the cats hopped carefully from the wall and walked unhesitatingly through the door into the kitchen. It was the first time they had been under our roof.

'Look at that!' Helen exclaimed. 'I can't believe it. They must be really ill. But what is it, Jim? Have they been poisoned?'

I shook my head. 'No, they've got cat flu.'

'You can tell?'

'Oh yes, this is classical.'

'And will they die?'

I rubbed my chin. 'I don't think so.' I wanted to sound reassuring, but I wondered. Feline virus rhinotracheitis had a fairly low mortality rate, but bad cases can die and these cats were very bad indeed. 'Anyway, close the door, Helen, and I'll see if they'll let me examine them.'

But at the sight of the closing door, both cats bolted back outside.

'Open up again,' I cried and, after a moment's hesitation, the cats walked back into the kitchen.

I looked at them in astonishment. 'Would you believe it? They haven't come in here for shelter, they've come for help!'

And there was no doubt about it. The two of them sat there, side by side, waiting for us to do something for them.

'The question is,' I said, 'will they allow their *bête noire* to get near them? We'd better leave the back door open so they don't feel threatened.'

I approached inch by inch until I could put a hand on them, but they did not move. With a feeling that I was dreaming, I lifted each of them, limp and unresisting, and examined them.

Helen stroked them while I ran out to my car which held my stock of drugs and brought in what I'd need. I took their temperatures; they were both over 104, which was typical. Then I injected them with oxytetracycline, the antibiotic which I had always found best for treating the secondary bacterial infection which followed the initial virus attack. I also injected vitamins, cleaned away the pus and mucus from the eyes and nostrils with cotton wool and applied an antibiotic ointment. And all the time I marvelled that I was lifting and handling these yielding little bodies which I hadn't even been able to touch before apart from when they had been under the anaesthetic for the neutering ops.

When I had finished I couldn't bear the thought of turning them out into that cruel wind. I lifted them up and tucked them one under each arm.

'Helen,' I said, 'let's have another try. Will you just gently close the door.'

She took hold of the knob and began to push very slowly, but immediately both cats leaped like uncoiled springs from my arms and shot into the garden. We watched them as they trotted out of sight.

'Well, that's extraordinary,' I said. 'Ill as they are, they won't tolerate being shut in.'

Helen was on the verge of tears. 'But how will they stand it out there? They should be kept warm. I wonder if they'll stay now or will they leave us again?'

'I just don't know.' I looked at the empty garden. 'But we've got to realise they are in their natural environment. They're tough little things. I think they'll be back.'

I was right. Next morning they were outside the window, eyes closed against the wind, the fur on their faces streaked and stained with the copious discharge.

Again Helen opened the door and again they walked calmly inside and made no resistance as I repeated my treatment, injecting them, swabbing out eyes and nostrils, examining their mouths for ulcers, lifting them around like any long-standing household pets.

This happened every day for a week. The discharges became more purulent and their racking sneezing seemed no better; then, when I was losing hope, they started to eat a little food and, significantly, they weren't so keen to come into the house.

When I did get them inside, they were tense and unhappy as I handled them and finally I couldn't touch them at all. They were by no means cured, so I mixed oxytet soluble powder in their food and treated them that way.

The weather was even worse, with fine flakes of snow spinning in the wind, but the day came when they refused to come inside and we watched them through the window as they ate. But I had the satisfaction of knowing they were still getting the antibiotic with every mouthful.

As I carried on this long-range treatment, observing them daily from the kitchen, it was rewarding to see the sneezing abating, the discharges drying up and the cats gradually regaining their lost flesh.

It was a brisk sunny morning in March and I was watching Helen putting their breakfast on the wall. Olly and Ginny, sleek as seals, their faces clean and dry, their eyes bright, came arching along the wall, purring like outboard motors. They were in no hurry to eat; they were clearly happy just to see her.

As they passed to and fro, she ran her hand gently along their heads and backs. This was the kind of stroking they liked – not overdone, with them continually in motion.

I felt I had to get into the action and stepped from the open door.

'Ginny,' I said and held out a hand. 'Come here, Ginny.' The little creature stopped her promenade along the wall and regarded me from a safe distance, not with hostility but with all the old wariness. As I tried to move nearer to her, she skipped away out of reach.

'Okay,' I said, 'and I don't suppose it's any good trying with you either, Olly.' The black-and-white cat backed well away from my outstretched hand and gave me a non-committal gaze. I could see he agreed with me.

Mortified, I called out to the two of them. 'Hey, remember me?' It was clear by the look of them that they remembered me all right – but not in the way I hoped. I felt a stab of frustration. Despite my efforts I was back where I started.

Helen laughed. 'They're a funny pair, but don't they look

marvellous! They're a picture of health, as good as new. It says a lot for fresh air treatment.'

'It does indeed,' I said with a wry smile, 'but it also says something for having a resident veterinary surgeon.'

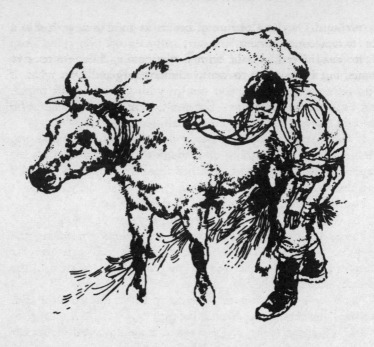

45

'Get back home to bed, James!' Siegfried was at his most imperious, chin jutting, arm outstretched, pointing to the door.

'No, I'm fine,' I said, 'honestly I am.'

'Well, you don't look so damn fine to me. About ready for Mallock's yard if you ask me. You're not fit to be out.'

His reference to the local knacker man was not inapposite. I had trailed into the surgery the day after one of my brucellosis attacks in the hope that a bit of work and exercise would make me feel better, but I knew that the weak, shivery object I had seen in my mirror didn't look much good for anything.

I dug my hands into my pockets and tried to stop shaking. 'I soon recover from these things, Siegfried, my temperature's normal and lying in bed gives me the willies. I'll be okay, I assure you.'

'James, maybe you'll be okay tomorrow but if you go out into the frozen country now and start stripping off you could drop down dead. I've got to be on my way now and I've no time to argue, but I *forbid* you to work! Understand? I tell you what. If you refuse to go home, you can go with Calum on his round. Just sit in the car with him – but don't do anything!' He lifted his medical bag and left the room at a half trot.

It didn't seem a bad idea. Better than lying in bed listening to the household noises going on through the closed door with the depressing feeling of being detached from the workaday world. I had always hated that.

I turned to our assistant. 'Is that all right, Calum?'

'Of course, Jim. I'll enjoy your company.'

I wasn't such bright company as I sat silently watching the drystone walls and the snow-covered hills roll past the car windows. When we arrived at the first farm, however, the gateway was blocked.

'We'll have to walk over a couple of fields, Jim,' Calum said. 'Perhaps you should stay here in the car.'

'No, I'll come with you.' I dragged myself out and we set off across the smooth unbroken blanket of white.

Even that short journey held something for my colleague. 'Look Jim, a fox has been along here. See his pad marks and the long trailing groove made by his brush. And those little holes – there are mice down there. The heat from their bodies melts the snow above them.' He identified the tracks of the various birds which had landed on the snow. They were just marks to me but a whole thrilling book to him.

The farmer, Edgar Stott, was waiting for us in the yard. Calum had never been to his farm and I introduced him. 'I'm not too grand today, so Mr Buchanan is going to see to your cow.'

Mr Stott was known as a 'clever bugger' among the local farmers. This didn't mean that they regarded him as intellectually superior, but rather as an aggressive know-all. In his own eyes, he was an outstanding wit and he did not endear himself to his neighbours by his propensity for taking people down a peg.

He was a big man and his bright little eyes in the fleshy face twinkled maliciously at Calum. 'Oh, we've got the reserve man

on the job today. Vet wi' t'badger, eh? I've heard about you.
We'll soon see how much ye know.'

In the byre, I sank down on a bale of straw, relishing the sweet
bovine warmth. Mr Stott led Calum along the line of cows and
pointed to a roan animal. 'Well, there she is. What d'ye make of
her?'

Calum scratched the root of her tail and looked along the
shaggy flank. 'Well now, what's the trouble, Mr Stott?'

'Ah, you're t'vitnery. I want *you* to tell *me*.'

My colleague smiled politely at the ancient joke. 'Let's put it
another way. What are her symptoms? Is she off her food?'

'Aye.'

'Taking anything at all?'

'Just a bit.'

'How long has she been calved?'

'About a month.'

Calum took the temperature. Auscultated stomach and lungs.
Pulled the head round and smelt the breath. Drew some milk on
to his palm and smelt that, too, but he was clearly baffled. His
enquiries about the animal's history were answered by grunts
from Mr Stott and several times when Calum stood back and
gazed blankly at the animal the farmer's mouth twisted in a
sneer.

'Will you bring me a bucket of hot water, soap and a towel,
please?' the young man asked.

He took off his shirt and thrust his arm first into the vagina,
then deeply up into the rectum where I knew he was palpating
the abdominal organs. Then he turned to the farmer who was
standing, hands in pockets, observing him with sardonic interest.

'You know, this is very strange. Everything seems normal. Is
there anything you haven't told me, Mr Stott?'

The big man hunched his shoulders and chuckled. 'Aye, there
is summat I haven't told ye. There's nowt wrong wi' that beast.'

'Eh?'

'I said there's nowt wrong with 'er. She's as healthy as thee
and me. I just wanted to see if you know owt about the job.'
Then he burst into a roar of laughter and slapped his knee in
glee.

As Calum, naked to the waist, his arm covered in faeces, looked back at him expressionlessly, the farmer tapped him on the shoulder.

'Now then, ah know you can take a joke, young man, Ha-ha-ha! There's nowt like a good laugh! Heh-heh-heh-heh!'

For several long seconds, Calum continued to stare at him, then his face relaxed slowly into a smile, and as he soaped and washed his arm in the bucket and pulled on his shirt, he began to giggle gently and finally he threw back his head and gave a great peal of mirth. 'Yes, you're right. Mr Stott! Ha-ha-ha! There's nowt like a good laugh. You're right, so right.'

The farmer led him along the byre. 'This is the cow you 'ave to see.'

As expected, he had already diagnosed the illness. Mr Stott knew everything. 'She's just got a touch o' slow fever.' This was the local name for acetonaemia, a metabolic disease easily cured. 'There's that sweet smell about 'er and she's losin' flesh.'

'Ah yes, Mr Stott, it sounds like it. I'll just check her over.' Still chuckling, he drew a few squirts from the udder, smelt the breath, took the temperature. All the time he kept murmuring, 'How funny, what a good joke,' then he began to whistle cheerfully. It was when he had his stethoscope on the stomach that the whistling slowed down and then stopped. He began to listen intently, grave-faced, moving from the left side of the cow to the right, then back again.

Finally he straightened up. 'Can you get me a spoon from the house, please.'

The grin faded from the farmer's face. 'A spoon? What the 'ell for? Is there summat wrong?'

'Oh, it's probably nothing. I don't want to worry you. Just get me the spoon.'

When the farmer returned, Calum recommenced his listening at the left side of the cow, only this time he kept tapping the lower ribs with the spoon.

'My God, it's there!' he exclaimed.

'What's there?' gasped the farmer. 'What are you talkin' about?'

'The tinkle.'

'The tinkle?'

'Yes, Mr Stott, it's the tinkling sound you hear in displacement of the abomasum.'

'Displacement . . . what the 'ell's that?'

'It is a condition where the fourth stomach or abomasum slips round from the right side to the left. I'm awfully sorry, but it's a very serious ailment.'

'But how about the sweet smell?'

'Well, yes, you do get that acetonaemia smell with a displacement. It's very easy to confuse the two things.'

'What's goin' to happen, then?'

Calum sighed. 'She'll have to undergo a very large operation. It requires two vets – one to open up the left side of the cow, the other to open the right. I'm afraid it's a very big job.'

'And it'll cost a lot of money, too, ah reckon!'

'Afraid so.'

The farmer took off his cap and began to churn his hair about. Then he swung round at me, slumped on my bale. 'Is all this I'm hearin' right? About this tinkle?'

'I'm sorry to have to tell you, Mr Stott, but it is,' I replied. 'That tinkling noise is classical. We get quite a lot of these cases now.'

He rounded on Calum again. 'Bloody 'ell! And will she be all right after the operation?'

The young man shrugged. 'Can't guarantee anything, I'm sorry to say. But most of them do quite well.'

'Most of 'em . . . and what if she doesn't have the operation?'

'She'll waste away and die. You can see she's losing flesh now. I'm really very sorry.'

The farmer stared, open mouthed and wordless, at the young man.

'I know how you feel, Mr Stott,' Calum said. 'A lot of farmers hate the idea of the big operation. It's a gory, messy business. You could send her in for slaughter if you like.'

'Send her in . . . ? She's a bloody good cow!'

'All right, then, let's go ahead with the job. Mr Herriot is quite ill and unfit to do anything, but I'll telephone Mr Farnon to come out with the equipment.'

The farmer, totally shattered, dropped down on my bale and his head sank on his chest. As he sat there, staring at the ground, Calum's face broke into a grin which almost reached his ears.

'It's okay, Mr Stott. I'm only kidding.'

'What?' the farmer gaped up at him uncomprehendingly.

'Only kidding. Just a little joke. Ha-ha! She's only got acetonaemia. I'll get some steroid from the car. A couple of shots and she'll be fine.'

As Mr Stott rose slowly from the bale, Calum wagged a finger at him.

'I know you like a joke. Ha-ha-ha-ha! As you say, there's nowt like a good laugh!'

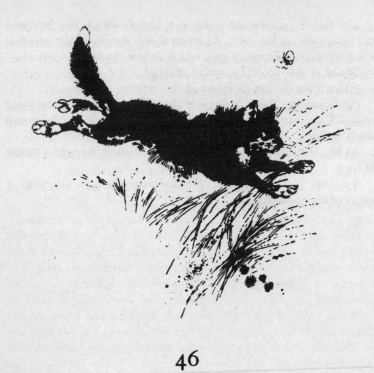

46

As a cat lover, it irked me that my own cats couldn't stand the sight of me. Ginny and Olly were part of the family now. We were devoted to them and whenever we had a day out the first thing Helen did on our return was to open the back door and feed them. The cats knew this very well and were either sitting on the flat top of the wall, waiting for her, or ready to trot down from the log shed which was their home.

We had been to Brawton on our half-day and they were there as usual as Helen put out a dish of food and a bowl of milk for them on the wall.

'Olly, Ginny,' she murmured as she stroked the furry coats. The days had long gone when they refused to let her touch them. Now they rubbed against her hand in delight, arching and purring and, when they were eating, she ran her hand repeatedly along their backs. They were such gentle little animals, their wildness expressed only in fear, and now, with her, that fear had gone. My children and some from the village had won their confidence, too, and were allowed to give them a careful caress, but they drew the line at Herriot.

Like now, for instance, when I quietly followed Helen out and moved towards the wall. Immediately they left the food and retreated to a safe distance where they stood, still arching their backs but, as ever, out of reach. They regarded me without hostility but as I held out a hand they moved further away.

'Look at the little beggars!' I said. 'They still won't have anything to do with me.'

It was frustrating since, throughout my years in veterinary practice, cats had always intrigued me and I had found that this helped me in my dealings with them. I felt I could handle them more easily than most people because I liked them and they sensed it. I rather prided myself on my cat technique, a sort of feline bedside manner, and was in no doubt that I had an empathy with the entire species and that they all liked me. In fact, if the truth were told, I fancied myself as a cats' pin-up. Not so, ironically, with these two – the ones to whom I had become so deeply attached.

It was a bit hard, I thought, because I had doctored them and probably saved their lives when they had cat flu. Did they remember that, I wondered, but if they did it still didn't give me the right apparently to lay a finger on them. And, indeed, what they certainly did seem to remember was that it was I who had netted them and then shoved them into a cage before I neutered them. I had the feeling that whenever they saw me, it was that net and cage which was uppermost in their minds.

I could only hope that time would bring an understanding between us but, as it turned out, fate was to conspire against me for a long time still. Above all, there was the business of Olly's coat. Unlike his sister, he was a long-haired cat and as such was subject to constant tangling and knotting of his fur. If he had been an ordinary domesticated feline, I would have combed him out as soon as trouble arose but since I couldn't even get near him I was helpless. We had had him about two years when Helen called me to the kitchen.

'Just look at him!' she said. 'He's a dreadful sight!'

I peered through the window. Olly was indeed a bit of a scarecrow with his matted fur and dangling knots in cruel contrast with his sleek and beautiful little sister.

'I know, I know. But what can I do?' I was about to turn away when I noticed something. 'Wait a minute, there's a couple of horrible big lumps hanging below his neck. Take these scissors and have a go at them – a couple of quick snips and they'll be off.'

Helen gave me an anguished look. 'Oh, we've tried this before. I'm not a vet and anyway, he won't let me do that. He'll let me pet him, but this is something else.'

'I know that, but have a go. There's nothing to it, really.' I pushed a pair of curved scissors into her hand and began to call instructions through the window. 'Right now, get your fingers behind that big dangling mass. Fine, fine! Now up with your scissors and –'

But at the first gleam of steel, Olly was off and away up the hill. Helen turned to me in despair. 'It's no good, Jim, it's hopeless – he won't let me cut even one lump off and he's covered with them.'

I looked at the dishevelled little creature standing at a safe distance from us. 'Yes, you're right. I'll have to think of something.'

Thinking of something entailed doping Olly so that I could get at him, and my faithful nembutal capsules sprang immediately to mind. This oral anaesthetic had been a valued ally on countless occasions where I had to deal with unapproachable animals, but this was different. With the other cases, my patients had been behind closed doors but Olly was outside with all the wide countryside to roam in. I couldn't have him going to sleep somewhere out there where a fox or other predator might get him. I would have to watch him all the time.

It was a time for decisions, and I drew myself up. 'I'll have a go at him this Sunday,' I told Helen. 'It's usually a bit quieter and I'll ask Siegfried to stand in for me in an emergency.'

When the day arrived, Helen went out and placed two meals of chopped fish on the wall, one of them spiked with the contents of my nembutal capsule. I crouched behind the window; watching intently as she directed Olly to the correct portion, and holding my breath as he sniffed at it suspiciously. His hunger soon overcame his caution and he licked the bowl clean with evident relish.

Now we started the tricky part. If he decided to explore the fields as he often did I would have to be right behind him. I stole out of the house as he sauntered back up the slope to the open log shed and to my vast relief he settled down in his own particular indentation in the straw and began to wash himself.

As I peered through the bushes I was gratified to see that very soon he was having difficulty with his face, licking his hind paw then toppling over as he brought it up to his cheek.

I chuckled to myself. This was great. Another few minutes and I'd have him.

And so it turned out. Olly seemed to conclude that he was tired of falling over and it wouldn't be a bad idea to have a nap. After gazing drunkenly around him, he curled up in the straw.

I waited a short time, then, with all the stealth of an Indian brave on the trail, I crept from my hiding place and tiptoed to the shed. Olly wasn't flat out – I hadn't dared give him the full anaesthetic dose in case I had been unable to track him – but he was deeply sedated. I could pretty well do what I wanted with him.

As I knelt down and began to snip away with my scissors, he opened his eyes and made a feeble attempt to struggle, but it was no good and I worked my way quickly through the ravelled fur. I wasn't able to make a particularly tidy job because he was wriggling slightly all the time, but I clipped off all the huge unsightly knots which used to get caught in the bushes, and must have been horribly uncomfortable, and soon had a growing heap of black hair by my side.

I noticed that Olly wasn't only moving, he was watching me. Dazed as he was, he knew me all right and his eyes told me all. 'It's you again!' he was saying. 'I might have known!'

When I had finished, I lifted him into a cat cage and placed it on the straw. 'Sorry, old lad,' I said, 'but I can't let you go free till you've wakened up completely.'

Olly gave me a sleepy stare, but his sense of outrage was evident. 'So you've dumped me in here again. You don't change much, do you?'

By teatime he was fully recovered and I was able to release him. He looked so much better without the ugly tangles but he didn't seem impressed, and as I opened the cage he gave me a single disgusted look and sped away.

Helen was enchanted with my handiwork and she pointed eagerly at the two cats on the wall next morning. 'Doesn't he look smart! Oh, I'm so glad you managed to do him, it was really worrying me. And he must feel so much better.'

I felt a certain smug satisfaction as I looked through the window. Olly indeed was almost unrecognisable as the scruffy animal of yesterday and there was no doubt I had dramatically altered his life and relieved him of a constant discomfort, but my burgeoning bubble of self-esteem was pricked the instant I put my head round the back door. He had just started to enjoy his breakfast but at the sight of me he streaked away faster than ever before and disappeared far over the hill-top. Sadly, I turned back into the kitchen. Olly's opinion of me had dropped several more notches. Wearily I poured a cup of tea. It was a hard life.

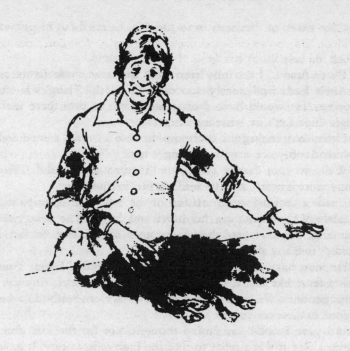

47

The little dog stared straight ahead, immobile, as if glued to the kitchen table. He was trembling, apparently afraid even to move his head, and his eyes registered something akin to terror.

I had first seen him when Molly Minican, one of my neighbours in Hannerly, got him from Sister Rose's dog sanctuary a few months before and I had been instantly charmed by his shaggy mongrel appeal and his laughing-mouthed friendliness. And now this.

'When did Robbie start with this, Molly?' I asked.

The old lady put out a hand towards her pet, then drew back.

'Just found 'im this morning. He was running around, last night, right as a bobbin.' She turned a worried face to me. 'You know, he seems frightened you're going to touch 'im.'

'He really does,' I said. 'His whole body is rigid. It looks like an acute attack of rheumatism to me. Has he cried out in pain at all?'

The old lady shook her head. 'No, not a sound.'

'That's funny.' I ran my hand over the tense musculature of the little body and gently squeezed the neck. There was no response. 'He would have shown some sign of pain there with rheumatism. Let's see what his temperature says.'

It was like inserting the thermometer into a stuffed animal and I whistled softly as I saw the reading – 105.

'Well, we can forget about the rheumatism,' I said. 'The temperature is nearly always dead normal in those cases.'

I made a thorough examination of the little animal, palpating his abdomen, auscultating his heart and lungs. The heart was pounding, but that was almost certainly due to fear. In fact I couldn't find any abnormality.

'He must have picked up some infection, Molly,' I said. 'And with a fever like that it could possibly be his kidneys. Anyway, thank goodness we have antibiotics now. We can really do a bit of good in these conditions.'

As I gave Robbie his shot, I thought, not for the first time, that in a way it was a relief to find the high temperature. It gave us something to get at with our new drugs. A puzzling case with a normal temperature was inclined to make me feel a bit helpless, and at the moment I felt reasonably confident, even though I wasn't at all sure of my diagnosis.

'I'll leave these tablets for you. Give him one at midday, another at bedtime and another first thing in the morning. I'll have a look at him some time tomorrow.' I had the reassuring conviction that I was really blasting that temperature with the antibiotic. Robbie would be a lot better after twenty-four hours.

Molly seemed to think so too. 'Ah, we'll soon have 'im right.' She bent her white head over the dog and smiled. 'Silly feller. Worrying us like this.'

She was a spinster in her seventies, and had always struck me as the archetypal Yorkshire woman; self-contained and unfussy, but with a quiet humour which was never far away. I had been called when her last dog had been run over by a farm tractor and had arrived just as he was dying, and although it must have been a savage blow to a lone woman to lose her only companion, there had been no tears, just a fixed expression and a repeated slow stroking of the little body. Molly was strong.

She had taken my advice and visited Sister Rose's kennels where she found Robbie.

I lifted the dog from the table and put him down by his bed, but he just stood there and made no attempt to lie down. I felt another wave of bafflement as I looked at him.

I went over to the sink by the window to wash my hands and had to duck my head to see out into the garden. There was a rabbit there, sunning himself by a gnarled apple tree and when he spotted me through the glass he hopped away and disappeared through a hole in the ancient stone wall.

Everything about the tiny cottage was old; the low, beamed ceilings, the weathered stonework with its climbing ivy and clematis, the once red roof tiles which sagged dangerously above the two bedroom windows which could not have measured more than eighteen inches square.

I had to bend my head again under the door lintel as I took my leave, and I glanced back at Robbie, still standing motionless by the side of his bed. A little wooden dog.

Molly was in her garden when I visited next day.

'Well now, how's Robbie?' I asked, rather more breezily than I felt.

My spirits dropped as the old lady hesitated and then was clearly trying to find something encouraging to say.

'Maybe a little better . . . but not much.'

He wasn't a bit better, he was just the same, standing in the kitchen in the same attitude as the previous day. Still rigid, still trembling, and the frightened look in his eyes was replaced by a great lassitude.

I bent and stroked him. 'Can't he lie down at all?'

'Yes, but it's difficult for 'im. He's been in his bed for a few hours but when he gets out he's like this.'

I took the temperature. Still exactly 105. I hadn't even dented it with my antibiotic injection and tablets. With a feeling of bewilderment I repeated the injection, then I turned to Molly.

'I'd like to test his urine. When you carry him out to the garden to cock his leg, try to catch a little in a clean soup plate and put it in this bottle.'

Typically, Molly laughed. 'Aye, I'll try, but I might have a job.'

'Yes,' I said. 'It can be tricky, but I'm sure you'll manage. I'll only need very little.'

On the following day, Robbie was unchanged. Even the temperature was resolutely stuck on 105. The urine test was normal – no protein, nothing to indicate kidney trouble.

I switched to another antibiotic and took a blood sample which I sent to the investigation laboratory. The lab telephoned back that the sample was normal and after five daily visits and a negative X-ray examination the little dog had not improved.

I stood in the kitchen, looking down at my baffling patient. He was the picture of misery; utterly dejected, stiff and trembling. The grim reality was there before me. Unless I could pull something out of the bag, Robbie was going to die.

'I'll have to try something else, Molly,' I said. I had with me one of the new steroid drugs, dexamethasone, and I injected 1 cc.

'You must be sick of the sight of me, but I'll call tomorrow morning to see if this new stuff has done any good.'

Molly didn't wait until the next day. Her cottage was only about a hundred yards from my house and she was on my doorstep the same afternoon.

She was out of breath. 'There's a wonderful improvement, Mr Herriot!' she gasped. 'He's like another dog. I wish you'd come and see 'im!'

I was only too eager and practically trotted along the road. Robbie looked almost like the little dog I used to know so well. He was still stiff, but he could walk carefully over the kitchen floor and his tail gave a slow wag as he saw me. The trembling was gone and he had lost his terrified look.

My relief was tremendous. 'Has he eaten anything?'

'Yes, he had his nose in his bowl about two hours after you left.'

'Well, that's wonderful.' I took the temperature and it was 102 – on the way down at last. 'I'll still come tomorrow, because I think one more shot will put him absolutely right.'

It did indeed, and a week later it was good to see the little animal leaping around in his garden, playing with a stick. He was full of life, back to normal, and although it niggled me that I still had no idea what had ailed him, I was able to file away the whole episode comfortably in my mind as just another happy ending.

I was wrong. A month later, Molly arrived at my door, looking distressed. 'He's starting again, Mr Herriot!'

'What do you mean?'

'Same as before. Tremblin' and can't move!'

Once again, an injection of the steroid brought a rapid recovery, but it wasn't the end of the affair, it was only the beginning of a saga.

Over the next two years I fought a long battle with the mysterious condition. Robbie would be a normal, healthy look-ing animal for a few weeks, then the dreaded symptoms would suddenly reappear and Molly would rush along to my house, and when I opened the door she would be on the step, head on one side and an anxious half-smile on her face, saying, 'SOS, Mr Herriot, SOS.' Desperately worried though she was, she always tried to brighten the situation with a wry humour.

Each time it happened, I dashed to the cottage with my steroids. Sometimes the symptoms were very severe, being accom-panied by gasping respiration, and I felt that I was saving the dog's life every time I treated him. I adopted various tactics along the way, the most successful being to supplement the injection with steroid tablets given regularly for a few days, then tailing off gradually before finally stopping. Then we would wait breath-lessly until the next recurrence.

Sometimes nothing happened for many weeks and we relaxed, thinking we had won and the whole thing could be forgotten like a bad dream. Then Molly would be back again at my door, head on one side. 'SOS, Mr Herriot, SOS.'

It became part of our lives. Being a near neighbour I had always known Molly well, but now, during those frantic visits she talked about her life as I cradled a cup of tea in the kitchen by the tiny window with its trailing ivy and the branches of the apple tree beyond.

She had been in domestic service as a young girl and had lived in the cottage for over thirty years. She had been very ill some time ago and would have died but for a life-saving operation carried out in Brawton by the brilliant surgeon, Sir Charles Armitage.

Her face became radiant when she talked about Sir Charles. 'Eee, he's that clever and world famous, but he was so kind to me. I'm only a poor old body with no money, but I might 'ave been a queen. He couldn't do enough for me.'

There was another hero in her life – the actor, John Wayne. Whenever one of his films came to the little cinema in Darrowby, Molly would be there and when she discovered that I too was a Wayne fan, we had long discussions about his films. 'Oh, he's such a lovely man,' she would say, giggling at her own infatuation.

It was a warm friendship, but hanging over it at all times was the spectre of Robbie's recurring illnesses. I was at her cottage scores of times and of course I never charged her. She had only her old age pension and previously I had made a nominal charge, but now even that went out of the window. Often she pleaded with me to accept something, but it was obviously unthinkable. In return, she knitted little things for Helen and the children and gave us jars of her home-made tomato chutney.

When I look back over the years, that part of my life shines like a vivid thread running through the busy routine of my veterinary practice. Robbie's unique illness, Sir Charles Armitage, John Wayne and SOS.

At all times, I wondered at the little dog's forgiving nature. Every time I met him, I stuck a hypodermic needle into him. He must have felt like a pin cushion, but when he had recovered he always wagged his tail furiously when he saw me and rushed up, planting his paws on my legs and looking up at me in delight.

There came a time, however, when the attacks became more violent and more frequent. The little animal's distress on those occasions was pitiful to see and although I always managed to pull him round I was gradually having to face the grim fact that the battle was going to be a losing one.

The climax came at 3 a.m. one morning. I heard the bell ringing, pulled on a dressing-gown and went to the door. Molly was on the step again but this time she was unable to summon her half-humorous password of SOS.

'Will you come, Mr Herriot?' she gasped. 'Robbie's real bad.'

I didn't bother to dress, but grabbed my bag and hurried with her to the cottage. The little dog was in a terrible rigor, shaking, panting, hardly able to breathe. It was the worst attack yet.

'Will you put him to sleep, please,' Molly said quietly.

'You really want that?'

'Aye, it's the end of the road for 'im. I just know it. And I can't stand any more of it, Mr Herriot. I've not been too well myself, and it's getting me down.'

I knew she was right. As I injected the barbiturate into the vein and saw the little dog relax into his last repose, there was no doubt in my mind that I was doing the best thing in ending his suffering for ever.

As before, there were no tears. Just a quiet, 'Oh, Robbie, Robbie,' as she patted the shaggy little body.

I slumped into the kitchen chair where I had drunk so many cups of tea. Sitting there, in dressing-gown and slippers, I could hardly believe that the long struggle had ended this way.

'Molly,' I said after a minute, 'I'd really like to get to the bottom of this.'

She looked at me. 'You mean a post mortem?' She shook her head. 'No, no, nothing like that.'

There didn't seem to be anything I could do or say. I went out, leaving the mystery behind me, and as I walked through the moonlit garden, sick with failure and frustration, I reflected that it was a mystery which would never be solved.

I was soon swept along in the rush of my everyday work, but I found it difficult to put Robbie out of my mind. Inevitably, some patients of every vet die and, with dogs, heartache is always round the corner; their lives are too short. I knew I would not survive if I suffered along with the bereaved owners every time and I did my best to preserve a professional attitude. But it didn't always work and it didn't work with Robbie.

The association had gone on too long and the memories of

that little dog wouldn't go away. And what made it worse was that I had to pass Molly's cottage every day of my life, seeing her white head bobbing about in her garden where she used to play with Robbie. She looked very alone.

I had withheld my usual advice to 'get another dog', because the old lady's health was obviously failing and I knew she could not bring herself to start all over again.

Sadly, my fears were confirmed, and Molly died a few weeks after Robbie. That chapter was finally closed.

It was late afternoon, some time later that I came into the surgery and found Siegfried making up some medicine in the dispensary.

'Hullo, Siegfried,' I said, 'I've had a damned awful day.'

He put down the bottle he had filled. 'In what way, James?'

'Well, every damn thing seems to have gone wrong. Every case I revisited has got worse – none has improved – and a few people more or less suggested that I was a bloody awful vet.'

'Surely not. You're imagining things.'

'I don't think so. It started first thing this morning when I was examining Mrs Cowling's dog. It is a rather obscure case and I tried to spell out the various possibilities to her. She gave me a frosty look and said, "Well, the long and short of it is that you simply have no idea what is wrong with the animal!"'

'I shouldn't worry about that, James. She probably didn't mean anything.'

'You didn't see her face. But then I went out to see a ewe at George Grindley's. It was a pregnancy toxaemia and I was taking its temperature when, out of the blue, George said, "You know, you've never cured a single animal on my place. I hope you'll do better with this 'un."'

'But that's not true, James, I know it's not.'

'Maybe so, but he said it.' I ran my fingers through my hair. 'And after that I drove out to cleanse a cow at old Hawkin's. I'd just got out of the car when he looked at me under his brows and grunted, "Oh, it's you. My wife says it's always fatal when Mr Herriot comes." I must have looked a bit shattered because he patted me on the shoulder and said, "Mind you, she likes you as a man."'

'Oh dear. I'm sorry, James.'

'Thank you, Siegfried. I won't bore you any more, but it's been like that all day. And then right in the middle of it, I had to go through my own village and past poor old Molly Minican's cottage. There was an auctioneer there, selling off her furniture and her bits and pieces. There were all sorts of things piled up in her garden and it hit me again that her dog died without my having any idea what was wrong with him even though I treated him for two years. She knew I didn't know and she must have thought I was a dead loss. I think that was the lowest point of my hellish day.'

Siegfried spread his hands. 'Look, how many vets and doctors have lost patients without ever being sure of their diagnosis? You're not the only one. Anyway, we all have days like today, James, when nothing goes right. Every vet runs up against them now and then. You'll have a lot of good days to make up for it.'

I nodded good-bye and set off for home. My partner was trying to be kind, but I still felt low when I got to High Field and as I sat down at the tea table, Helen gave me a questioning look.

'What's the matter, Jim? You're very quiet.'

'Sorry, Helen, I'm afraid I won't be a barrel of laughs tonight.' I poured out my story.

'I thought it must be something to do with your work,' she said, 'but what's really getting you down is Molly Minican, isn't it?'

I nodded. 'That's right. She was a bit special. Seeing all her things lying in her garden brought everything back to me, and I don't like the thought that Molly died convinced I was a bit of a chump.'

'But she was always nice to you, Jim.'

'She was nice to everybody, me included. But I know that she must have felt that I had let her down. She's gone now, but I have this rotten feeling that in her heart she had a poor opinion of me and that's something I can never alter.'

Helen gave me a quizzical smile. 'I think I have something here that will make you feel better.' She left the room and I waited, mystified, until she came back with what looked like a framed picture under her arm.

'Peggy Ford in the village was at Molly's sale,' she said. 'She handed this in to me because it was hanging in the old lady's bedroom and she thought you'd be interested in it. Here, have a look.'

It wasn't a picture. It was a framed square of cardboard and across the top, in Molly's spidery writing, I read: 'My three favourite men.'

Underneath, gummed to the cardboard, were three photographs in a row. There was Sir Charles Armitage, John Wayne ... and me.

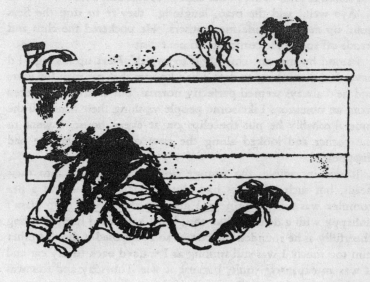

48

It was the first time I had ever seen a man coming out of a house and *then* removing bicycle clips from his trouser legs.

I had been called to this cottage by a Mr Colwell to attend his dog and as I got out of the car I was surprised to see this man emerge, then, after looking back carefully, bend down to take off the clips. There was no sign of a bike anywhere.

'Excuse me,' I said, 'I hope you don't mind my asking, but why the clips?'

The man looked back again, grinned and spoke quietly. 'Now then, Mr Herriot, it's you, is it. I've just been in to read t'gas meter and I'm takin' precautions.'

'Precautions?'

'Aye, against the fleas.'

'Fleas!'

'Aye, that's right. They're canny folks, the Colwells, but the missus isn't ower particular and there's a lot of fleas in there.'

I stared at him. 'But . . . the clips . . . I still don't see . . .'

'Aye well,' said the man, laughing, 'they're to stop the fleas goin' up me legs inside me trousers.' He pocketed the clips and strode off round the corner to his next visit.

I stood by my car, chuckling to myself. Fleas up his legs! I'd never heard anything so daft. I had known that gas man for years and he'd always seemed perfectly normal, but clearly he suffered from an obsession. Like some people washing their hands all the time. Probably he put the clips on at every house. I went to the corner and looked along the row of cottages but he had disappeared.

It was incredible, the strange notions people got into their heads, but such whimsies had always fascinated me and a flea complex was something new. I just hoped the poor chap wasn't unhappy with a delusion like this, but I had heard him whistling cheerfully as he rounded the corner so I supposed it didn't bother him too much. I was still smiling as I walked back to my car and it was an expansive smile, because it was Thursday and this was my last visit before starting my half-day.

Though veterinary surgery was my life and I wouldn't have wanted to do anything else, the snag was that it never stopped – except on Thursday afternoons. On that special day I invariably felt lighthearted as soon as I awoke, knowing that by midday Helen and I would be off to Brawton, free as birds. A leisurely lunch at one of the town's splendid cafés then we would meet my pal, Gordon Rae the vet from Boroughbridge and his wife, Jean, fellow escapees from the telephone and the wellington boots. We would spend the afternoon shopping, followed by tea and the cinema. It doesn't sound much but to us it was a blessed relief.

The evening would be different this time since Helen had been given tickets for a concert by the Hallé Orchestra from the Miss Whitlings, pillars of the Darrowby Music Society. We would be returning home to change and then be making up a four with them for the concert. The conductor was my old hero, Sir John Barbirolli and the programme was mouth-watering. Coriolanus, Elgar Violin Concerto and Brahms' First.

I took a long contented breath as I knocked on the Colwells' door – in about an hour's time, we'd be off.

It was opened by the man of the house; sixtyish, collarless and unshaven, but with a welcoming smile.

'Come in, Mr 'erriot,' he cried, waving a courtly arm. 'I'm sorry we had to call you out, but we 'aven't no transport and our awd dog needs attention.'

'That's all right, Mr Colwell. I understand he's had a bump with a car?'

'Aye, he ran out in front of the post office van this mornin' and it sent him flyin'.' The smile vanished from his face and his eyes widened with anxiety. 'We hope it's nowt serious. Poor awd Roopy – we call 'im that because he's got a funny bark.'

The front door opened directly into the living room and the atmosphere was stuffier and more odoriferous than a cow byre. Dust lay thickly on the furniture and a colourful miscellany of newspapers, articles of clothing and food scraps littered the table and floor. Mrs Colwell was indeed not ower particular.

The lady herself appeared from the kitchen and greeted me with the same affability as her husband, but her eyes were red and swollen with weeping.

'Eee, Mr Herriot,' she quavered, 'we're that worried about Roopy. He's never ailed a thing all 'is life, but we're frightened we might lose 'im now.'

I looked at the dog stretched in a basket against the wall. He seemed to be a spaniel cross and he gazed at me with terrified eyes.

'Did he manage to walk inside after the accident?' I asked.

'Nay,' replied Mr Colwell. 'We had to carry 'im in.' He gulped. 'We think he might have a broken back.'

'Mmm, let's have a look.' I knelt by the basket and the Colwells knelt on either side of me. I pulled down Roopy's lower eyelid and saw a pink conjunctiva.

'He's a good colour. No sign there of internal injury.' I felt my way over all four legs, ribs and pelvis and found no fractures.

'Let's see if you can stand, old boy,' I said.

Gently I eased my hand underneath the dog's body and very carefully started to lift. He responded with a yowling protest which brought exclamations of anguish from his owners. 'Aw, poor awd Roopy!' 'Never mind, lad!' 'Oh, he's such a brave boy!' as they patted and caressed him.

I persevered and kept lifting until I had him standing shakily for a moment, then I let him down.

'Well, it seems he's got away with it,' I said. 'He's a bit bruised and you can see his pads are scuffed and sore, but I'm sure he's not seriously injured.'

Cries of joy went up from the Colwells and they redoubled their strokings and cooings while Roopy, his big spaniel eyes liquid and pathetic, gazed around him at each of us in turn. He was clearly milking the situation to its full.

The three of us got to our feet and I reached for my bag. 'I'm going to give him a couple of injections to relieve his discomfort and to help the sores on his pads.' I administered steroid and antibiotic and counted out some penicillin tablets. 'He's suffering from shock, too, but I think he's making the most of it.' I laughed and patted the shaggy head. 'You're an old soldier, Roopy.'

The Colwells joined in happily. 'Aye, you're right, Mr Herriot. He allus puts it on!' But again a tear stole down the lady's cheek. 'Eee, but it's such a relief to know we're not going to lose 'im.'

Then she quickly wiped her face with the back of her hand. 'We must celebrate with a cup o'tea. You've got time, Mr Herriot?'

Brawton beckoned but I couldn't say no. 'Right, thank you very much but it will have to be a quickie.'

The kettle was soon boiling and Mrs Colwell used both arms to make a sort of clearing in the table-top jungle where she deposited the cups. As I sipped my tea and looked at the friendly people laughing and gazing with love at their dog, I knew that the gas man had been right again. They were canny folks.

My departure had a triumphant quality as they ushered me out with repeated thanks and wavings of arms.

I shouted back as I boarded my car, 'Give me a ring in a couple of days and let me know how he's going on. I'm sure he'll be fine.'

I had only just driven round the corner when I felt a prickling round my ankles. Maybe those new socks were irritating me and I began to push them down. But the strange tingling and itching began to spread to my calves and I pulled in to the roadside and rolled up a trouser leg. My flesh was sprinkled with little black dots, but they were dots which hopped and jumped and bit, and they were working their way rapidly up my thighs. Oh my God, that gas man hadn't been so daft!

I wanted to get home with all speed but I got behind a couple of farm tractors with wide loads and was unable to overtake. By the time I reached High Field, the invasion had reached my chest and back and the maddening itch was setting me afire, making me wriggle around in my seat.

Helen was changing in readiness for Brawton and she turned in surprise as I galloped in to our bedroom.

'I have to get into the bath!' I shouted.

'Oh . . . had a dirty job?'

'No, I've got fleas!'

'*What!*'

'Fleas! Millions of them – they're all over me!'

'But . . . but . . . how . . .?'

'I'll tell you later. Please come and get my clothes and dump them in the washer. I'll need a complete change.'

In the bathroom I undressed and submerged myself, plunging my head repeatedly under the water. Helen came in and looked with horror at my heap of clothes with the agile insects leaping against the white of the shirt.

'Oooo . . . yuk-yuk-yuk!' she gasped as she grimaced and lifted each article by one corner and disappeared to the wash.

I felt as if I could have stayed in that bath for ever. The relief was enormous as I lay there, freed from the torture of the itch, watching in disbelief as the dark tormentors floated on the surface of the water. I wasn't going to take any chances. I emptied the bath and refilled it before having another long steep. I washed and scrubbed my hair again and again and when I finally climbed out and donned a completely new set of clothes I thanked heaven that my troubles were over. It was my first experience of such a thing and I hadn't realised how shattering it could be. I had often read about the suffering of people in foreign prisons lying on flea-ridden mattresses but I had never fully comprehended it until now.

When we at last set off for Brawton, it was difficult to recapture the carefree feeling which always settled on us each Thursday. The bizarre events of the morning were still too fresh in our minds. However, as we left the hills and began to bowl along the great plain of York with the familiar Thursday scenes rolling past the car windows, we began gradually to relax. Soon we would be at lunch, out of reach of our pressures, then, this evening, the particular joy of the Hallé Orchestra.

As a schoolboy in Glasgow I had actually met the legendary Barbirolli – it was before he was Sir John – and in rather odd circumstances. I was attending a special schools concert by the Scottish Orchestra in St Andrew's Hall. I went to the toilet in the interval and became aware that a white-tie and tailed figure was standing in the next stall to me. I looked up and was amazed and delighted to see that it was the great man himself. It was a strange place to meet, but he asked me how I was enjoying the music, what I had liked best and about myself. He was indeed the gracious, kindly man who became such a beloved figure throughout the world.

Since our meeting, I had followed his career through the years, from when he had succeeded Toscanini as conductor of the New York Philharmonic until now when he had been, since 1942, in charge of the great Hallé Orchestra. Over the years I had gone to his concerts whenever they were in reach and had watched him shrinking in size. He had always been small but now he was tiny and frail – but totally inspiring on the rostrum.

I was sharing these thoughts with Helen as our half-day euphoria mounted, and we were within a mile of Brawton when I stiffened in my seat and fell silent.

After a minute or so my wife looked at me. 'What's wrong? You've gone very quiet.'

I shifted position carefully. 'Oh, it's probably nothing, but I have a daft feeling that I've still got some fleas on me.'

'What! You can't have – not after two baths and a complete change! It's impossible!'

'I know it's impossible, but I tell you – I've got that same feeling.'

'Oh, it's just the after effects, Jim. Remember you were bitten all over.'

'I know, I know,' I grunted, 'but I'm pretty sure there's some fresh activity going on.'

She took my hand and smiled encouragingly. 'It's all in your mind. Try to think of something else.'

I did my best, but I was still wriggling when I mounted the stairs to Brown's café. The mingled cooking smells, the clatter of cutlery, the cheerful bustle and the welcoming smiles of the waitresses we knew so well had always sent my spirits soaring as though a great gong was signalling the beginning of our happy few hours, but today was different.

As we took our places and read through the good old-fashioned Yorkshire menu which had always delighted me – roast beef with Yorkshire pudding, plaice and chips, steak and kidney pie, steamed jam sponge, spotted dick and custard – my mind was churning and my smile was a fixed mask as I ordered.

Sipping my way through the delicious soup and toying with the meal, I was like a man in a bad dream as I tried to ignore the torture under my shirt.

Around the halfway stage, a couple threaded their way between the crowded tables and the man approached us.

'May we join you?' he asked politely. 'There's not a seat anywhere.'

'Of course,' I replied, digging up another smile. 'By all means.'

As they sat down it was easy to label them. A farmer and his wife out for the day like ourselves. They were in their fifties, with scrubbed, weathered faces and the man's bright tie and smart tweed jacket sat uneasily upon him. He reached a huge hand for the menu and studied it with his wife.

'Aye well,' he said, looking up at us. 'That were a good rain last night.'

That settled it, I thought as we nodded agreement. I didn't know them. Brawton was rather far for most of my farmers. They would probably be from Wharfedale.

My conjectures were cut short by Helen pressing her knee against mine. I turned to her and saw a look of horror on her face.

'There's one on your collar,' she muttered, then, 'Ooo, it's jumped!'

It had indeed jumped, right onto the middle of the white table cloth. As I sat helplessly, another one hopped out then another.

The farmer and his wife, who were clearly on the point of starting a friendly conversation, stared in amazement at the leaping objects. There was a terrible silence then the man spoke again.

'Ah, there's a table by the window, Eva,' he said, rising to his feet. 'That's where we usually sit. You'll excuse us, won't you.'

After they had gone we raced through our meal. I don't know how many more of the flitting creatures appeared on the table. I was too stunned to count and, looking back now, I have only the terrifying memory of the first few. We abandoned all idea of our dessert and instead of a happy discussion of the relative merits of ginger pudding and apple pie we called for our bill and fled.

We couldn't stay in Brawton to see Jean and Gordon. The bathroom at home was our only goal and, as I drove at top speed, images of the little terrors on that table cloth rose again and again in my mind. How could it possibly have happened? How had that second wave of fleas escaped all my precautions? To this day I have no answer, I only know it was so.

Back home, we repeated the morning's performance: the total submersion in the bath, Helen's finger-tip bearing away of my contaminated clothing and a complete change.

It was fortunate that I had reserved my 'good suit' for the concert because my limited wardrobe was running low. When I finally stood freshly arrayed and ready to go I turned despairingly to my wife. 'Surely I'll be all right this time.'

'Oh, you must be. There can't possibly be any of those things left now.'

I shifted gloomily under my fresh shirt. 'That's what we thought before.'

We had to pick up the Miss Whitlings, Harriet and Felicity, and we found them, as usual, bursting with vitality and good humour. They were in their late forties, large, busty ladies, and though some people might have called them fat, I had always considered them extremely comely and had been mystified that neither of them was married.

The journey back to Brawton passed quickly, aided by the non-stop conversation and, for me, the blissful knowledge that at last nothing was eating me alive. In the concert hall our two friends stationed themselves on either side of me, which I took as a compliment. In fact I was tightly squeezed between them because they both overflowed their seats to some extent.

As I drank in the familiar sounds of the concert hall, the orchestra tuning, the expectant buzz of conversation with my two attractive neighbours chattering on either side, I decided that, after my traumatic day, things had taken an upturn. Life was pretty good.

I joined in the wave of applause which greeted the slight figure of Barbirolli as he almost tiptoed across the platform. The people of Yorkshire loved him as much as anybody and the clapping went on and on. As he finally mounted the rostrum and raised his baton in the sudden hush, I settled back in happy anticipation.

It was just as the first majestic bars of Coriolanus sounded that I felt the prickle on my right shoulder blade. Oh, my God, no, it couldn't be. But the growing irritation was only too familiar. I tried to ignore it but, after a minute, I had to lean hard against the back of my seat to try to relieve the itch, and then, as it spread across my back, I had to execute the slightest of wriggles to transfer my weight the other way.

I realised suddenly and to my horror, that in my squashed-in situation even the slightest movement was transmitted instantly to one or other of my neighbours. As the maddening tickle mounted I wanted to scratch, throw myself about, fight the thing in every way, but that was unthinkable. I had to accept the frightening reality that for the next several hours I would have to sit still.

This involved a supreme effort of will on my part but I would have had to have been some sort of yogi to succeed. I did my best to concentrate on the music, but was forced to settle for short periods of inaction then a careful shifting of position, sometimes to brace my back against the seat or move my clothes against my skin by side-to-side shufflings.

I reckoned that there was only one flea at work now. After my experiences, I had become an authority on the species and I was positive that I could track his progress over my person. As Beethoven thundered around me, I had the feverish idea that I might trap him in the act and squash him and whenever I felt a fresh bite I tried to exert a fierce pressure against the hard wood and move slowly from side to side.

These manoeuvres inevitably involved encroachment on my partners' territory. I had expected during the evening to get to know the nice sisters better, to find out more about their personalities, but in fact I learned much more about their anatomies than anything else. Rounded arms, well-fleshed ribs, yielding hips – all were contacted and repeatedly explored in my helpless squirmings but, like the well-bred ladies that they were, neither of them showed any outward reactions to my incursions beyond an occasional clearing of the throat or sharp intake of breath. However, on two occasions, when I found my right knee deeply buried in the softness of Harriet's thigh, there was a definite withdrawal of the limb, and when my left elbow inadvertently but relentlessly nudged aside a weighty bosom I saw Felicity's eyebrows climb up her forehead.

I would rather say no more about that unhappy evening except that the pattern did not change. The divine Elgar Violin Concerto which, more than any other musical work, has the power to transport me to a perfect world, was only a background noise to my private battle. It was the same with the beloved Brahms' First Symphony. All I wanted was to get home.

During the interval and as we bade them goodnight at the end of the evening, there were a lot of fixed smiles and darting glances from the Miss Whitlings and the old saying about wanting the ground to swallow me was never so true.

And when it was all over and Helen and I were sitting on the edge of our bed going over the night's events I still felt terrible.

'My God, what a night!' I groaned, and as I dredged through my embarrassments with the sisters yet again Helen managed to keep a straight face but I could see that it was costing her dearly. Twitchings of the mouth, fierce frowns and an occasional sinking of her face in her hands betrayed her inner struggle.

At the end of my recital of woe, I threw out my hands in despair. 'And, do you know, Helen, I am convinced that all that agony I went throught tonight was caused by a single flea. Think of that! Just one flea!'

My wife suddenly dropped her chin on her chest, thrust out her lips and made a creditable attempt to sink her voice down a few octaves to basso-profundo pitch.

'A flea!' she intoned in true Chaliapin fashion. 'Ha-ha-ha-haaa, a flea!'

'Ah yes, very funny,' I replied, 'but Mussorgsky would never have put all the laughter in that song if he had suffered like me.'

Two days later Mr Colwell telephoned. 'Roopy's grand!' he cried in delight. 'Runnin' round, good as new, but 'e has a bit of broken nail sort of hangin' from his paw, and it's catchin' on things. I wish you'd come and cut it off.'

I didn't answer for a few seconds. 'You . . . you couldn't take it off yourself . . . just a little snip with scissors?'

'Nay, nay, I'm no good at that sort o' thing. I'd be right grateful if you'd drop in if you're out this way.'

'Right . . . right, Mr Colwell. I'll see you later this morning.'

'Helen,' I cried as I left the house, 'that was another call from the Colwells.'

'What!' she looked round the kitchen door in alarm.

'Yes . . . afraid so, but I'm calling first to see young Jack Arnold along the road.'

'Farmer Arnold's son?'

'Yes, that's right. The lad who does all that bicycle racing.'

'Why?'

'I'm going to borrow his clips.'

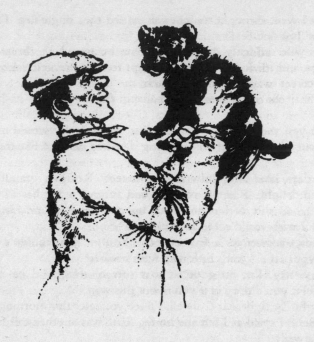

49

Sister Rose gently lifted the trembling dog on to the table. He was a tiny cross-bred terrier and he looked at me with terrified eyes.

'Poor little beggar,' I said, 'no wonder he's frightened. This is the one that was found on the road in Helvington, isn't it?'

Sister Rose nodded. 'Yes, running about aimlessly, looking for his owners. You've seen it all before.'

I had indeed. The desperate search for the people he had loved and trusted but who had dumped him and driven away. The dashing up, open-mouthed to somebody who looked familiar then turning away in bewilderment. To me it was an almost unbearable sight, evoking feelings of rage and pity which almost choked me.

'Never mind, old lad,' I said, stroking the shaggy head, 'there are better days ahead.'

There were always better days ahead for the abandoned dogs at Sister Rose's little animal sanctuary. It was amazing how soon her care and affection reassured and transformed the helpless creatures, and through the open door of the treatment room I could see the wagging tails and hear the joyous barking of the dogs in the row of wire-fronted pens.

I was here to do the usual duties. Check up on the health and condition of the new arrivals and give them their shots against distemper, hepatitis and leptospirosis, remove the stitches from the spay incisions (all bitches were spayed on arrival) and generally attend to any illness I might find.

'I see he's holding up a hind leg,' I said.

'Yes, he doesn't seem to be able to use that leg at all and I want you to have a look at it. I hope it's just a temporary thing.'

I examined the foot and claws. Normal. But as I felt my way up the leg, I soon found the cause of the trouble.

I turned to Sister Rose. 'He's had a fractured femur and it's never been set. The bone has formed a sort of callus but there's no real healing.'

'So this little thing had a broken leg and his owners just didn't bother about it?'

'That's right.' I ran my hand over the little body, feeling the jutting backbone, the almost fleshless ribs. 'He's emaciated too, just about skin and bone. This is a neglected dog if ever I saw one.'

'And I'll bet he's never had any affection either,' she said softly. 'Look how he trembles when we speak. He seems to be afraid of people.' She gave a long sigh. 'Ah well, we'll do what we can. How about that leg?'

'I'll have to X-ray it later today to see what can be done.' I gave the dog his inoculations and then Sister Rose carried him out and placed him in a pen on his own. 'By the way,' I said, 'what have you called this one?'

She smiled. 'I've called him Titch. Not a very elegant name, but he's so little.'

'Yes, I agree. Very suitable.' As I spoke, the thought recurred that finding names for her constant flow of rescued animals was only one of Sister Rose's problems. She was the radiologist at a big hospital but still found time to care for her ever-changing doggy family, and still was able to find the money by running events for her 'biscuit fund' and by dipping into her own pocket.

I was bandaging another dog's infected foot when I saw a man walking up and down the row of pens. He had his hands behind his back as he looked intently at the eager faces behind the wire.

'I see you've got a customer,' I said.

'I hope so. I like the look of him. He arrived just before you and he's making a very thorough search.'

As she spoke, the man half-turned to have a closer look. There was something familiar about that stocky frame.

'That's Rupe Nellist,' I exclaimed. 'I know him.'

A few years ago he had run a large grocery shop in Darrowby but he had expanded and opened another bigger business in the bustling town of Hargrove, thirty miles away, and had moved away to live there, but he was still a faithful client and had brought his dog to me regularly until it had died at the age of fifteen only a week ago.

I finished my bandaging and went out to him with Sister Rose.

'Hello, Rupe,' I said.

He turned in surprise. 'Now then, Mr Herriot. I didn't expect to see you.' His blunt-featured face, slightly pugnacious in repose, was attractive when he smiled. 'I've been miserable since I lost t'awd dog and I'm takin' your advice. I'm looking for another.'

'It's the only way, Rupe, and you've come to the right place. There are some lovely dogs here.'

'Aye, you're right.' He took off his trilby hat and smoothed back his hair. 'But I've had a heck of a job makin' up my mind. It sounds daft, but if I pick one out I'm goin' to feel sorry for all the other poor little blighters I'm leaving behind.'

Sister Rose laughed. 'A lot of people feel like that, Mr Nellist, but you needn't worry. I find good homes for all my dogs. I don't care how long I have to keep them – none is ever put to sleep. The only exceptions are in cases of extreme old age or incurable disease.'

'Aye, well, that's wonderful. I'll just have another stroll along here.' He recommenced his inspection of the pens, walking with a pronounced limp in his right leg, a relic of childhood polio.

Sister Rose hadn't been exaggerating when she said he was thorough. Up and down he went, talking to the animals, pushing a finger through the wire to tickle their noses. Many of the dogs were handsome specimens with a pedigree look about them – noble labradors, majestic golden retrievers, and a German shepherd which could have been a Crufts winner, and as I watched them all, tails wagging, leaping up at Rupe, I wondered as I often did how they could possibly have been abandoned. Each time he passed Titch's pen the little dog hopped along the other side of the wire on this three legs, keeping pace with him, looking up into his face.

Finally he stopped and gazed for a long time at the little creature. 'You know, I fancy that 'un,' he murmured.

'Really?' Sister Rose was surprised. 'He's only just arrived. We haven't had a chance to do anything for him. He's in a shocking state. Very lame, too.'

'Aye, I can see that. But let's have a look at 'im, will you?'

Sister Rose opened the door of the pen and Rupe Nellist reached in and lifted the little animal up until he was head high, gazing at him, eyeball to eyeball. 'Now, little feller,' he said softly, 'how would you like to come home wi' me?' The frightened eyes in the shaggy face regarded him for a few moments then the tail twitched and a pink tongue reached for his face.

The man smiled. 'I reckon this is a right good-natured little dog. We'll get on fine together.'

'You want him, then?' asked Sister Rose, wide-eyed.

'I do that. Right now.'

'Oh, I do wish we'd been able to get him straightened up for you first.'

'Don't worry. I'll do all that.' He put the dog down and pushed a note into the donation box. 'Thank ye, Sister, for letting me look round. What have you called this little bloke?'

'Titch, I'm afraid. Probably you'll want to change that.'

He laughed. 'Not at all. Come on, Titch.' He limped away toward his car with his new pet limping beside him. After a few steps he looked back with a grin. 'Walks like me, doesn't he? Same leg, too.'

*

I saw man and dog a fortnight later at my surgery when they came in for the booster inoculation. The difference in Titch was dramatic. He had filled out and, more striking still, the trembling and fear had gone.

'He's a different dog, Rupe,' I said. 'He looks as though he's had some good food at last, and he's happy, too.'

'Aye, by gum, he did eat for the first few days and he's settled down grand at home, too. My missus thinks the world of 'im.'

I noticed that as he spoke, the tiny animal's gaze was fixed unwaveringly on his new master. He was a shaggy little thing of baffling breeding, but his face had a scruffy appeal which was undeniably attractive and his eyes shone with devotion. Titch had found somebody else to love and this time I knew he wasn't going to be let down. Rupe Nellist was not a demonstrative man, but the way he looked at his new pet and gently stroked his head made it very clear that there was something in the little creature to which he responded deeply.

I took the opportunity to X-ray the lame leg and the picture was as I expected.

'It's too late to set the broken bone in plaster, Rupe,' I said. 'The only hope would be to plate the leg – bring the ends of the bone together and hold them there for a few weeks with a metal plate, and even then I couldn't guarantee he'd ever be sound. These things are best done at the time of the injury.'

'Yes, I understand that, but, you know, I'd give a lot to see the little feller goin' around on all four legs. He never puts that bad leg to the ground, and it upsets me. Think about it, and I'll do whatever you advise.'

Plating fractures was going deeper into orthopaedic surgery than I had ever done, but two things motivated me to have a go. Firstly, Rupe Nellist had a steadfast faith in my ability and, secondly, Calum Buchanan was determined to drag me into the modern world of small animal practice.

There was another thing, too. I kept hearing from people I knew who lived in Hargrove about Rupe's extraordinary affection for his new dog. It seemed that he took him everywhere with him, socially and in his work, showing him off proudly as if he was of the highest pedigree instead of, as most people would say, just a little mongrel. Rupe's business had continued to prosper with the opening of another large shop and he was active, too, on the town council and in local government. It caused some surprised comment that he actually took Titch into the council meetings with him, and had he not been a formidable personality, growing in power, he'd never have got away with it. There was no doubt about it, I'd have to try to fix that leg.

I found myself in a very familiar situation – having to perform an operation which I had never done, never even seen. I had received a good, scientific education at the veterinary college, but I had qualified at a time when a great wave of new drugs and procedures was sweeping over the profession and I was breathlessly trying to keep up with it all. All I could do was read up the new findings in our professional journals and this had enabled me to do a lot of bovine surgery such as Caesarean operations and rumenotomies which had never been performed in our district before. In my modest way, I was a pioneer in that field.

However, these things had been forced upon me, an unavoidable part of my life as a large animal practitioner. It had been only too easy to side-step the small animal surgery by sending our problem cases to the brilliant Granville Bennett, but it was time to face up to the fact that dog and cat work was going to occupy more and more of our lives. This was another revolution.

Calum was an enthusiastic advocate of the new ideas. He would tackle any kind of surgery with courage and determination, and he was enchanted at the opportunity to repair Titch's leg. And, unlike me, he had seen many of these orthopaedic operations done. The modern veterinary colleges had fine clinics where all the latest procedures were carried out – something undreamed of in my time.

We had to get in some new instruments and equipment but we were ready to start by the following Sunday morning. We picked that day because the practice would be quiet and we'd have more time.

I found, as with all new operations, that the actuality was ten times more difficult and frightening than I had expected from my reading. I seemed to spend an age, head to head with Calum, bending over Titch's sleeping form. Digging our way through the muscles down to the damaged bone, removing the partial callus and a seemingly endless mass of fibrous tissue, tying off the spurting blood vessels, freshening the ends of the bone, drilling, screwing in the plates which would hold the broken ends together. I was sweating and exhausted by the time the last skin suture was inserted and all that could be seen was the line of stitches. Thinking of what lay underneath, I breathed a silent prayer.

Over the next few weeks, Rupe Nellist kept bringing Titch in for examination. The wound had healed well with no reaction, but there was no attempt by the little dog to put the leg to the ground.

After two months we removed the plate. The bone had united beautifully, but Titch was still a three-legged dog.

'Doesn't he ever try to touch the ground with it?' I asked.

Rupe shook his head. 'Nay, he's as you see 'im. Never any different. Maybe he's been lame so long that he just holds the leg up out of habit?'

'Could be, but it's disappointing.'

'Never mind, Mr Herriot. You chaps have done your best and I'm grateful. And the little feller's grand in every other way.'

As he took his leave with his pet limping by his side, Calum turned to me with a wry smile. 'Ah well, some you lose.'

It was several months later when Calum read out a piece in the *Darrowby and Houlton Times*.

'Listen to this. "On Saturday there will be a civic reception for Rupert Nellist, newly elected Mayor of Hargrove, followed by an appearance outside the Town Hall."'

'Well, good old Rupe,' I said. 'He deserves it after all he's done for the town. I like that man.'

Calum nodded. 'So do I. And I wouldn't mind seeing him in his moment of glory. Do you think we could sneak through to Hargrove for half an hour?'

I looked at him thoughtfully. 'That would be nice, wouldn't it? And there's nothing much fixed for Saturday. I'll speak to Siegfried – I'm sure he'll hold the fort for us.'

Saturday morning found Calum and me among the crowd

standing in bright sunshine outside Hargrove Town Hall. At the top of the steps, several large pots of flowers had been placed on either side of the big doors and the multi-coloured blooms added to the festive air and the feeling of expectancy. A group of BBC men stood with their television cameras at the ready.

We hadn't long to wait. The doors swung open and as Rupe emerged, wearing his chain of office and with the Lady Mayoress by his side, a swelling cheer arose from the crowd. His popularity was reflected in the smiling faces and waving arms around us, then the sound increased suddenly in volume as Titch trotted out from behind his master. Everybody knew about Rupe's relationship with his dog.

However, the sound was as nothing compared to the great roar of laughter when Titch strolled to the front, cocked his leg, and relieved himself against one of the flower pots, a gesture which was to make him famous among TV audiences throughout the country.

Everybody was still laughing as the little procession came down the steps and began to pass through the crowd who opened up to make an avenue down which the Mayor and Mayoress walked, with Titch bringing up the rear.

It was a happy sight but Calum and I had eyes for only one thing.

Calum nudged me in the ribs. 'Do you see what I see?'

'I do,' I breathed, 'I certainly do.'

'He's sound. On four legs. Absolutely no signs of a limp.'

'Yes . . . great . . . marvellous!' The feeling of triumph made the sun shine more brightly.

We couldn't wait any longer, and as we got into the car, Calum turned to me. 'There was something else. When Titch was watering those flowers, did you notice anything?'

'Yes. He was cocking his good leg. All his weight was on the bad one.'

'Which means . . .' said Calum grinning.

'That he'll never be lame again.'

'That's right.' Calum settled behind the wheel and as he started the engine, he sighed contentedly. 'Ah well, some you win.'

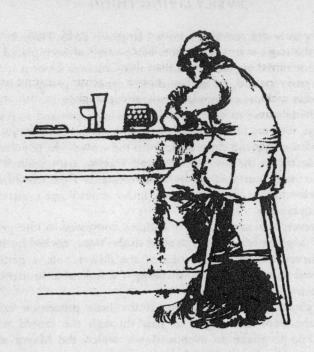

50

Bob Stockdale was the sole survivor of the cataclysm which had struck the Lord Nelson Inn. In dirty wellington boots and flat cap, he sat there on a high stool at the end of the bar counter, seemingly oblivious of the endless torrent of piped music and the babel of voices from the jostling pack of smart young people.

I fought my way to the bar, collected a pint of bitter and, as I stood surveying the scene from a space against the wall, my thoughts drifted sadly back to the old days. A year ago the Lord Nelson was a typical Yorkshire country pub and I remembered an evening when I dropped in there with a friend from Glasgow, the city of my youth. There was just one big room then, rather like a large kitchen, with a log fire burning in a black cooking range at one end and a dozen farm men sitting on high-backed oak settles, their pints resting on tables of pitted wood. Those settles were a draught-proof refuge from the cold winds which whistled along the streets of the village outside and over the high pastures where those men spent their days.

The conversation never rose above a gentle murmur over which the ticking of a wall clock and the click of dominoes added to the atmosphere of rest and quiet.

'Gosh, it's peaceful in here,' my friend said. Wonderingly, he watched the proprietor, in shirt and braces, proceed unhurriedly down to the cellar and emerge with a long enamel jug from which he replenished the glasses, regulating the flow expertly to achieve the required head of froth.

'A bit different from West Nile Street,' I said.

He grinned. 'It certainly is. In fact, it's unbelievable. How does a place like this pay? Only a few chaps here, and they aren't drinking much.'

'I think it hardly pays at all. Maybe a few pounds a week, but the owner has a smallholding — there are cows, calves and pigs just through that wall — and he looks on this as a pleasant sideline.'

My friend took a pull at his glass, stretched out his legs and half closed his eyes. 'Anyway, I like it. You can relax here. It's lovely.'

It was indeed lovely and most of the pubs around Darrowby were still attractive, but as I looked at the modernised Lord Nelson I wondered how long they would stay that way.

When the new owner took over he didn't waste any time in starting his revolution. He wasn't a farmer, he was an experienced landlord and he could see rich possibilities in the old inn in the pretty village of Welsby tucked among the fells. The kitchen range disappeared and was replaced by a smart bar counter with a background of mirrors and gleaming bottles; the antique settles and tables were swept away, and horse brasses, hunting horns and sporting prints appeared on the walls. The end wall was knocked down and people ate in an elegant dining room where once I calved the cows and tended the pigs.

Two things happened almost at once; droves of young people swarmed out to Welsby in their cars from the big Yorkshire towns, and the old clientele melted away. I never knew where those farm men went, probably to pubs in the neighbouring villages – just Bob Stockdale stayed. I couldn't understand why, but he was a quiet man, a bit of a loner, and maybe he felt that he had sat in that room several nights a week for years and, despite all the changes, he didn't want to leave it. Anyway, whenever I called in, he was there, perched on the same stool, with his old bitch, Meg, tucked underneath. Welsby was part of the long long road up the dale which I had travelled a thousand times and when I had had a night call up there I sometimes dropped in for a beer. Tonight I had replaced a prolapsed uterus in a cow, and as I sipped at my glass I had the warm feeling of satisfaction after a successful operation.

I spotted a gap in the crush round the bar and pushed my way to Bob's side. 'Hello, Bob,' I said, 'can I top up your glass? It's getting a bit low.'

'Aye, thank ye, Mr Herriot. It's gettin' far down, right enough.' He drained the last few inches and pushed the glass across the counter.

He spoke slowly, articulating with care. It was nearing closing time and he would have been there a long time, quietly lowering the pints. He had reached a state of detachment from the world which I had seen before.

I looked down at Meg's nose protruding from between the legs of the stool and bent down to stroke the greying muzzle of the old bitch who was Bob's helper and friend. By day she brought the cows in for him, skirting eagerly around them, nipping at their heels if they strayed, and in the evenings they relaxed together.

I looked at the growing opacity in the friendly eyes. 'She's getting on a bit now, Bob.'

'Aye, she'll be ten come Easter, but she's still right active.'

'Oh yes, I've seen her at work. She'll go on for a long time yet.'

He nodded solemnly.

We talked for a few minutes. I had a great fellow feeling for men like Bob, the hardy farm workers who were part of my life – catching and holding the big beasts for me, sweating side by side with me at tough calvings and lambings. It was a pleasure to be able to meet them off the job and I could see that Bob was enjoying our reminiscing together. He smiled gently at the memories even though his speech was slurring and his eyes half closed.

I finished my drink and looked at my watch. 'Got to go now, Bob. Take care of yourself till I see you again.'

In reply he slid off the stool. 'Ah'm off 'ome, too.' He tacked his way carefully to the door, followed by Meg.

Outside in the summer dusk, he went over to his bicycle which was resting against the wall. I paused by my car. I had seen this ritual before and found it fascinating.

He pulled the bike from the wall and took some time about lining it up to his satisfaction, then he made an attempt to throw a wellingtoned leg over the saddle. He didn't make it first time and stood for a few seconds apparently breathing deeply, then with great care he got the bike into position before jerking his leg up again. Once more he missed and I thought for a moment that he was going to finish up, bike and all, on the ground, but he regained his balance and stood with bowed head, communing with himself. Then he squared his shoulders decisively, peered along cross bar and handlebars and this time with a convulsive leap he landed in the saddle.

For a tense period he sat there, moving only a few inches forward, feet working on the pedals, hands pulling the handlebars from side to side in his struggle to stay upright. Then at last he took off and began to move an inch at a time, almost imperceptibly along the road. After a few yards, he stopped and was stationary for several seconds keeping the bike vertical by some mystical means. I thought, not for the first time, that it was a pity that Bob had never entered for the annual slow bicycle race at Darrowby Gala. He would have carried the prize off every year.

Leaning on my car, I watched his progress. Old Meg, obviously familiar with the routine, stepped along patiently by his side, dropping on her chest whenever he carried out one of his miraculously balanced pauses. Bob's cottage was about a mile along the road and I wondered how long it would take him to get there. His erstwhile companions before the old pub was modernised were always adamant that he never ever fell off and I personally had never seen him come to grief. When man and dog finally disappeared in the growing darkness I got into my car and drove home.

As I said, I seemed to spend half my life on the road through Welsby, and I dropped into the Lord Nelson several times over the next few months. As always, I spotted Bob's flat cap perched incongruously among the modish jackets and dresses but one night as I peered through the crush I noticed something different.

I pushed my way to the corner of the bar. 'Hello, Bob. I see you haven't got Meg with you.'

He glanced down to the space under his stool, then took a sip at his glass before looking at me with a doleful expression. 'Nay . . . nay . . .' he murmured. 'Couldn't bring 'er.'

'Why not?'

He didn't reply for a few moments and when he spoke his voice was husky, almost inaudible. 'She's got cancer.'

'What!'

'Cancer. Meg's got cancer.'

'How do you know?'

'There's a big growth on 'er. It's been comin' on for a bit.'

'Why didn't you tell me?'

'You'd 'ave put her down. Ah don't want her put down yet.'

'But . . . but . . . you're jumping to conclusions, Bob. All growths aren't cancerous.'

'This 'un must be. It's a bloody great thing as big as a cricket ball.'

'And where is it?'

'Underneath 'er belly. Hangin' right down nearly to t'ground. It's awful.' He rubbed his eyes as though to blot out the memory. His face was a mask of misery.

I grasped his arm. 'Now, look, Bob, this sounds to me like a simple mammary tumour.'

'A what?'

'A growth on the bitch's udder. These things are very common and they're very often benign and quite harmless.'

'Oh not this 'un,' he quavered. 'It's a bloody big . . .' He demonstrated with his hands.

'Size doesn't matter. Come on, Bob, we'll go along to your house and have a look at it.'

'Nay . . . nay . . . Ah know what you'll do.' His eyes took on a hunted expression.

'I'll not do anything, I promise you.' I looked at my watch. 'It's nearly closing time. Let's go.'

He gave me a final despairing look, then got off his stool and made his careful way to the door.

Outside I watched the usual ceremony with the bike, but this time, at the third attempt at mounting, man and bike crashed to the ground. A bad sign. And on the interminable journey to the cottage Bob went down several times and as I looked at him, sprawled face down on top of his machine, I realised that the heart had gone out of him.

At the cottage, Bob's brother, Adam, looked up from his work on a hookey rug. Neither of the men had married and, though entirely different personalities, lived together in complete harmony. I hastened to Meg's basket and gently rolled the old bitch on to her side. It was indeed a huge tumour, but it was rock hard, confined to the skin and not attached to the mammary tissue.

'Look, Bob,' I said, 'I can get my fingers right behind it. I'm sure I can take it off with every chance of complete recovery.'

He dropped into a chair and Meg ambled across to greet him. He slowly stroked her ears. There was something pathetic about the waving tail, the open, panting mouth and the monstrous growth dangling almost to the floor.

There was no reply, and Adam broke in. 'You can see what 'e's like, Mr Herriot. I've been telling 'im for weeks to come to you but he takes no notice. I've lost patience with him.'

'How about it, Bob?' I said. 'Will you bring her to the surgery as soon as possible? The quicker it's done the better. You can't let her go on like this.'

He went on with his stroking for some time, then nodded his head. 'All right.'

'When?'

'Ah'll let ye know.'

Adam came in again. 'You see. He won't say, because I can tell you now that 'e never will bring her in to you. He's made up 'is mind that Meg's going to die.'

'That's daft, Bob,' I said. 'I tell you I'm pretty sure I can put her right. Will I take her away with me now? How about that?'

Still looking down, he shook his head vigorously. I decided on shock tactics.

'Well, let me do the operation now.'

He shot me a startled glance. 'What . . . right here?'

'Why not? It's not as big a job as you think. It doesn't involve any vital organs, and I always carry an operating kit in my car.'

'Good idea!' burst out Adam. 'It's the only way we'll get it done!'

'Just one thing,' I said, 'when did she last eat?'

'She had a few biscuits this morning,' Adam replied. 'But that's all. Bob always gives her her main meal last thing at night.'

'Fine, fine. She'll be just right for the anaesthetic.'

Bob seemed stupefied and he didn't say a word or make a move as Adam and I began to bustle about with our preparations. I had always been interested in the relationship between these two middle-aged brothers. They were opposites. Adam had never had an alcoholic drink in his life but seemed totally uncritical of Bob's beer-orientated lifestyle and when Bob was at the Lord Nelson he was usually attending night classes at the village school, rug-making being his latest interest. Adam wasn't a farm worker and was employed by the big dairy which collected the milk from the Dales farms. He was small and slightly built, finicky and fussy in his manner, unlike his burly, stolid brother.

After I had boiled the instruments, we lifted Meg on to the table and a quick injection of intravenous barbiturate sent the old bitch into deep anaesthesia. I made her fast on her back with bandages to the table legs and then all three of us scrubbed up at the kitchen sink. Bob, still wearing his cap, displayed a growing lack of enthusiasm and when I handed the brothers an artery forceps apiece and poised my scalpel he closed his eyes tightly.

My system with these tumours was to cut out an ellipse on the skin, then proceed by blunt dissection with my fingers. It looked a bit crude, but greatly reduced the amount of haemorrhage. I made my first incision and started to peel back the skin, and it was just at the moment when I had taken the forceps from the brothers and was clamping a couple of spurting vessels that Bob opened his eyes. He gave a hollow groan and tottered to an old horsehair sofa where he slumped and buried his head in his hands. His frail brother, however, was made of sterner stuff, and although he lost a little colour he set his lips firmly and gripped both the forceps on the vessels with a steady hand as I tied them off.

Once started, I went about my job with gusto, working my way with my fingers round the spherical growth, pushing back the adhering fascia from the skin. Some of these things almost popped out, and although this one wasn't quite as easy as that, I was doing fine. Soon I had the whole tumour in my hand except for a mass right at the bottom and I knew from experience that there would be a big vessel down there. 'Get ready with your forceps, Adam,' I said, tearing carefully at the tissue, but almost as I spoke a crimson jet fountained up into his face.

Bob chose this moment to uncover his eyes and after one appalled glance at his brother's blood-spattered spectacles he gave a strangled grunt and flopped onto his back on the sofa, pulling his cap over his eyes with a limp hand.

'Well done, Adam,' I said to the little man as he stood resolutely at his post, the forceps clamped on that final vessel while I ligated it and removed the tumour. 'We're about finished now. Just a few stitches to put in.' I inserted a row of nylon sutures and stood back, well satisfied.

'The old girl looks a lot better without that horrible thing,' I said and swept my hand across the unsullied abdomen. Unfortunately my fingers struck the tumour which was lying on the table and it fell to the floor with a bump and rolled towards the sofa.

Bob turned a startled face toward the source of the noise and his mouth fell open as he spotted the grisly object bowling in his direction. 'Oh, bloody 'ell,' he moaned, then turned his face to the wall.

There he stayed, immobile, while I helped his brother carry Meg over to her basket, scrub the table and generally clear up the debris.

When all signs of our operation had disappeared Adam took the kettle to the kitchen sink. 'I don't know about you, Mr Herriot, but I could do wi' a cup of tea.'

'I'd love one,' I said gratefully and dropped onto one of the oaken chairs.

Adam turned to the prone form on the sofa. 'How about you, Bob? Are you goin' to have a cup?'

Bob stirred, sat up and looked warily round the room. 'Nay ... nay ...' He got to his feet and went across to a cupboard from which he extracted a bottle of brown ale. He poured a glassful and took a long swallow, then he went over to the dog basket and peered in at the flat abdomen and the neat row of stitches. He crouched there for some minutes, stroking the sleeping animal and fondling her ears. Then he turned and looked at us and a slow smile of utter contentment spread over his face.

'Well,' he said, 'we did it.'

'Aye, Bob lad,' said his brother, smiling back at him. 'We did it.'

When I removed the stitches ten days later, I was able to reassure Bob that microscopic examination had shown the tumour to be benign and that his worries were over.

After that I didn't see him for nearly a month until, one evening, I spotted his cap above the crowd in the Lord Nelson. It was nearly closing time and as I pushed my way towards him he rose from his stool and Meg appeared from below and began to amble after him to the door. She looked younger and brighter without her disfiguring appendage. I watched the pair through the pub window, and once outside Meg flopped down with her nose on her paws waiting for her master to go through the time-honoured routine.

Bob seized his bike and gave it a good shake as though to let it know who was boss. He took only two efforts to get astride, and although he was poised there immobile, working the handlebars from side to side, there was an authoritative look about his movements and it wasn't long before he took off on his journey home. I watched man and dog until they were out of sight and although there were frequent pauses I could see that there was no danger of a catastrophe.

Bob wasn't going to fall off tonight. He was himself again.

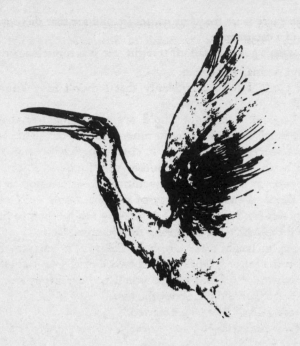

51

Calum inserted the last stitch after one of his dextrous operations and looked down at the sleeping cat for a few seconds.

'Jim', he said, without raising his head, 'I'm afraid I'm going to leave you.'

'Oh.' My heart gave a lurch, and I couldn't think of anything else to say at that moment. Calum had been with us for two years and, like all young vets, there had to come a time when he wanted to branch out on his own. But there was only one thought in my mind – I didn't want him to go.

Receiving no further reply, Calum went on. 'Yes, I've had the chance of a job which I think will suit me.'

'Oh . . .' My restricted vocabulary was making me feel like an idiot. 'Well . . . I understand, of course, Calum. Where will you be going?' My brain was starting to work again and one certainty loomed large – it would be somewhere isolated, somewhere in the wilds. Most likely the north of Scotland ... maybe in the Western Isles.

'Nova Scotia,' he replied.

'My God!' I realised suddenly that I didn't fully know him after all.

He laughed. 'I thought you'd say something like that. I've been in touch with a chap who runs a practice out there, and the prospect seems right for me. It covers a wide area of a rural district with some quite primitive conditions – a lot of the countryside is in its natural uncultivated state; unmade roads, rough farms, wonderful variety of wildlife. Some quite desolate country nearby, I understand.' A faraway look crept into his dark eyes as though he were glimpsing the promised land.

I began to laugh, too. 'Oh, hell, Calum, I'm sorry to be like this. It was a bit of a shock, in fact two shocks, but it does sound like your cup of tea and I hope you'll be very happy out there. What does Deirdre think about the idea?'

'Loves it. Can't wait to get started.'

'I don't doubt it. I think I hear Siegfried coming in. We'd better tell him.'

We met my partner in the passage. He looked a bit solemn as we gave him the news, then, like me, he put on a cheerful face and thumped Calum on the shoulder. 'I'm so glad you've found something you really want, my boy. I'm sure it will be the very thing for you and I wish you and Deirdre every happiness and success. But damn it, I'm going to miss you.'

He stopped suddenly and pointed wordlessly at an enormous feathered creature stalking past him. 'What ...? What ...?' In the darkness of the passage it looked as big as an ostrich.

The young man smiled happily. 'Just a heron. I picked it up a few days ago, down by the river. Wandering around, couldn't fly. Obviously damaged a wing, but seems to be improving.' As he spoke, the great bird spread its wings and flapped round the corner and out of sight. 'Ah, look. Soon be completely recovered.'

'I hope so ... I do hope so.' Siegfried stared at him, then cocked an ear at the scrabbling of a couple of recently adopted tortoises on the tiles further along the passage. Then he grinned suddenly. 'Yes, I'm going to miss you all right.'

The few weeks before Calum's departure fled past and after he and Deirdre had gone, I had that empty feeling again as I went into the deserted flat. John Crooks and now Calum – they had become my friends and both had left a gap, but with Calum the change was even more traumatic. The silence in the absence of the menagerie was almost palpable and as I looked out of the window where he had demolished that cake on his first day, many things rose and lingered in my mind. 'Permission to eat, sir', 'I'll just put Deirdre up a tree', Herriot's duct and, most emotive of all, the picture of his rapt face and dark eyes as he squeezed 'Shenandoah' from my children's little concertina.

Calum had been an acutely interesting man during his stay in Darrowby, but it was nearly as interesting to follow his career after he had left. I received regular letters telling me about his growing practice among the dirt roads and untamed countryside of Nova Scotia. His bursting energy led him to start the first auction mart in the district and he was trying to develop small animal work. A sentence sticks in my mind, 'Doing quite a few cat spays – Herriot's duct much in evidence.' The letters often ended, 'Permission to fall out, sir' which pulled me back to the old days.

Training Border collies was another of his passions and he gave frequent public demonstrations of his skill, several generations of his dogs being descended from prize winning sheep dogs which he bought from a farmer friend during his stay in Darrowby. He bought a farm, too, in Cape Breton, as though he didn't have enough to occupy him.

I also was kept abreast of the regular arrival of his children, noting with growing wonder as they mounted up to six. He brought up all of them in his own image, to love the outdoors and the wild creatures which abounded, to scorn the soft things of life as he had always done, and to camp and back-pack in the forests and mountains.

Often as I read those letters from Calum, the thought recurred that at last he had found his ideal environment, but I was wrong.

Twenty years after he left Darrowby, I was treating a cow for his farmer friend, Alan Beech. Alan, who was holding the animal's nose, spoke to me over his shoulder. 'Have you heard the latest about Calum?'

'No, what's that?'

'He's leaving Nova Scotia.'

'Never!'

'It's right. And where d'you think he's going?'

A jumble of thoughts spun in my mind. At last, with the advance of middle age, he was finding it too rough and tough out there. Felt it necessary to take his family to somewhere which offered a more gentle life. Maybe he was coming back here.

'I've no idea.' I said, 'tell me.'

'Papua New Guinea.'

'What!'

'Absolutely right.' Alan's face broke into a wide grin. 'Would you believe it!'

'My God, from cold and snows to steamy heat. It could only be Calum! Maybe Nova Scotia was too soft and sophisticated for him?'

'That could be it. He doesn't seem satisfied there – wants a place where there's still a lot o' cannibals about from what I've heard. By heck, he's a rum feller!'

I'd heard that description of Calum a thousand times from the farmers around Darrowby and now it seemed to be more strikingly proven than ever. I looked up Papua New Guinea in the public library and read that it wasn't until 1930 that the first white man had made contact with the million inhabitants of the unexplored highlands where Calum had gone. It was a whole intact civilisation which had had no connection with the outside world.

I looked at pictures of fierce-looking, almost naked men with slivers of bone transfixing their nostrils and brandishing bows and arrows as they glared into the camera. These frightening people would be his neighbours and there was nothing more certain than that he would love them all, especially those wide-eyed little black children.

In due course, letters started to arrive from Mendi in the Southern Highlands. Calum, as expected, was utterly entranced by it all. The agriculture was Stone Age in character with pigs the only livestock, most of the settlements unchanged from when the first whites discovered them, and the primitive farmers, although a bit careless about keeping appointments when he tried to teach them animal husbandry, were charming chaps. Deirdre and he were already firm friends with all of them.

As the months and years passed, he was clearly absorbed in the development and improvement of the country. I learned how he introduced cattle, sheep and poultry into the local agriculture, educated the farmers and immersed himself in the life there with all his energy.

In 1988, his daughter, Sarah, wrote to me. She said: 'Dad still amazes me with his knowledge of the local vegetation and wild life. On his station farm he has 11 Border Collies, 2 pig dogs (labrador crosses), 2 water buffalo, 5 horses, many cattle, sheep, goats, an assortment of chickens, ducks, guinea fowl and a huge flock of homing pigeons.'

As I put down her letter I thought of Calum's little menagerie at Skeldale House. It had been only a rehearsal for this. The vet wi' t'badger would be happy now.

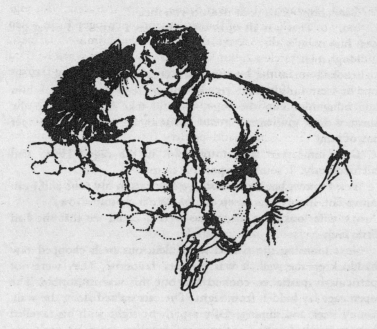

52

Months passed without any thawing of relations between me and our two wild cats and I noticed with growing apprehension that Olly's long coat was reverting to its previous disreputable state. The familiar knots and tangles were reappearing and within a year it was as bad as ever. It became more obvious every day that I had to do something about it. But could I trick him again? I had to try.

I made the same preparations, with Helen placing the nembutal-laden food on the wall, but this time Olly sniffed, licked, then walked away. We tried at his next meal time but he examined the food with deep suspicion and turned away from it. It was very clear that he sensed there was something afoot.

Hovering in my usual position at the kitchen window I turned to Helen. 'I'm going to have to try to catch him.'

'Catch him? With your net, do you mean?'

'No, no. That was all right when he was a kitten. I'd never get near him now.'

'How, then?'

I looked out at the scruffy black creature on the wall. 'Well, maybe I can hide behind you when you feed him and grab him and bung him into the cage. I could take him down to the surgery then, give him a general anaesthetic and make a proper job of him.'

'Grab him? And then fasten him in the cage?' Helen said incredulously. 'It sounds impossible to me.'

'Yes, I know, but I've grabbed a few cats in my time and I can move fast. If only I can keep hidden. We'll try tomorrow.'

My wife looked at me, wide-eyed. I could see that she had little faith.

Next morning she placed some delicious fresh chopped raw haddock on the wall. It was the cats' favourite. They were not particularly partial to cooked fish but this was irresistible. The open cage lay hidden from sight. The cats stalked along the wall, Ginny sleek and shining, Olly a pathetic sight with his ravelled hair and ugly knotted appendages dangling from his neck and body. Helen made her usual fuss of the two of them, then, as they descended happily on the food she returned to the kitchen where I was lurking.

'Right, now,' I said. 'I want you to walk out very slowly again and I am going to be tucked in behind you. When you go up to Olly he'll be concentrating on the fish and maybe won't notice me.'

Helen made no reply as I pressed myself into her back in close contact from head to toe.

'Okay, off we go.' I nudged her left leg with mine and we shuffled off through the door, moving as one.

'This is ridiculous,' Helen wailed. 'It's like a music hall act.'

Nuzzling the back of her neck I hissed into her ear. 'Quiet, just keep going.'

As we advanced on the wall, double-bodied, Helen reached out and stroked Olly's head, but he was too busy with the haddock to look up. He was there, chest-high, within a couple of feet of me. I'd never have a better chance. Shooting my hand round Helen, I seized him by the scruff of his neck, held him, a flurry of flailing black limbs, for a couple of seconds then pushed him into the cage. As I crashed the lid down, a desperate paw appeared at one end but I thrust it back and slotted home the steel rod. There was no escape now.

I lifted the cage on to the wall with Olly and me at eye level and I flinched as I met his accusing stare through the bars. 'Oh no, not again! I don't believe this!' it said. 'Is there no end to your treachery?'

In truth, I felt pretty bad. The poor cat, terrified as he was by my assault, had not tried to scratch or bite. It was like the other occasions – his only thought was to get away. I couldn't blame him for thinking the worst of me.

However, I told myself, the end result was going to be a fine handsome animal again. 'You won't know yourself, old chap,' I said to the petrified little creature, crouched in his cage on the car seat by my side as we drove to the surgery. 'I'm going to fix you up properly, this time. You're going to look great and feel great.'

Siegfried had offered to help me and when we got him on the table, a trembling Olly submitted to being handled and to the intravenous anaesthetic. As he lay sleeping peacefully, I started on the awful tangled fur with a fierce pleasure, snipping and trimming and then going over him with the electric clippers followed by a long combing until the last tiny knot was removed. I had only given him a make-shift hair-do before, but this was the full treatment.

Siegfried laughed when I held him up after I had finished. 'Looks ready to win any cat show,' he said.

I thought of his words next morning when the cats came to the wall for their breakfast. Ginny was always beautiful, but she was almost outshone by her brother as he strutted along, his smooth, lustrous fur gleaming in the sunshine.

Helen was enchanted at his appearance and kept running her hand along his back as though she couldn't believe the transformation. I, of course, was in my usual position, peeking furtively from the kitchen window. It was going to be a long time before I even dared to show myself to Olly.

*

It very soon became clear that my stock had fallen to new depths, because I had only to step out of the back door to send Olly scurrying away into the fields. The situation became so bad that I began to brood about it.

'Helen,' I said one morning, 'this thing with Olly is getting on my nerves. I wish there was something I could do about it.'

'There is, Jim,' she said. 'You'll really have to get to know him. And he'll have to get to know you.'

I gave her a glum look. 'I'm afraid if you asked him, he'd tell you that he knows me only too well.'

'Oh, I know, but when you think about it, over all the years that we've had these cats, they've hardly seen anything of you, except in an emergency. I've been the one to feed them, talk to them, pet them, day in day out. They know me and trust me.'

'That's right, but I just haven't had the time.'

'Of course you haven't. Your life is one long rush. You're no sooner in the house than you're out again.'

I nodded thoughtfully. She was so right. Over the years I had been attached to those cats, enjoyed the sight of them trotting down the slope for their food, playing in the long grass in the field, being fondled by Helen, but I was a comparative stranger to them. I felt a pang at the realisation that all that time had flashed past so quickly.

'Well, probably it's too late. Do you think there is anything I can do?'

'Yes,' she said. 'You have to start feeding them. You'll just have to find the time to do it. Oh, I know you can't do it always, but if there's the slightest chance, you'll have to get out there with their food.'

'So you think it's just a case of cupboard love with them?'

'Absolutely not. I'm sure you've seen me with them often enough. They won't look at their food until I've made a fuss of them for quite a long time. It's the attention and friendship they want most.'

'But I haven't a hope. They hate the sight of me.'

'You'll just have to persevere. It took me a long time to get their trust. Especially with Ginny. She's always been the more timid one. Even now if I move my hand too quickly, she's off.'

Despite all that's happened, I think Olly might be your best hope
– there's a big well of friendliness in that cat.'

'Right,' I said. 'Give me the food and milk. I'll start now.'

That was the beginning of one of the little sagas in my life. At
every opportunity, I was the one who called them down, placed
the food on the wall top and stood there waiting. At first I
waited in vain. I could see the two of them watching me from
the log shed – the black-and-white face and the yellow, gold and
white one observing me from the straw beds – and for a long
time they would never venture down until I had retreated into
the house. Because of my irregular job, it was difficult to keep
the new system going and sometimes when I had an early
morning call they didn't get their breakfast on time, but it was
on one of those occasions when breakfast was over an hour late
that their hunger overcame their fear and they came down
cautiously while I stood stock still by the wall. They ate quickly
with nervous glances at me then scurried away. I smiled in
satisfaction. It was the first breakthrough.

After that, there was a long period when I just stood there as
they ate until they became used to me as part of the scenery.
Then I tried a careful extension of a hand. To start with, they
backed away at that but, as the days passed, I could see that my
hand was becoming less and less of a threat and my hopes rose
steadily. As Helen had prophesied, Ginny was the one who shied
right away from me at the slightest movement, whereas Olly,
after retreating, began to look at me with an appraising eye as
though he might possibly be willing to forget the past and revise
his opinion of me. With infinite patience, day by day, I managed
to get my hand nearer and nearer to him and it was a memorable
occasion when he at last stood still and allowed me to touch his
cheek with a forefinger. As I gently stroked the fur, he regarded
me with unmistakably friendly eyes before skipping away.

'Helen,' I said, looking round at the kitchen window, 'I've
made it! We're going to be friends at last. It's a matter of time now
till I'm stroking him as you do.' I was filled with an irrational
pleasure and sense of fulfilment. It did seem a foolish reaction in a
man who was dealing every day with animals of all kinds, but I
was looking forward to years of friendship with that particular cat.

I was wrong. At that moment I could not know that Olly would be dead within forty-eight hours.

It was the following morning when Helen called to me from the back garden. She sounded distraught. 'Jim, come quickly! It's Olly!'

I rushed out to where she was standing near the top of the slope near the log shed. Ginny was there, but all I could see of Olly was a dark smudge on the grass.

Helen gripped my arm as I bent over him. 'What's happened to him?'

He was motionless, his legs extended stiffly, his back arched in a dreadful rigor, his eyes staring.

'I . . . I'm afraid he's gone. It looks like strychnine poisoning.' But as I spoke he moved slightly.

'Wait a minute!' I said. 'He's still alive, but only just.' I saw that the rigor had relaxed and I was able to flex his legs and lift him without any recurrence. 'This isn't strychnine. It's like it, but it isn't. It's something cerebral, maybe a stroke.'

Dry-mouthed, I carried him down to the house where he lay still, breathing almost imperceptibly.

Helen spoke through her tears. 'What can you do?'

'Get him to the surgery right away. We'll do everything we can.' I kissed her wet cheek and ran out to the car.

Siegfried and I sedated him because he had begun to make paddling movements with his limbs, then we injected him with steroids and antibiotics and put him on an intravenous drip. I looked at him as he lay in the big recovery cage, his paws twitching feebly. 'Nothing more we can do, is there?'

Siegfried shook his head and shrugged. He agreed with me about the diagnosis – stroke, seizure, cerebral haemorrhage, call it what you like, but certainly the brain. I could see that he had the same feeling of hopelessness as I had.

We attended Olly all that day and, during the afternoon, I thought for a brief period that he was improving, but by evening he was comatose again and he died during the night.

I brought him home and as I lifted him from the car, his smooth, tangle-free fur was like a mockery now that his life was ended. I buried him just behind the log shed a few feet from the straw bed where he had slept for so many years.

Vets are no different from other people when they lose a pet, and Helen and I were miserable. We hoped that the passage of time would dull our unhappiness, but we had another poignant factor to deal with. What about Ginny?

Those two cats had become a single entity in our lives and we never thought of one without the other. It was clear that to Ginny the world was incomplete without Olly. For several days she ate nothing. We called her repeatedly but she advanced only a few yards from the log house, looking around her in a puzzled way before turning back to her bed. For all of those years, she had never trotted down that slope on her own and over the next few weeks her bewilderment as she gazed about her continually, seeking and searching for her companion, was one of the most distressing things we had ever had to witness.

Helen fed her in her bed for several days and eventually managed to coax her on to the wall, but Ginny could scarcely put her head down to the food without peering this way and that, still waiting for Olly to come and share it.

'She's so lonely,' Helen said. 'We'll have to try to make a bigger fuss of her now than ever. I'll spend more time outside talking with her, but if only we could get her inside with us. That would be the answer, but I know it will never happen.'

I looked at the little creature, wondering if I'd ever get used to seeing only one cat on the wall, but Ginny sitting by the fireside or on Helen's knee was an impossible dream. 'Yes, you're right, but maybe I can do something. I'd just managed to make friends with Olly – I'm going to start on Ginny now.'

I knew I was taking on a long and maybe hopeless challenge because the tortoiseshell cat had always been the more timid of the two, but I pursued my purpose with resolution. At meal times and whenever I had the opportunity, I presented myself outside the back door, coaxing and wheedling, beckoning with my hand. For a long time, although she accepted the food from me, she would not let me near her. Then, maybe because she needed companionship so desperately that she felt she might as well even resort to me, the day came when she did not back away but allowed me to touch her cheek with my finger as I had done with Olly.

After that, progress was slow but steady. From touching I moved week by week to stroking her cheek then to gently rubbing her ears, until finally I could run my hand the length of her body and tickle the root of her tail. From then on, undreamed of familiarities gradually unfolded until she would not look at her food until she had paced up and down the wall top, again and again, arching herself in delight against my hand and brushing my shoulders with her body. Among these daily courtesies one of her favourite ploys was to press her nose against mine and stand there for several moments looking into my eyes.

It was one morning several months later that Ginny and I were in this posture – she on the wall, touching noses with me, gazing into my eyes, drinking me in as though she thought I was rather wonderful and couldn't quite get enough of me – when I heard a sound from behind me.

'I was just watching the veterinary surgeon at work,' Helen said softly.

'Happy work, too,' I said, not moving from my position, looking deeply into the green eyes, alight with friendship, fixed on mine a few inches away. 'I'll have you know that this is one of my greatest triumphs.'